VOLUME **2**

Intrathecal Drug Delivery for Pain and Spasticity

VOLUME

2 Intrathecal Drug Delivery for Pain and Spasticity

Volume Editors

Sudhir Diwan, MD, DABIPP, FIPP

Executive Director
The Spine & Pain Institute of New York
Staten Island University Hospital
New York, New York

Asokumar Buvanendran, MD

Professor
Department of Anesthesiology
Rush University Medical Center
Chicago, Illinois

Series Editor

Timothy R. Deer, MD, DABPM, FIPP

President and CEO
The Center for Pain Relief
Clinical Professor of Anesthesiology
West Virginia University School of Medicine
Charleston, West Virginia

ELSEVIER
SAUNDERS

1600 John F. Kennedy Blvd.
Ste 1800
Philadelphia, PA 19103-2899

INTRATHECAL DRUG DELIVERY FOR PAIN AND SPASTICITY   ISBN: 978-1-4377-2217-8
(Volume 2: A Volume in the Interventional and Neuromodulatory Techniques
for Pain Management Series by Timothy Deer)

Library of Congress Cataloging-in-Publication Data
Interventional and neuromodulatory techniques for pain management.
    p. ; cm.
    Includes bibliographical references and indexes.
    ISBN 978-1-4377-3791-2 (series package : alk. paper)—ISBN 978-1-4377-2216-1 (hardcover, v. 1 : alk. paper)—ISBN 978-1-4377-2217-8 (hardcover, v. 2 : alk. paper)—ISBN 978-1-4377-2218-5 (hardcover, v. 3 : alk. paper)—ISBN 978-1-4377-2219-2 (hardcover, v. 4 : alk. paper)—ISBN 978-1-4377-2220-8 (hardcover, v. 5 : alk. paper)
    1. Pain—Treatment.   2. Nerve block.   3. Spinal anesthesia.   4. Neural stimulation.   5. Analgesia.
I. Deer, Timothy R.
    [DNLM: 1. Pain—drug therapy.   2. Pain—surgery.   WL 704]
    RB127.I587 2012
    616'.0472—dc23

                                                                    2011018904

Acquisitions Editor: Pamela Hetherington
Developmental Editor: Lora Sickora
Publishing Services Manager: Jeff Patterson
Project Manager: Megan Isenberg
Design Direction: Lou Forgione

For Missy for all your love and support.

For Morgan, Taylor, Reed, and Bailie for your inspiration.

To those who have taught me a great deal: John Rowlingson, Richard North, Giancarlo Barolat, Sam Hassenbusch, Elliot Krames, K. Dean Willis, Peter Staats, Nagy Mekhail, Robert Levy, David Caraway, Kris Kumar, Joshua Prager, and Jim Rathmell.

To my team: Christopher Kim, Richard Bowman, Matthew Ranson, Doug Stewart, Wilfredo Tolentino, Jeff Peterson, and Michelle Miller.

Timothy R. Deer

I dedicate this book to my mother Late Raniba Diwan for teaching me the meaning of life; my family, Indira, Sneh, Kaushal and Shira for believing in me; and my granddaughter Belen Rani for bringing happiness to our lives.

Sudhir Diwan

This book is dedicated to my family, including my wife, Gowthamy; my two children, Dhanya and Arjun; and my loving and supportive parents who taught me the value of hard work and perseverance.

Asokumar Buvanendran

Contributors

Michael A. Ashburn, MD, MPH
Professor of Anesthesiology and Critical Care; Director, Pain Medicine and Palliative Care, Department of Anesthesiology and Critical Care, University of Pennsylvania, Philadelphia, Pennsylvania
Chapter 4, Principles of Patient Management for Intrathecal Analgesia

Ignacio Badiola, MD
Fellow, UCLA Pain Management Center, Department of Anesthesiology, David Geffen School of Medicine at UCLA, Los Angeles, California
Chapter 24, Perioperative Management of Patients with Intrathecal Drug Delivery Systems

Rajpreet Bal, MD
Assistant Professor of Anesthesiology and Pain Medicine, Department of Anesthesiology and Pain Medicine, Weill Cornell Medical Center, New York Presbyterian Hospital, Pain Medicine Center, New York, New York
Chapter 12, SynchroMed EL versus SynchroMed II

Shannon L. Bianchi, MD
Penn Pain Medicine Center, Department of Anesthesiology and Critical Care, University of Pennsylvania, Philadelphia, Pennsylvania
Chapter 4, Principles of Patient Management for Intrathecal Analgesia

Allen W. Burton, MD
Houston Pain Associates, Houston, Texas
Chapter 23, Trialing for Ziconotide Intrathecal Analgesic Therapy

Asokumar Buvanendran, MD
Professor, Department of Anesthesiology, Rush University Medical Center, Chicago, Illinois
Chapter 1, Basic Science of Spinal Receptors
Chapter 10, Techniques of Implant Placement for Intrathecal Pumps

Kenneth D. Candido, MD
Chairman and Professor, Department of Anesthesiology, Advocate Illinois Masonic Medical Center, Chicago, Illinois
Chapter 15, Management of Intrathecal Drug Delivery Systems in Patients with Co-Morbidities

Sukdeb Datta, MD
Associate Professor, Department of Anesthesiology, Vanderbilt University Medical Center, Nashville, Tennessee; Medical Director, Laser Spine & Pain Institute, LLC, New York, New York
Chapter 18, Anticoagulation Guidelines and Intrathecal Drug Delivery Systems

Miles Day, MD, DABA, FIPP, DABIPP
Professor, Pain Management Fellowship Director, Department of Anesthesiology and Pain Management, Texas Tech University Health Sciences Center, Lubbock, Texas
Chapter 5, Patient Selection for Intrathecal Infusion to Treat Chronic Pain

Timothy R. Deer, MD, DABPM, FIPP
President and CEO, The Center for Pain Relief; Clinical Professor of Anesthesiology, West Virginia University, School of Medicine, Charleston, West Virginia
Chapter 10, Techniques of Implant Placement for Intrathecal Pumps
Chapter 17, Neuroaugmentation by Stimulation versus Intrathecal Drug Delivery Systems

Allen Dennis, MD, MS
Assistant Professor, Department of Anesthesiology and Pain Management, Oklahoma University Health Sciences Center, Oklahoma City, Oklahoma
Chapter 5, Patient Selection for Intrathecal Infusion to Treat Chronic Pain

Sudhir Diwan, MD, DABIPP, FIPP
Executive Director, The Spine & Pain Institute of New York, Staten Island University Hospital, New York, New York
Chapter 2, Pharmacological Agents and Compounding of Intrathecal Drugs
Chapter 11, Programmable versus Fixed-Rate Pumps for Intrathecal Drug Delivery
Chapter 12, SynchroMed EL versus SynchroMed II
Chapter 17, Neuroaugmentation by Stimulation versus Intrathecal Drug Delivery Systems

Daniel M. Doleys, PhD
Director, Pain and Rehabilitation Institute, Birmingham, Alabama
Chapter 7, Psychological Considerations in Intrathecal Drug Delivery

F. Michael Ferrante, MD
Director, UCLA Pain Management Center, Professor of Clinical Anesthesiology and Medicine, David Geffen School of Medicine at UCLA, Los Angeles, California
Chapter 24, Perioperative Management of Patients with Intrathecal Drug Delivery Systems

Corey W. Hunter, MD
Clinical Fellow, Department of Anesthesiology and Pain Medicine, Tri-Institute Pain Medicine Fellowship, Weill Cornell Medical College, New York, New York
Chapter 17, Neuroaugmentation by Stimulation versus Intrathecal Drug Delivery Systems

Matthew Jaycox, MD
Department of Anesthesiology and Pain Management, Rush University Medical Center, Chicago, Illinois
Chapter 10, Techniques of Implant Placement for Intrathecal Pumps
Chapter 14, Complications Associated with Intrathecal Drug Delivery Systems

Tarun Jolly, MD
Director, Southern Pain Relief, LLC, New Orleans, Louisiana
Chapter 6, Patient Preparation

Maruti Kari, MD
Department of Anesthesiology and Pain Management, Rush University Medical Center, Chicago, Illinois
Chapter 14, Complications Associated with Intrathecal Drug Delivery Systems

Jeffrey S. Kroin, PhD
Department of Anesthesiology, Rush University Medical Center, Chicago, Illinois
Chapter 1, Basic Science of Spinal Receptors

Erin R. Lawson, MD
Assistant Clinical Professor, Division of Pain Medicine, Department of Anesthesiology, University of California, San Diego
Chapter 22, Future of Intrathecal Drug Delivery Systems (Including New Devices)

Jeffrey Loh, MD
Senior Resident, Department of Anesthesiology and Pain Medicine, Weill Cornell Medical Center, New York Presbyterian Hospital, Pain Medicine Center, New York, New York
Chapter 12, SynchroMed EL versus SynchroMed II

Timothy R. Lubenow, MD
Department of Anesthesiology and Pain Management, Rush University Medical Center, Chicago, Illinois
Chapter 14, Complications Associated with Intrathecal Drug Delivery Systems

Devin Peck, MD
Assistant Professor of Anesthesiology and Pain Medicine, Department of Anesthesiology and Pain Medicine, Weill Cornell Medical Center, New York Presbyterian Hospital, Pain Medicine Center, New York, New York
Chapter 11, Programmable versus Fixed-Rate Pumps for Intrathecal Drug Delivery

Joshua P. Prager, MD, MS
Clinical Assistant Professor of Medicine, Clinical Assistant Professor of Anesthesiology, David Geffen School of Medicine at UCLA; Director, California Pain Medicine Centers, Center for Rehabilitation of Pain Syndromes (CRPS), Los Angeles, California
Chapter 13, Minimizing the Risks of Intrathecal Therapy

Steven M. Rosen, MD
Fox Chase Pain Management Associates, Jenkintown, Pennsylvania; Doylestown, Pennsylvania; Marlton, New Jersey
Chapter 16, Cost-Effectiveness of Implanted Drug Delivery Systems

Eric Royster, MD
Clinical Director, Section of Pain Management, Ochsner Medical Center, New Orleans, Louisiana
Chapter 6, Patient Preparation

Michael Saulino, MD, PhD
Physiatrist, MossRehab; Assistant Professor, Department of Rehabilitation Medicine, Jefferson Medical College, Philadelphia, Pennsylvania
Chapter 20, Intrathecal Baclofen Trialing
Chapter 21, Baclofen Pump Management

David Schultz, MD
Medical Director, MAPS Medical Pain Clinics; Adjunct Professor, Department of Anesthesiology, University of Minnesota, Minneapolis, Minnesota
Chapter 8, Intrathecal Drug Delivery: Medical Necessity, Documentation, Coding, and Billing

Shalini Shah, MD
Senior Resident, Department of Anesthesiology and Pain Medicine, Weill Cornell Medical Center, New York Presbyterian Hospital, Pain Medicine Center, New York, New York
Chapter 2, Pharmacological Agents and Compounding of Intrathecal Drugs

Peter S. Staats, MD, MBA
Adjunct Associate Professor, Department of Anesthesiology and Critical Care Medicine, Johns Hopkins University, Baltimore, Maryland; Partner, Premier Pain Centers, Shrewsbury, New Jersey
Chapter 2, Pharmacological Agents and Compounding of Intrathecal Drugs

Lisa Jo Stearns, MD
Medical Director, Center for Pain and Supportive Care, Scottsdale, Arizona
Chapter 19, Intrathecal Therapy for Malignant Pain

Thuong D. Vo, MD
Fellow, UCLA Pain Management Center, Department of Anesthesiology, David Geffen School of Medicine at UCLA, Los Angeles, California
Chapter 24, Perioperative Management of Patients with Intrathecal Drug Delivery Systems

Mark S. Wallace, MD
Professor of Clinical Anesthesiology; Chair, Division of Pain Medicine, Department of Anesthesiology, University of California, San Diego, San Diego, California
Chapter 22, Future of Intrathecal Drug Delivery Systems (Including New Devices)

Joshua Wellington, MD, MS
Assistant Professor of Clinical Anesthesia and Physical Medicine and Rehabilitation, Medical Director, Indiana University Pain Medicine Center, Indiana University, Indianapolis, Indiana
Chapter 9, Methods of Trials for Consideration of Intrathecal Drug Delivery Systems

Bryan S. Williams, MD, MPH
Assistant Professor of Anesthesiology, Division of Pain Medicine, Rush Medical College, Rush University Medical Center, Chicago, Illinois
Chapter 3, Polyanalgesia for Implantable Drug Delivery Systems

Preface

It is my privilege and honor to write a preface to Volume 2 of the *Interventional and Neuromodulatory Techniques for Pain Management* series. Dr. Timothy Deer has been motivated to compile this volume by his deep feeling for those who are afflicted by intractable pain and intense desire to contribute something towards the alleviation of their suffering.

Volume 2 focuses on intrathecal drug delivery for pain and spasticity and covers a very important facet of the field of pain. It describes the recent advances in diagnosing and managing various pain states and presents procedures and strategies to combat chronic pain. Despite the impressive advances and optimistic outlook, pain remains intractable for some of our patients. The continued suffering of millions indicates that we have a long way to go. Dr. Deer endeavors to fill this gap.

This authoritative volume is divided into five sections and twenty-four chapters authored by experts in the field. It elegantly captures the full scope of therapy from basic pathophysiology to clinical practice, technological advancement, and future potential. It is a product of a diverse group of multidisciplinary individuals who share the vision of relieving the burden of chronic pain through the judicious use of technology.

It details the methods used for trialing, techniques of implantation, and various hardware solutions. The chapters on risk management, complications, and cost-effectiveness augment the book's practical relevance. Last, but not least, section five covers the future of intrathecal drug therapy, succinctly highlighting both the promise and challenge inherent to this field.

This volume will be of interest to pain physicians, scientists, students, biomedical engineers, the medical device industry, insurers, and others working in the exciting field of neuromodulation. This is a must-read for those who invest in these devices and aim to restore quality of life.

K. Kumar
Member Order of Canada, Saskatchewan Order of Merit
MBBS, MS, LLD (hon), FRCSC
Clinical Professor of Neurosurgery, University of Saskatchewan,
Regina, Canada

Acknowledgments

I would like to acknowledge Jeff Peterson for his hard work on making this project a reality, and Michelle Miller for her diligence to detail on this and all projects that cross her desk.

I would like to acknowledge Lora Sickora, Pamela Hetherington, and Megan Isenberg for determination, attention to detail, and desire for excellence in bringing this project to fruition.

Finally, I would like to acknowledge Samer Narouze for his diligent work filming and reviewing the procedural videos associated with all of the volumes in the series.

Timothy R. Deer

I would like to congratulate Timothy Deer, MD for producing a very educational series of volumes. I am grateful for the opportunity to work with him and Dr. Buvanendran.

Sudhir Diwan

Contents

SECTION I General Considerations

1 Basic Science of Spinal Receptors   3
Jeffrey S. Kroin and Asokumar Buvanendran

2 Pharmacological Agents and Compounding of Intrathecal Drugs   14
Shalini Shah, Peter S. Staats, and Sudhir Diwan

3 Polyanalgesia for Implantable Drug Delivery Systems   25
Bryan S. Williams

4 Principles of Patient Management for Intrathecal Analgesia   30
Shannon L. Bianchi and Michael A. Ashburn

5 Patient Selection for Intrathecal Infusion to Treat Chronic Pain   37
Allen Dennis and Miles Day

6 Patient Preparation   42
Tarun Jolly and Eric Royster

7 Psychological Considerations in Intrathecal Drug Delivery   48
Daniel M. Doleys

8 Intrathecal Drug Delivery: Medical Necessity, Documentation, Coding, and Billing   56
David Schultz

SECTION II Implant Devices

9 Methods of Trials for Consideration of Intrathecal Drug Delivery Systems   69
Joshua Wellington

10 Techniques of Implant Placement for Intrathecal Pumps   78
Asokumar Buvanendran, Matthew Jaycox, and Timothy R. Deer

11 Programmable versus Fixed-Rate Pumps for Intrathecal Drug Delivery   84
Devin Peck and Sudhir Diwan

12 SynchroMed EL versus SynchroMed II   90
Rajpreet Bal, Sudhir Diwan, and Jeffrey Loh

13 Minimizing the Risks of Intrathecal Therapy   96
Joshua P. Prager

14 Complications Associated with Intrathecal Drug Delivery Systems   102
Maruti Kari, Matthew Jaycox, and Timothy R. Lubenow

SECTION III Evidence-Based Practice

15 Management of Intrathecal Drug Delivery Systems in Patients with Co-Morbidities   113
Kenneth D. Candido

16 Cost-Effectiveness of Implanted Drug Delivery Systems   122
Steven M. Rosen

17 Neuroaugmentation by Stimulation versus Intrathecal Drug Delivery Systems   129
Corey W. Hunter, Sudhir Diwan, and Timothy R. Deer

18 Anticoagulation Guidelines and Intrathecal Drug Delivery Systems   139
Sukdeb Datta

19 Intrathecal Therapy for Malignant Pain   146
Lisa Jo Stearns

SECTION IV Intrathecal Drug Delivery Systems for Spasticity

20 Intrathecal Baclofen Trialing   159
Michael Saulino

21 Baclofen Pump Management   166
Michael Saulino

SECTION V Future of Intrathecal Drug Delivery Systems

22 Future of Intrathecal Drug Delivery Systems (Including New Devices)   175
Erin R. Lawson and Mark S. Wallace

23 Trialing for Ziconotide Intrathecal Analgesic Therapy   179
Allen W. Burton

24 Perioperative Management of Patients with Intrathecal Drug Delivery Systems   187
Thuong D. Vo, Ignacio Badiola, and F. Michael Ferrante

Index   195

I General Considerations

Chapter 1 Basic Science of Spinal Receptors

Chapter 2 Pharmacological Agents and Compounding of Intrathecal Drugs

Chapter 3 Polyanalgesia for Implantable Drug Delivery Systems

Chapter 4 Principles of Patient Management for Intrathecal Analgesia

Chapter 5 Patient Selection for Intrathecal Infusion to Treat Chronic Pain

Chapter 6 Patient Preparation

Chapter 7 Psychological Considerations in Intrathecal Drug Delivery

Chapter 8 Intrathecal Drug Delivery: Medical Necessity, Documentation, Coding, and Billing

1 Basic Science of Spinal Receptors

Jeffrey S. Kroin and Asokumar Buvanendran

CHAPTER OVERVIEW

Chapter Synopsis: In many ways, the spinal cord acts as a master integrator of information coming from the body's periphery on its way to the brain. In turn, descending pathways provide input from the brain. The many proteins that regulate this information exchange, including receptors, ion channels, and enzymes, may be used as therapeutic targets for maladies, including chronic pain and spasticity. This chapter provides a brief overview of these many spinal targets—some currently in use and others with future potential. γ-Aminobutyric acid (GABA) receptors, the most plentiful inhibitory receptors in the central nervous system, can be used to control pain and spasticity. Glycine receptors, for the other major inhibitory neurotransmitter, seem to contribute to some pathological conditions. Adrenergic receptors have emerged as a major target of descending inhibition of pain, which is still poorly understood. Excitatory glutamate receptors appear particularly important for setting up central sensitization. The many glutamate receptor subtypes provide a rich variety of pain mediators and targets. Cholinergic, cannabinoid, and prostanoid receptors represent other potential pathways that are under investigation. Although opioid receptors have been major targets for some time now, many other peptides have not been fully appreciated. Ion channels form a huge and diverse group of molecular targets as well. This rich and diverse cast together orchestrates both healthy and pathological sensory conditions, including pain states.

Important Points: Preclinical studies in animal models have yielded much data on spinal cord receptors, ion channels, enzymes, transporters, and glia that relate to mechanisms of pain and spasticity. These basic studies of spinal receptors provide a rationale foundation for choosing intrathecal drugs to relieve symptoms in patients while minimizing side effects. Continued study of spinal mechanisms can lead to the development of new compounds with better specificity for existing receptors and even the possibility of finding novel receptors systems.

Introduction

The spinal cord is the primary integrating network for sensory receptors from our legs and arms. Afferent signals entering the spinal cord can be synaptically coupled to ascending pathways to the brain or undergo processing that influences other spinal input pathways. In turn, the brain has descending pathways that can influence sensory input. Just as important, the spinal cord mediates descending efferent pathways associated with motor performance. In addition, homeostatic mechanisms such as shivering or blood pressure depend on reliable spinal cord circuits. Hundreds of receptor, ion channel, and enzyme systems essential for spinal cord function have been identified. However, only a small number have been exploited to date for therapeutic purposes. As more knowledge expands in the pharmacology of spinal receptors, potentially more compounds can be developed for treating conditions such as chronic pain and spasticity. There are two main limitations on how successfully any receptor system can be used for therapeutic purposes: (1) with systemic delivery, similar receptors in the brain may cause untoward effects that negate any advantages of improved spinal control, and (2) within the spinal cord, the same receptor may have opposite functions depending on its pathological state or anatomical location. With intrathecal drug delivery, the first problem may be reduced, although most spinally delivered compounds will have some access to the brain, either by vascular absorption and recirculation, or by ascending cerebrospinal fluid (CSF) flow that can transport a drug from the lumbar spinal cord to the brainstem in humans. In this introductory chapter, we discuss the spinal receptors that are believed to play important roles in normal function and disease and emphasize pharmacologic strategies that have already proven to be clinically successful and those that may enter clinical practice over the next few years (**Fig. 1-1**).

Nonpeptide Receptors

γ-Aminobutyric Acid Receptors

Receptors for the amino acid γ-aminobutyric acid (GABA) represent the main inhibitory neurotransmitter system of the central nervous system (CNS). GABA receptors are distributed at both presynaptic and postsynaptic locations, so they may inhibit both synaptic release of excitatory neurotransmitters and the response of second-order neurons to activation of their excitatory receptors. Spinal GABA receptors are divided into two important subtypes: GABA-A receptors, which appear to have an important role in pain pathways, and GABA-B receptors, which can be exploited therapeutically to control spasticity.

GABA-A Receptors Typically, activation of GABA-A receptors on the presynaptic binding site of neurons controls a ligand-gated chloride channel that depolarizes presynaptic endings, resulting in reduced excitatory neurotransmitter release (presynaptic inhibition). When GABA binds to postsynaptic GABA-A receptors, again chloride channels are activated, but because of ion gradients and transporters, the neuron hyperpolarizes, resulting in inhibition of action potential formation.[1] However, in some animal pain models, ion gradients and transporters may be altered so that activation of GABA-A receptors excites primary afferent nerve terminals[2] and

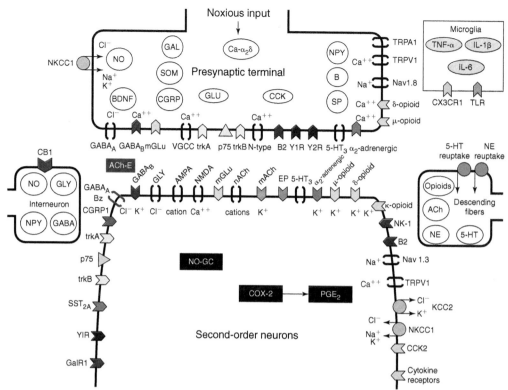

Fig. 1-1 Spinal cord receptors, ion channels, enzymes, transporters, and glial cells involved in pain and spasticity. *ACh*, acetylcholine; *mACh*, muscarinic acetylcholine; *nACh*, nicotinic acetylcholine; *Ach-E*, acetylcholine esterase; *AMPA*, α-amino-3-hydroxy-5-methylisoxazole-4-propionic acid; *B*, bradykinin; *BDNF*, brain-derived neurotrophic factor; *Bz*, benzodiazepine; *Ca-α₂δ*, calcium channel subunit α2δ; *CB1*, cannabinoid; *CCK*, cholecystokinin; *CGRP*, calcitonin gene-related peptide; *COX*, cyclooxygenase; *CX3CR1*, fractalkine receptor; *EP*, prostaglandin receptors; *GABA*, γ-aminobutyric acid; *GAL*, galanin; *GC*, guanylyl cyclase; *GLU*, glutamate; *mGLu*, metabotropic glutamate; *GLY*, glycine; *5-HT*, serotonin; *IL*, interleukin; *KCC*, potassium-chloride cotransporter; *Nav*, voltage-gated sodium channels; *NE*, norepinephrine; *NK*, neurokinin; *NKCC*, sodium-potassium-chloride cotransporter; *NMDA*, N-methyl-D-aspartate; *NO*, nitric oxide; *NPY*, neuropeptide Y; *p75*, low-affinity neurotrophin receptor; *PGE*, prostaglandin E; *SOM*, somatostatin; *SST*, somatostatin receptor; *SP*, substance P; *TLR*, toll-like receptor; *trk*, high-affinity neurotrophin receptor; *TNF*, tumor necrosis factor; *TRP*, transient receptor potential; *VGCC*, voltage-gated calcium channels; *Y*, neuropeptide Y.

depolarizes and excites dorsal horn neurons.[3] Although the plant-derived GABA-A receptor agonist muscimol has been available for many years, it has never been used intrathecally in patients to inhibit pain. Muscimol can inhibit neurons in the brain for therapeutic purposes.[4] Clinically, the benzodiazepine receptor binding site of the GABA-A receptor–chloride channel complex has been the therapeutic route to GABA-A inhibition. The prototype benzodiazepine agonist diazepam acts potently in the brain to terminate seizures and reduce anxiety. The sedative midazolam is a water-soluble benzodiazepine agonist that is widely used for anesthetic induction. Intrathecal midazolam has been shown to improve perioperative analgesia.[5] Preclinical studies with continuous intrathecal infusion in sheep showed no spinal cord pathology, although bolus injections in rabbits did produce toxicity, so issues of dosing may still be of concern.[6] Although there have been several studies of its long-term intrathecal use for chronic pain or spasticity,[6] intrathecal midazolam has not had widespread acceptance for chronic applications.

GABA-B Receptors In 1984, a new GABA receptor (GABA-B receptor) was characterized that was not sensitive to the prototype GABA-A antagonist bicuculline but instead was sensitive to the antispastic drug baclofen.[7] The GABA-B receptor is a G-protein coupled receptor that when activated presynaptically reduces

calcium influx and therefore neurotransmitter release and postsynaptically increases potassium influx, hyperpolarizing the neuron and decreasing impulse formation. In animal studies, intrathecal baclofen reduced nociception[8] and spinal reflexes.[9] As early as 1970, baclofen was used orally to treat spinal cord plasticity but was dose limited by sedation.[10] Bolus intrathecal injection of baclofen was demonstrated to rapidly ameliorate severe spinal cord spasticity in patients.[11] When given continuously with an implanted intrathecal catheter and infusion pump, baclofen treatment maintained spasticity control for years.[12-14] No studies have shown any long-term neuropathological sequelae to intrathecal baclofen use.

Glycine Receptors

Glycine is released by spinal cord interneurons and binds to postsynaptic ligand-gated chloride channels to increase chloride influx and by hyperpolarizing the neuron decreases action potential formation. Strychnine is a classical antagonist to the glycine receptor. Under pathological conditions (e.g. peripheral inflammation), prostaglandin E₂ (PGE₂) is released in the spinal cord and can affect the α₃ glycine receptor subtype to block chloride influx and thus reduce glycine inhibition.[15] This loss of glycine inhibition under pathological conditions may explain why intrathecal glycine given over 4 weeks in patients with complex regional pain syndrome is ineffective for pain or dystonia.[16]

α₂-Adrenergic Receptors

Descending noradrenergic fibers from neurons in brainstem sites such as the locus coeruleus have been shown to inhibit spinal cord nociception.[17] α₂-Adrenergic receptors are G-protein coupled[18] and exist on afferent terminals (presynaptic inhibition) and neuron cell bodies in the spinal cord where receptor stimulation activates potassium channels that hyperpolarize the cell.[19] Agonists at the α₂ subtype of adrenergic receptors, such as clonidine, produce analgesia when given intrathecally in animal models of acute and chronic pain.[20,21] There are limitations on how α₂ agonists can be used chronically for pain relief because excitation of α₂-adrenergic receptors can also produce sedation and sympathetic inhibition.

Clonidine is an effective analgesic acting on spinal cord α₂-adrenergic receptors,[22] but when given intrathecally in animals, it may cause hypotension by direct action on spinal cord sympathetic neurons.[23] Because intrathecal infusion of clonidine is dose limited by hypotension and sedation in clinical use, it is often used as an adjuvant to intrathecal opioids for long-term infusion.[24] Clonidine is also used in spinal anesthesia mixtures with local anesthetics and opioids during surgery, in which sedative side effects are not an issue.[25] Tizanidine is an α₂-adrenergic agonist that is used for treating spasticity.[26] Long-term intrathecal infusion of tizanidine also produces analgesia in animals[27] but has not been used clinically by the intrathecal route. Dexmedetomidine is another α₂ adrenergic agonist that produces analgesia with intrathecal administration in animals.[28] Intrathecal dexmedetomidine has been used in patients as an adjuvant medication to local anesthetics and opioids during surgery.[25]

Glutamate Receptors

Glutamate is the most important excitatory neurotransmitter in the CNS.[29] Virtually all primary afferent neurons release glutamate from their central terminals in the spinal cord. Glutamate is especially important in the development of chronic pain syndromes, particularly in mechanisms such as central sensitization.[30] With such a variety of roles in the CNS, it is not surprising that there are different subtypes of glutamate receptors.

α-Amino-3-Hydroxy-5-Methylisoxazole-4-Propionic Acid Receptors
α-Amino-3-hydroxy-5-methylisoxazole-4-propionic acid (AMPA) receptors respond rapidly when excited by glutamate. They are ligand-gated ion channel receptors that when activated open sodium and calcium channels that depolarize the postsynaptic neuron. In animal models, antagonists to the AMPA receptor can block acute pain[31] and postoperative pain[32] when given intrathecally. AMPA receptors, along with N-methyl-D-aspartate (NMDA) receptors, are involved with central sensitization in pathological settings, such as peripheral information.[30] Although there have been clinical trials with AMPA receptor antagonists and modulators (e.g. in epilepsy), no selective drug in this class is currently used to treat patients with chronic pain.

N-Methyl-D-Aspartate Receptors
Depolarization of the postsynaptic neuron allows glutamate to activate ligand-gated NMDA receptors. In particular, magnesium blocks the NMDA ion channel pore, and depolarization removes the magnesium ion and permits glutamate to open the pore. As such, the magnesium ion was the first identified NMDA antagonist,[33] and intrathecal magnesium sulfate potentiates morphine antinociception in animal models.[34] When the NMDA channel opens, calcium enters the cell and activates many intracellular pathways that contribute to central

sensitization, which is believed to be the first step in the development of neuropathic pain.[30] Although intrathecal NMDA antagonists do not inhibit postoperative pain in animal models,[32] they can inhibit neuropathic pain.[35]

Ketamine is an uncompetitive (i.e., does not act at the glutamate, or glycine, site) NMDA antagonist that binds to open NMDA channels. Systemic ketamine is widely used as a dissociative anesthetic but has also been used to treat neuropathic pain,[36] although its overall efficacy is moderate to weak.[37] Although there have been a few case reports of epidural ketamine for chronic pain, this route of administration is not widely used. Another uncompetitive NMDA channel blocker, memantine, may have efficacy when used early in chronic pain conditions.[38] New antagonist drugs being developed target subunits of the NMDA receptor, such as NR2B.[29]

Kainate Receptors
Although kainate receptors for glutamate have been identified, study of this class of ligand-gated channel receptors was hampered in the past by lack of selective antagonists.[29] Newer antagonists of the GluK1 subtype of kainate receptors have shown activity in animal pain models.[39,40] No selective kainate receptor antagonists are currently available for clinical use.

G-Protein Coupled (Metabotropic) Glutamate Receptors
To date, eight subtypes of G-protein coupled glutamate receptors have been identified and classified into three groups based on similarities in structure, second messengers, and pharmacology.[29,30] These receptors can be presynaptic to regulate neurotransmitter release or postsynaptic to stimulate neural activity. Several studies have shown that the mGluR1 and mGluR5 subtypes are active in rat neuropathic pain models, and intrathecal injection of an antagonist decreased hyperalgesia.[41] However, no mGluR antagonist is currently available for clinical use.

Cholinergic Receptors and Acetylcholine Esterase

Although cholinergic receptors are considered important in brain function (e.g., Alzheimer disease) and essential at the neuromuscular junction, their role in the spinal cord is less appreciated. Intrathecal injection of neostigmine, which blocks acetylcholine esterase and so increases acetylcholine concentration, inhibits nociception[42] and postoperative pain[42,43] in animals. Intrathecal neostigmine enhances postsurgical analgesia when combined with bupivacaine, but high neostigmine doses produce nausea.[44] In human volunteers, intrathecal neostigmine produces analgesia but also nausea, weakness, and sedation.[45] Therefore, as a single agent, intrathecal neostigmine infusion does not look promising for chronic pain therapy.

Nicotinic Acetylcholine Receptors
Neuronal nicotinic acetylcholine receptors are ligand-gated ion channels.[46] Agonist activation allows cations to enter the cell. Nicotine is a classic agonist at these receptors, but newer compounds such as epibatidine have been studied in pain models. However, even with intrathecal administration to limit systemic side effects, these agonists do not produce consistent analgesia.[46]

Muscarinic Acetylcholine Receptors
Muscarinic acetylcholine receptors are G-protein coupled receptors that are located in the dorsal horn, with the M2 subtype being the more prevalent and contributing to pain.[47] Intrathecal injection of muscarinic

acetylcholine agonists produces a potent antinociceptive effect in rats.[48] Although the muscarinic agonist bethanechol has been infused into the brain of patients with Alzheimer disease,[49] no selective M2 muscarinic agonists are currently available for testing in humans.

Cannabinoid Receptors

Although the effect of cannabis on the brain has been known for centuries, there is recent interest in cannabinoid analogs in pain research. Moreover, cannabinoids given intrathecally have analgesic effects even after brain influence is removed by spinal cord transsection.[50]

Cannabinoid CB1 Receptors   In the brain, CB1 receptors are G-protein coupled receptors that activate potassium channels and inhibit calcium currents and in the spinal cord are present on interneurons but not primary afferent terminals.[51] However, it is not clear yet what pharmacological characteristics CB1 selective drugs need to have to be useful as analgesics.[52]

Cannabinoid CB2 Receptors   CB2 receptors are also G-protein coupled receptors, but their localization in spinal cord neurons is controversial.[53] In animal studies, intrathecal administration of the CB2 agonist JWH015 reduced hypersensitivity in a postoperative pain model[54] and mechanical allodynia in a mouse neuropathic pain model.[55] No CB2 selective drug is available for human use.

Prostanoid Receptors and Cyclooxygenase Enzymes

After peripheral inflammation, there is upregulation of PGE_2 and cyclooxygenase-2 (COX-2) enzymes in the rat spinal cord,[56,57] and after surgical incision, spinal cord COX-1,[58] COX-2,[59] and PGE_2[60] are upregulated along with pain. After hip replacement surgery, CSF PGE_2 rapidly increased and was positively correlated with postoperative pain.[61]

PGE_2 exerts its effects by binding to G-protein coupled prostaglandin receptors of which there are four in the spinal cord, EP1 to EP4. Spinal application of agonists at EP1, EP2, and EP4 receptors enhanced responses of dorsal horn neurons to peripheral stimulation.[62] Intrathecal application of an EP1 receptor antagonist decreased mechanical hypersensitivity in a rat postoperative pain model.[63] Although EP subtype selective antagonists are under development, no compound is currently available for intrathecal use in the treatment of pain. Ketorolac is a water-soluble COX-1/COX-2 inhibitor that when given intrathecally reduces postoperative pain in rats.[64] However, in a recent study in patients with chronic pain or postoperative pain, intrathecal ketorolac did not reduce pain.[65]

Serotonin Receptors

Serotonin (5-HT) receptors are a diverse group with more than 15 receptor subtypes.[66] The $5-HT_3$ receptor is a ligand-gated cation channel, and the other 5-HT receptors are G-protein coupled. In pain research, the greatest interest in the spinal cord is in the $5HT_3$ receptor. A descending facilitatory pathway from the medulla releases 5-HT, and its effect is to activate $5HT_3$ receptors on afferent presynaptic endings and to excite $5HT_3$ receptors on spinal cord neurons.[66-68] In neuropathic pain models, intrathecal injection of the $5HT_3$ antagonist ondansetron attenuated tactile allodynia and thermal hyperalgesia.[68] Although ondansetron is water soluble and is available commercially in a

preservative-free isotonic formulation, there have been no reports of its intrathecal administration in patients.

Peptide Receptors

Opioid Receptors

Because opioids continue to be the most important class of drugs for controlling severe pain, interest in opioid receptors remains high. Descending supraspinal inhibitory pathways synapse on opioid receptors both on afferent terminals to reduce calcium influx and neurotransmitter release and on neurons to increase potassium conductance, thus hyperpolarizing the cell and reducing action potential formation.[22,69] All three major subtypes of opioid receptors are G-protein coupled.

μ-Opioid Receptors   Morphine is the classical agonist of the μ-opioid receptor, and intrathecal morphine has been shown to be a potent analgesic in acute pain models,[70] postoperative pain models,[71] and some neuropathic pain models.[72] The reduced effectiveness of morphine in animal neuropathic pain models may be related to down-regulation of μ-opioid receptor mRNA in injured dorsal root ganglions.[73] Infusion of intrathecal morphine from fixed-rate[74] or programmable infusion pumps[75] has been an effective way to treat intractable chronic pain. The main limitations of long-term intrathecal morphine infusion are clinically significant drug tolerance in some patients and the possibility of granuloma formation with high morphine doses.[76] For spinal anesthesia during surgery, short-acting lipophilic μ-opioids that have limited spread rostrally, such as fentanyl, are preferred because they produce less respiratory depression and sedation.

δ-Opioid Receptors   Because μ-opioid agonists have many side effects and tolerance can develop, other opioid subtypes have been investigated for analgesic efficacy. δ-Opioid agonists can reduce thermal hyperalgesia when given systemically in inflammatory pain models.[77] However, on intrathecal injection, they do not change the response to noxious heat, although mechanical hypersensitivity is reduced.[78] Although endogenous peptides (met- and leu-enkephalin) exist with high affinity for δ-opioid receptors, there are still no commercially available selective δ-opioid agonists.

κ-Opioid Receptors   Unlike the μ- and δ-opioid agonists, κ-opioid receptor agonists do not act presynaptically at Aδ or C fibers in the spinal cord to block neurotransmitter release.[79] Nevertheless, intrathecal selective κ-opioid agonists can reverse heat and pressure hyperalgesia as well as mechanical and cold allodynia in a rat neuropathic pain model.[80,81] Although selective κ-opioid agonists, including those acting on peripheral receptors to produce analgesia, are being developed, none are commercially available.

Tachykinin Receptors

In addition to releasing glutamate, small nociceptive primary afferents in the spinal cord release substance P (SP), which binds to the G-protein coupled receptor neurokinin-1 (NK1) and induces excitation in second-order neurons in laminae 1 and 2.[22] Intrathecal injection of SP causes hyperalgesia and pain-related behaviors.[82] In several animal pain models, hyperalgesia can be blocked by NK1 antagonists.[82] Unfortunately, clinical trials with SP antagonists as analgesics have been unsuccessful.[83] The endogenous peptide neurokinin-A and its neurokinin-2 (NK2) receptor have also been implicated in primary afferent neurotransmission, and an intrathecal NK2 antagonist blocked mechanical hyperalgesia in a rat neuropathic pain model.[84]

Calcitonin Gene-Related Peptide Receptors

Calcitonin gene-related peptide (CGRP) is released from terminals of small nociceptive primary afferents and excites G-protein coupled CGRP1 receptors on second-order spinal neurons.[22,85] The CGRP1 receptor is a complex of three proteins; however, the exact binding site of antagonists is not clear at present.[85] Intrathecal injection of a CGRP1 antagonist in rats reduces mechanical allodynia and hyperalgesia from a capsaicin skin injection[86] and inhibits pain-related responses to thermal and mechanical noxious stimulation in rats.[85] Although a CGRP antagonist has been successful in clinical trials of migraine pain relief, no CGRP antagonist has been evaluated for chronic pain involving spinal cord pathways.

Neurotrophin Receptors

Neurotrophins are secreted peptides that act as target-derived growth factors for specific neuronal populations.[87] However, they have a more immediate function in pain transmission. Neurotrophins bind to a high-affinity trk receptor as well as a low-affinity p75 receptor.[87]

Nerve Growth Factor Receptors: trkA

The high-affinity receptor for nerve growth factor (NGF) is the trkA receptor, and binding of NGF leads to phosphatidylation of receptor and second messengers. TrkA receptors are located both on nerve terminals and second-order neuron cell bodies in the rat dorsal horn.[88] A 7-day intrathecal infusion of NGF in rats with neuropathic pain caused by nerve injury reduced mechanical allodynia and thermal hyperalgesia.[89]

Brain-Derived Neurotrophic Factor Receptors: trkB

The high-affinity receptor for brain-derived neurotrophic factor (BDNF) is the trkB receptor and includes cell surface glycoproteins.[87] BDNF is released by primary afferent terminals in spinal cord lamina. TrkB receptors are present on both primary afferent terminals and on second-order neurons in the dorsal horn.[90] After peripheral nerve injury, BDNF is released from microglia and via trkB receptors on ion transporters reverses the chloride ion gradient so that GABA-A receptor activation in the dorsal horn no longer hyperpolarizes neurons.[91] Thus, the usual GABA-A inhibition is reduced, and this may contribute to neuropathic pain. Controversy exists in the literature on the effect of intrathecal BDNF or BDNF blockers in animal pain models, but in long-term clinical trials with intrathecal BDNF infusion in patients with amyotrophic lateral sclerosis, no pain syndromes were induced.[92]

Bradykinin Receptors

Bradykinin is an inflammatory mediator at periphery nerve terminals but also has a role in pain transmission in the spinal cord. Bradykinin is present in primary afferent terminals and spinal cord neurons in the dorsal horn, and after painful capsaicin skin injection, spinal cord bradykinin levels are greatly increased.[93] The bradykinin B_2 receptor is a G-protein coupled receptor that is expressed at primary sensory and second-order neurons. Intrathecal bradykinin increased mechanical and thermal hyperalgesia in this capsaicin model and potentiated NMDA receptor action.

Intrathecal administration of a B_2-selective antagonist reduced the late phase of the behavioral response to the painful irritant formalin, implying that the B_2 receptor contributes to central sensitization.[93] Icatibant acetate, a B_2-selective antagonist, has received approval in Europe, but even though it exists in an acceptable water-soluble preservative-free formulation, there is no report of its intrathecal use in patients. The G-protein coupled bradykinin B_1 receptor has a similar distribution, and intrathecal administration of an antagonist attenuated the response to noxious thermal stimulation.[94]

Somatostatin Receptors

Somatostatin (SST) is a peptide with widespread distribution throughout the body and is found in small primary afferent neurons, where it is released into the dorsal horn.[95] There are five major G-protein coupled types of SST receptors, with the SST_{2A} subtype the most prominent in the dorsal horn, and located on second-order neurons.[96,97] Most experimental studies show that SST applied locally to the spinal cord inhibits neuronal activity.[96,97] Octreotide is a stable SST analog that is compatible with implantable infusion pump systems and has not shown any neurodegenerative changes with chronic intrathecal infusion in dogs.[98] When delivered intrathecally for up to 3 months to patients with severe cancer pain, octreotide lowered pain scores and supplemental opioid use without central or systemic side effects.[98] In a prospective, randomized, double-blind, placebo-controlled trial, 18 noncancer patients received intrathecal octreotide without any evidence of adverse effects of intrathecal administration. There was an overall trend toward better analgesia in the octreotide arm, but it did not reach statistical significance.[99]

Neuropeptide Y Receptors

Neuropeptide Y (NPY) is found in dorsal horn interneurons and after peripheral nerve injury at presynaptic ending of large afferents.[100] There are two NPY receptors, Y1R and Y2R, in the spinal cord. Y1R is located in presynaptic endings, usually colocalized with CGRP and in many types of second-order neurons throughout the spinal cord; Y2R is on presynaptic terminals, but not cell bodies, in the dorsal horn. Studies with intrathecal administration of NPY or analogs have shown both anti- and pro-nociceptive actions, which may suggest different roles for Y1R (inhibits pain) and Y2R (excites pain).[100]

Cholecystokinin

Cholecystokinin (CCK) is widely distributed in the CNS, and intrathecal CCK reduces the antinociceptive effects of opioids.[101] There are two CCK receptor subtypes, CCK_1 (CCK-A) and CCK_2 (CCK-B), and intrathecal CCK_2 receptor antagonists enhance opioid-induced antinociception. Although a clinical trial with the nonspecific CCK antagonist proglumide administered systemically slightly enhanced morphine analgesia in chronic pain patients,[102] no intrathecal use of CCK receptor antagonists has been reported.

Galanin Receptors

Galanin is found in presynaptic terminals and second-order neurons in the dorsal horn, and galanin receptors subtypes, mainly GalR1, are found on second-order dorsal horn neurons.[103] After nerve injury, intrathecal galanin reduces hypersensitivity in neuropathic rats; an antagonist increases pain behavior. Intravenous galanin in patients had an acute antidepressant effect.[104] There have been no reports of intrathecal galanin use in humans.

Ion Channel Modulators

Voltage-Gated Calcium Channels

Depolarization of calcium channels at the central terminals of small primary afferents allows calcium inflow that leads to neurotransmitter release.[22] As discussed earlier, afferent terminal excitability can be decreased by opioid and α_2-adrenergic receptors that reduce calcium influx. However, voltage-gated calcium channels can also be modulated directly.

$\alpha_2\delta$ Subunit of Calcium Channel: Gabapentoid Receptor Presynaptic calcium channels are produced in the dorsal root ganglion (DRG) and transported to the central terminals of primary afferents.[105] After nerve injury that produces neuropathic pain, there is upregulation of the calcium channel subunit $\alpha_2\delta$ in the DRG and in the presynaptic terminals in the dorsal horn.[106] Calcium channels are complex proteins consisting of α_1 pore-forming units and modulatory subunits, including the $\alpha_2\delta$ subunit that regulates calcium current density and channel activation and inactivation.[107] The drug gabapentin and its related analog pregabalin bind with high affinity to the $\alpha_2\delta$ subunit[108] and decrease levels of $\alpha_2\delta$ calcium subunit in the presynaptic terminal. It is hypothesized that the binding occurs within the central axons that transport these voltage-gated calcium channels to the presynaptic endings.[105] Fewer presynaptic calcium channels means less presynaptic calcium current and reduced release of pain neurotransmitters. Intrathecal gabapentoids reduce neuropathic pain[109] and postoperative pain[43] in animal models. However, when gabapentin and pregabalin are given orally to treat chronic pain in patients, the main binding site for analgesic action may be brain $\alpha_2\delta$ calcium subunits. It has been suggested that oral gabapentoid drugs activate descending noradrenergic pathways to reduce pain in neuropathic and postsurgical pain models.[109,110] Therefore, although gabapentin and pregabalin are water-soluble compounds, intrathecal drug infusion may not offer any advantage over systemic administration for control of chronic pain.

N-Type Calcium Channels N-type calcium channels are composed of a α_1 subunit and are located on synaptic nerve terminals in the dorsal horn.[111] N-type calcium channels are upregulated in pathological states, and animals lacking these channels show less hypersensitivity in animal pain models.[107] Intrathecal administration of selective inhibitors of N-type calcium channels reduced pain behaviors in rats but with significant neurological side effects.[112] An initial clinical trial with intrathecal infusion of ziconotide, an N-type calcium channel blocker, showed analgesia but with severe neurological side effects.[113] Lower doses of intrathecal ziconotide showed less severe side effects but a weaker analgesic effect.[114]

Voltage-Gated Sodium Channels

Action potential generation and conduction of nerve impulses along nerves depend on voltage-gated sodium channels. In addition, these channels appear to have specific roles in pain pathways. All sodium channels have α-subunits that comprise four homologous domains that form a voltage-gated sodium-selective aqueous pore and are associated with accessory β-subunits that modify channel properties.[115] Sodium channels are usually divided into two categories, depending on their sensitivity to the potent sodium channel blocker tetrodotoxin (TTX). In the sensory system, the most important TTX-sensitive subtypes are the Nav1.1, Nav1.3, Nav1.6, and Nav1.7 channels, and the most relevant TTX-resistant channels are Nav1.8 and Nav1.9. All of the clinically used local anesthetics are nonselective sodium channel blockers.

Nav1.3 Sodium Channels After peripheral nerve injury, when hyperalgesia has developed, Nav1.3 channels are upregulated in second-order neurons in the dorsal horn.[1,116] Therefore, reducing Nav1.3 expression has a potential in the treatment of neuropathic pain. However, intrathecal administration of antisense selective for Nav1.3 failed to attenuate mechanical or cold allodynia.[117]

Nav1.7 Sodium Channels The Nav1.7 channel is of special interest because it has been associated with clinical pain disorders: patients with loss-of-function mutations are unable to detect noxious stimuli; patients with gain-of-function mutations have intense burning pain.[107] Nav1.7 is upregulated in the DRG in inflammatory, but not neuropathic, pain models.[107] It is not known if Nav1.7 channels are at presynaptic endings or second-order neurons, and there have been no reports of intrathecal administration of Nav1.7 selective blockers.

Nav1.8 Sodium Channels The Nav1.8 channel is expressed exclusively by primary afferent neurons, and animals lacking Nav1.8 display attenuated responses to noxious mechanical and cold stimuli.[107] Intrathecal injection of Nav1.8 antisense blocked inflammatory pain[115] and neuropathic pain in animal models.[118] Intrathecal injection of Nav1.8-selective snail conotoxins reversed inflammatory and neuropathic pain established in rats.[119] Immunostaining suggests that Nav1.8 channels also exist at presynaptic endings.[120]

Transient Receptor Potential Channels

Transient receptor potential (TRP) channels are nonselective cation channels that respond to noxious chemicals at peripheral nerve endings. However, recent studies show that these receptors also exist on the central terminals of primary afferents and on second-order neurons in the spinal cord.

TRPV1 Vanilloid Type 1 Channels TRPV1 channels have a high permeability to calcium ions. In the peripheral nerve, TRPV1 responds to capsaicin, heat, and protons by evoking painful sensation.[121] TRPV1 channels are also on the central axons of small DRG neurons, down to the presynaptic endings in the spinal cord.[122-124] In addition, TRPV1 channels are on second-order neurons in the dorsal horn,[125] and activation of TRPV1 in the spinal cord results in mechanical allodynia.[126] Intrathecal administration of antisense against TRPV1 reduced mechanical hypersensitivity in rats with peripheral nerve injury,[127] and intrathecal injection of a selective TPPV1 antagonist blocked mechanical allodynia and thermal hyperalgesia in a model of hindpaw inflammation.[128]

Although intrathecal injection of RTX, a capsaicin analog, can relieve pain in dogs with advanced cancer or arthritis, its mode of action is to destroy DRG neurons.[129]

TRPA1 Channels Exposure of the peripheral endings of primary afferents to volatile irritants excites the calcium permeable TRPA1 channel.[107] TRPA1 channels are also on presynaptic small afferent endings in the spinal cord.[130] Intrathecal injection of TRPA1 antagonists blocks mechanical and thermal hyperalgesia evoked by inflamed rat hindpaw[131] and reduce mechanical hypersensitivity in diabetic rats.[132]

Enzyme Systems

We have already discussed the role of intrathecal acetylcholine esterase inhibitors in producing analgesia and attempts to use intrathecal COX inhibitors as analgesics. Many other enzymes, including kinases, and second messenger systems have been associated with pain pathways; however, many have ubiquitous roles in the spinal cord so that a pain-selective effect without numerous side effects may make intrathecal delivery in humans difficult to achieve.

Nitric Oxide Synthase

Nitric oxide (NO) is a gas that can be released from precursor molecules such as L-arginine, when acted on by enzymes: neuronal NO synthase (nNOS) or inducible NOS (iNOS). nNOS is normally present in both presynaptic endings of primary afferents and postsynaptically in inhibitory interneurons and projection neurons in the dorsal horn.[133] In neuropathic pain models, iNOS can also be released in the spinal cord.[134] Intrathecal injection of nonspecific NOS inhibitors, such as L-NAME (L-nitro-arginine methyl ester), reduces nociceptive behavior in several animal models of neuropathic and inflammatory pain.[133] The primary route of NO action in pain pathways is activation of guanylyl cyclase and production of cGMP (cyclic guanosine monophosphate), and intrathecal injection of a guanylyl cyclase inhibitor reduces antinociception in animal pain models.[133] However, the overall role of NO in nociceptive transmission is still unclear because intrathecal injection of NO donors can also be antinociceptive.[133,134] Specific systemically delivered nNOS or iNOS inhibitors are being evaluated in clinical trials for migraine, inflammatory, and neuropathic pain, but no intrathecal formulations exist for clinical trials.

Transporters

The pharmacology of many neurotransmitters, such as norepinephrine and 5-HT, depend on transporters called *reuptake systems*. Reuptake inhibitors of norepinephrine and 5-HT form an important basis for antidepressants and are useful adjuvants in pain management. The effectiveness of intrathecal norepinephrine and 5-HT reuptake inhibitors varies depending on the animal pain model. An intrathecal 5-HT and noradrenaline reuptake inhibitor (but not selective 5-HT reuptake inhibitor) was antiallodynic in a nerve injury model of neuropathic pain, but both classes of drugs were effective in diabetic neuropathic pain.[135]

Ion transporters help to maintain ion gradients, such as those that drive chloride currents.[1,30,107] There are two transport systems that regulate chloride concentration gradients at second-order neurons and presynaptic terminals in the dorsal horn: (1) the potassium-chloride cotransporter, KCC2, which reduces intracellular chloride (opening chloride channel hyperpolarizes cell body), and (2) the sodium-potassium-chloride cotransporter, NKCC1, which increases intracellular chloride (opening chloride channel depolarizes presynaptic terminals, producing presynaptic inhibition).[1,2] Although pharmacological block of KCC2 in rats induces hyperalgesia,[136] the importance of chloride channels to all cells in the spinal cord makes intrathecal modulation of these cotransporters problematic in patients with chronic pain.

Glia

Although this review has emphasized neurons in the spinal cord, other spinal cord cells, specifically microglia and astrocytes, appear to have a role in chronic pain models.[137,138] In response to peripheral inflammation, microglia become activated and release inflammatory cytokines, such as tumor necrosis factor-α (TNF-α), interleukin-1β (IL-1β), and IL-6, that contribute to persistent pain. Soon after the start of peripheral inflammation in rats, IL-1β is upregulated in CSF and precedes COX-2 upregulation.[139] After hip replacement surgery, IL-6, IL-8, and later PGE$_2$ increase in the patient's CSF.[61] After peripheral nerve injury that produces neuropathic pain, microglia are activated, but pre-injury administration of an inhibitor of microglia activation, minocycline, inhibits production of TNF-α, IL-1β, and IL-6, and prevents development of neuropathic pain.[140] The chemokine fractalkine is released by neurons, and after peripheral nerve injury, its CX3CR1 receptor is upregulated in microglia; intrathecal injection of a neutralizing antibody to block CX3CR1 prevents persistent pain.[141,142] Recent interest has been in the toll-like receptor (TLR) subtypes, which are activated in the very earliest stages of pain development, and may decrease opioid potency.[138] Clinical trials have begun in the United States with the orally available, blood–brain barrier permeable glial activation inhibitor ibudilast (an asthma drug used in Japan) for the treatment of neuropathic pain.[138] The main caution about targeting glial cells is that they also have important roles in immune function and homeostasis in the CNS, and so chronically inhibiting their activity, or even the release or binding of one cytokine, for pain management may have unforeseen side effects.

Summary and Conclusions

Knowledge of spinal receptors should be a consideration in selecting existing drugs or new compounds for intervention in pain or spasticity. This is especially true for intrathecal drug delivery, in which the spinal receptors and the neurophysiologic mechanisms that they mediate can provide a rationale basis for drug therapy. Although efficacy in preclinical models does not always predict clinical success, these basic science studies can at least warn of potential side effects. In addition, formulation issues are better addressed at this earlier stage. As more information is obtained about the normal and pathological roles of spinal receptors, improved targeted development of drugs can proceed rather than a more traditional trial-and-error approach. Novel analgesics are still much needed in pain management, and although this chapter presents a myriad of potential receptor binding sites, there may still be unexploited spinal mechanisms that will lead to the drugs of the future.

References

1. Sandkühler J: Models and mechanisms of hyperalgesia and allodynia. *Physiol Rev* 89:707-758, 2009.
2. Price TJ, Cervero F, de Koninck Y: Role of cation-chloride-cotransporters (CCC) in pain and hyperalgesia. *Curr Top Med Chem* 5:547-555, 2005.
3. Coull JA, Boudreau D, Bachand K, et al: Trans-synaptic shift in anion gradient in spinal lamina I neurons as a mechanism of neuropathic pain. *Nature* 424:938-942, 2003.
4. Penn RD, Kroin JS, Reinkensmeyer A, et al: Injection of GABA-agonist into globus pallidus in patient with Parkinson's disease. *Lancet* 351:340-341, 1998.
5. Ho KM, Ismail H: Use of intrathecal midazolam to improve perioperative analgesia: a meta-analysis. *Anaesth Intensive Care* 36:365-373, 2008.

6. Yaksh TL, Allen JW: The use of intrathecal midazolam in humans: a case study of process. *Anesth Analg* 98:1536-1545, 2004.

7. Price GW, Wilkin GP, Turnbull MJ, et al: Are baclofen-sensitive GABAB receptors present on primary afferent terminals of the spinal cord? *Nature* 307:71-74, 1984.

8. Wilson PR, Yaksh TL: Baclofen is antinociceptive in the spinal intrathecal space of animals. *Eur J Pharmacol* 51:323-330, 1978.

9. Kroin JS, Penn RD, Beissinger RL, et al: Reduced spinal reflexes following intrathecal baclofen in the rabbit. *Exp Brain Res* 54:191-194, 1984.

10. Knutsson E, Lindblom U, Mårtensson A: Plasma and cerebrospinal fluid levels of baclofen (Lioresal) at optimal therapeutic responses in spastic paresis. *J Neurol Sci* 23:473-484, 1974.

11. Penn RD, Kroin JS: Intrathecal baclofen alleviates spinal cord spasticity. *Lancet* 1(8385):1078, 1984.

12. Penn RD, Kroin JS: Continuous intrathecal baclofen for severe spasticity. *Lancet* 2(8447):125-127, 1985.

13. Penn RD, Kroin JS: Long-term intrathecal baclofen infusion for treatment of spasticity. Long-term intrathecal baclofen infusion for treatment of spasticity. *J Neurosurg* 66:181-185, 1987.

14. Penn RD, Savoy SM, Corcos D, et al: Intrathecal baclofen for severe spinal spasticity. *N Engl J Med* 320:1517-1521, 1989.

15. Harvey RJ, Depner UB, Wässle H, et al: GlyR alpha3: an essential target for spinal PGE2-mediated inflammatory pain sensitization. *Science* 304:884-887, 2004.

16. Munts AG, van der Plas AA, Voormolen JH, et al: Intrathecal glycine for pain and dystonia in complex regional pain syndrome. *Pain* 146:199-204, 2009.

17. Jones SL: Descending noradrenergic influences on pain. *Prog Brain Res* 88:381-394, 1991.

18. Pertovaara A: Noradrenergic pain modulation. *Prog Neurobiol* 80:53-83, 2006.

19. Ishii H, Kohno T, Yamakura T, et al: Action of dexmedetomidine on the substantia gelatinosa neurons of the rat spinal cord. *Eur J Neurosci* 27:3182-3190, 2008.

20. Reddy SV, Maderdrut JL, Yaksh TL: Spinal cord pharmacology of adrenergic agonist-mediated antinociception. *J Pharmacol Exp Ther* 213:525-533, 1980.

21. Yaksh TL, Pogrel JW, Lee YW, et al: Reversal of nerve ligation-induced allodynia by spinal alpha-2 adrenoceptor agonists. *J Pharmacol Exp Ther* 272:207-214, 1995.

22. Yaksh TL: Spinal systems and pain processing: development of novel analgesic drugs with mechanistically defined models. *Trends Pharmacol Sci* 20:329-337, 1999.

23. Eisenach JC, Lavand'homme P, Tong C, et al: Antinociceptive and hemodynamic effects of a novel alpha2-adrenergic agonist, MPV-2426, in sheep. *Anesthesiology* 91:1425-1436, 1999.

24. Bennett G, Deer T, Du Pen S, et al: Future directions in the management of pain by intraspinal drug delivery. *J Pain Symptom Manage* 20(suppl):S44-S50, 2000.

25. Axelsson K, Gupta A: Local anaesthetic adjuvants: neuraxial versus peripheral nerve block. *Curr Opin Anaesthesiol* 22:649-654, 2009.

26. Malanga G, Reiter RD, Garay E: Update on tizanidine for muscle spasticity and emerging indications. *Expert Opin Pharmacother* 9:2209-2215, 2008.

27. Kroin JS, McCarthy RJ, Penn RD, et al: Continuous intrathecal clonidine and tizanidine in conscious dogs: analgesic and hemodynamic effects. *Anesth Analg* 96:776-782, 2003.

28. Sabbe MB, Penning JP, Ozaki GT, et al: Spinal and systemic action of the alpha 2 receptor agonist dexmedetomidine in dogs. Antinociception and carbon dioxide response. *Anesthesiology* 80:1057-1072, 1994.

29. Kew JN, Kemp JA: Ionotropic and metabotropic glutamate receptor structure and pharmacology. *Psychopharmacology (Berl)* 179:4-29, 2005.

30. Latremoliere A, Woolf CJ: Central sensitization: a generator of pain hypersensitivity by central neural plasticity. *J Pain* 10:895-926, 2009.

31. Nishiyama T, Yaksh TL, Weber E: Effects of intrathecal NMDA and non-NMDA antagonists on acute thermal nociception and their interaction with morphine. *Anesthesiology* 89:715-722, 1998.

32. Zahn PK, Umali E, Brennan TJ: Intrathecal non-NMDA excitatory amino acid receptor antagonists inhibit pain behaviors in a rat model of postoperative pain. *Pain* 74:213-223, 1998.

33. Ault B, Evans RH, Francis AA, et al: Selective depression of excitatory amino acid induced depolarizations by magnesium ions in isolated spinal cord preparations. *J Physiol* 307:413-428, 1980.

34. Kroin JS, McCarthy RJ, Von Roenn N, et al: Magnesium sulfate potentiates morphine antinociception at the spinal level. *Anesth Analg* 90:913-917, 2000.

35. Xiao WH, Bennett GJ: Magnesium suppresses neuropathic pain responses in rats via a spinal site of action. *Brain Res* 666:168-172, 1994.

36. Backonja M, Arndt G, Gombar KA, et al: Response of chronic neuropathic pain syndromes to ketamine: a preliminary study. *Pain* 56:51-57, 1994.

37. Hocking G, Cousins MJ: Ketamine in chronic pain management: an evidence-based review. *Anesth Analg* 97:1730-1739, 2003.

38. Buvanendran A, Kroin JS: Early use of memantine for neuropathic pain. *Anesth Analg* 107:1093-1094, 2008.

39. Wu LJ, Ko SW, Zhuo M: Kainate receptors and pain: from dorsal root ganglion to the anterior cingulate cortex. *Curr Pharm Des* 13:1597-1605, 2007.

40. Jane DE, Lodge D, Collingridge GL: Kainate receptors: pharmacology, function and therapeutic potential. *Neuropharmacology* 56:90-113, 2009.

41. Li JQ, Chen SR, Chen H, et al: Regulation of increased glutamatergic input to spinal dorsal horn neurons by mGluR5 in diabetic neuropathic pain. *J Neurochem* 112:162-172, 2010.

42. Chiari AI, Eisenach JC: Intrathecal adenosine: interactions with spinal clonidine and neostigmine in rat models of acute nociception and postoperative hypersensitivity. *Anesthesiology* 90:1413-1421, 1999.

43. Kroin JS, Buvanendran A, Nagalla SK, et al: Postoperative pain and analgesic responses are similar in male and female Sprague-Dawley rats. *Can J Anaesth* 50:904-908, 2003.

44. Lauretti GR, Hood DD, Eisenach JC, et al: A multi-center study of intrathecal neostigmine for analgesia following vaginal hysterectomy. *Anesthesiology* 89:913-918, 1998.

45. Eisenach JC, Hood DD, Curry R: Phase I human safety assessment of intrathecal neostigmine containing methyl- and propylparabens. *Anesth Analg* 85:842-846, 1997.

46. Decker MW, Rueter LE, Bitner RS: Nicotinic acetylcholine receptor agonists: a potential new class of analgesics. *Curr Top Med Chem* 4:369-384, 2004.

47. Cai YQ, Chen SR, Han HD, et al: Role of M2, M3, and M4 muscarinic receptor subtypes in the spinal cholinergic control of nociception revealed using siRNA in rats. *J Neurochem* 111:1000-1010, 2009.

48. Yaksh TL, Dirksen R, Harty GJ: Antinociceptive effects of intrathecally injected cholinomimetic drugs in the rat and cat. *Eur J Pharmacol* 117:81-88, 1985.

49. Harbaugh RE: Intracerebroventricular bethanechol chloride administration in Alzheimer's disease. *Ann N Y Acad Sci* 531:174-179, 1988.

50. Lichtman AH, Martin BR: Spinal and supraspinal components of cannabinoid-induced antinociception. *J Pharmacol Exp Ther* 258:517-523, 1991.

51. Farquhar-Smith WP, Egertová M, Bradbury EJ, et al: Cannabinoid CB(1) receptor expression in rat spinal cord. *Mol Cell Neurosci* 15:510-521, 2000.

52. Pernía-Andrade AJ, Kato A, Witschi R, et al: Spinal endocannabinoids and CB1 receptors mediate C-fiber-induced heterosynaptic pain sensitization. *Science* 325:760-764, 2009.

53. Beltramo M: Cannabinoid type 2 receptor as a target for chronic pain. *Mini Rev Med Chem* 9:11-25, 2009.

54. Romero-Sandoval A, Eisenach JC: Spinal cannabinoid receptor type 2 activation reduces hypersensitivity and spinal cord glial activation after paw incision. *Anesthesiology* 106:787-794, 2007.

55. Yamamoto W, Mikami T, Iwamura H: Involvement of central cannabinoid CB2 receptor in reducing mechanical allodynia in a mouse model of neuropathic pain. *Eur J Pharmacol* 583:56-61, 2008.

56. Beiche F, Scheuerer S, Brune K, et al: Up-regulation of cyclooxygenase-2 mRNA in the rat spinal cord following peripheral inflammation. *FEBS Lett* 390:165-169, 1996.

57. Ebersberger A, Grubb BD, Willingale HL, et al: The intraspinal release of prostaglandin E2 in a model of acute arthritis is accompanied by an up-regulation of cyclo-oxygenase-2 in the spinal cord. *Neuroscience* 93:775-781, 1999.

58. Zhu X, Conklin D, Eisenach JC: Cyclooxygenase-1 in the spinal cord plays an important role in postoperative pain. *Pain* 104:15-23, 2003.

59. Kroin JS, Ling ZD, Buvanendran A, et al: Upregulation of spinal cyclooxygenase-2 in rats after surgical incision. *Anesthesiology* 100: 364-369, 2004.

60. Kroin JS, Buvanendran A, Watts DE, et al: Upregulation of cerebrospinal fluid and peripheral prostaglandin E2 in a rat postoperative pain model. *Anesth Analg* 103:334-343, 2006.

61. Buvanendran A, Kroin JS, Berger RA, et al: Upregulation of prostaglandin E2 and interleukins in the central nervous system and peripheral tissue during and after surgery in humans. *Anesthesiology* 104:403-410, 2006.

62. Bär KJ, Natura G, Telleria-Diaz A, et al: Changes in the effect of spinal prostaglandin E2 during inflammation: prostaglandin E (EP1-EP4) receptors in spinal nociceptive processing of input from the normal or inflamed knee joint. *J Neurosci* 24:642-651, 2004.

63. Omote K, Yamamoto H, Kawamata T, et al: The effects of intrathecal administration of an antagonist for prostaglandin E receptor subtype EP(1) on mechanical and thermal hyperalgesia in a rat model of postoperative pain. *Anesth Analg* 95:1708-1712, 2002.

64. Zhu X, Conklin DR, Eisenach JC: Preoperative inhibition of cyclooxygenase-1 in the spinal cord reduces postoperative pain. *Anesth Analg* 100:1390-1393, 2005.

65. Eisenach JC, Curry R, Tong C, et al: Effects of intrathecal ketorolac on human experimental pain. *Anesthesiology* 112:1216-1224, 2010.

66. Suzuki R, Rygh LJ, Dickenson AH: Bad news from the brain: descending 5-HT pathways that control spinal pain processing. *Trends Pharmacol Sci* 25:613-617, 2004.

67. Svensson CI, Tran TK, Fitzsimmons B, et al: Descending serotonergic facilitation of spinal ERK activation and pain behavior. *FEBS Lett* 580:6629-6634, 2006.

68. Dogrul A, Ossipov MH, Porreca F: Differential mediation of descending pain facilitation and inhibition by spinal 5HT-3 and 5HT-7 receptors. *Brain Res* 1280:52-59, 2009.

69. Ossipov MH, Lai J, King T, et al: Antinociceptive and nociceptive actions of opioids. *J Neurobiol* 61:126-148, 2004.

70. Yaksh TL, Rudy TA: Analgesia mediated by a direct spinal action of narcotics. *Science* 192:1357-1358, 1976.

71. Brennan TJ, Vandermeulen EP, Gebhart GF: Characterization of a rat model of incisional pain. *Pain* 64:493-501, 1996.

72. Zhao C, Tall JM, Meyer RA, et al: Antiallodynic effects of systemic and intrathecal morphine in the spared nerve injury model of neuropathic pain in rats. *Anesthesiology* 100:905-911, 2004.

73. Kohno T, Ji RR, Ito N, et al: Peripheral axonal injury results in reduced mu opioid receptor pre- and post-synaptic action in the spinal cord. *Pain* 117:77-87, 2005.

74. Onofrio BM, Yaksh TL, Arnold PG: Continuous low-dose intrathecal morphine administration in the treatment of chronic pain of malignant origin. *Mayo Clin Proc* 56:516-520, 1981.

75. Penn RD, Paice JA, Gottschalk W, et al: Cancer pain relief using chronic morphine infusion. Early experience with a programmable implanted drug pump. *J Neurosurg* 61:302-306, 1984.

76. Coffey RJ, Burchiel K: Inflammatory mass lesions associated with intrathecal drug infusion catheters: report and observations on 41 patients. *Neurosurgery* 50:78-86, 2002.

77. Codd EE, Carson JR, Colburn RW, et al: JNJ-20788560 [9-(8-azabicyclo[3.2.1]oct-3-ylidene)-9H-xanthene-3-carboxylic acid diethylamide], a selective delta opioid receptor agonist, is a potent and efficacious antihyperalgesic agent that does not produce respiratory depression, pharmacologic tolerance, or physical dependence. *J Pharmacol Exp Ther* 329:241-251, 2009.

78. Scherrer G, Imamachi N, Cao YQ, et al: Dissociation of the opioid receptor mechanisms that control mechanical and heat pain. *Cell* 137:1148-1159, 2009.

79. Ikoma M, Kohno T, Baba H: Differential presynaptic effects of opioid agonists on Adelta- and C-afferent glutamatergic transmission to the spinal dorsal horn. *Anesthesiology* 107:807-812, 2007.

80. Eliav E, Herzberg U, Caudle RM: The kappa opioid agonist GR89,696 blocks hyperalgesia and allodynia in rat models of peripheral neuritis and neuropathy. *Pain* 79:255-264, 1999.

81. Caram-Salas NL, Reyes-García G, Bartoszyk GD, et al: Subcutaneous, intrathecal and periaqueductal grey administration of asimadoline and ICI-204448 reduces tactile allodynia in the rat. *Eur J Pharmacol* 573:75-83, 2007.

82. Hua XY, Chen P, Marsala M, et al: Intrathecal substance P-induced thermal hyperalgesia and spinal release of prostaglandin E2 and amino acids. *Neuroscience* 89:525-534, 1999.

83. Hill R: NK1 (substance P) receptor antagonists—why are they not analgesic in humans? NK1 (substance P) receptor antagonists—why are they not analgesic in humans? *Trends Pharmacol Sci* 21:244-246, 2000.

84. Coudoré-Civiale MA, Courteix C, et al: Effect of tachykinin receptor antagonists in experimental neuropathic pain. *Eur J Pharmacol* 361:175-184, 1998.

85. Yu LC, Hou JF, Fu FH, et al: Roles of calcitonin gene-related peptide and its receptors in pain-related behavioral responses in the central nervous system. *Neurosci Biobehav Rev* 33:1185-1191, 2009.

86. Sun RQ, Lawand NB, Willis WD: The role of calcitonin gene-related peptide (CGRP) in the generation and maintenance of mechanical allodynia and hyperalgesia in rats after intradermal injection of capsaicin. *Pain* 104:201-208, 2003.

87. Mufson EJ, Kroin JS, Sendera TJ, et al: Distribution and retrograde transport of trophic factors in the central nervous system: functional implications for the treatment of neurodegenerative diseases. *Prog Neurobiol* 57:451-484, 1999.

88. Pezet S, Onténiente B, Grannec G, et al: Chronic pain is associated with increased TrkA immunoreactivity in spinoreticular neurons. *J Neurosci* 19:5482-5492, 1999.

89. Cirillo G, Cavaliere C, Bianco MR, et al: Intrathecal NGF administration reduces reactive astrocytosis and changes neurotrophin receptors expression pattern in a rat model of neuropathic pain. *Cell Mol Neurobiol* 30:51-62, 2010.

90. Salio C, Lossi L, Ferrini F, et al: Ultrastructural evidence for a pre- and postsynaptic localization of full-length trkB receptors in substantia gelatinosa (lamina II) of rat and mouse spinal cord. *Eur J Neurosci* 22:1951-1966, 2005.

91. Coull JA, Beggs S, Boudreau D, et al: BDNF from microglia causes the shift in neuronal anion gradient underlying neuropathic pain. *Nature* 438:1017-1021, 2005.

92. Ochs G, Penn RD, York M, et al: A phase I/II trial of recombinant methionyl human brain derived neurotrophic factor administered by intrathecal infusion to patients with amyotrophic lateral sclerosis. *Amyotroph Lateral Scler Other Motor Neuron Disord* 1:201-206, 2000.

93. Wang H, Kohno T, Amaya F, et al: Bradykinin produces pain hypersensitivity by potentiating spinal cord glutamatergic synaptic transmission. *J Neurosci* 25:7986-7992, 2005.

94. Conley RK, Wheeldon A, Webb JK, et al: Inhibition of acute nociceptive responses in rat spinal cord by a bradykinin B1 receptor antagonist. *Eur J Pharmacol* 527:44-51, 2005.

95. Hökfelt T, Elde R, Johansson O, et al: Immunohistochemical evidence for separate populations of somatostatin-containing and substance P-containing primary afferent neurons in the rat. *Neuroscience* 1:131-136, 1976.

96. Schulz S, Schreff M, Schmidt H, et al: Immunocytochemical localization of somatostatin receptor sst2A in the rat spinal cord and dorsal root ganglia. *Eur J Neurosci* 10:3700-3708, 1998.

97. Gamboa-Esteves FO, McWilliam PN, Batten TF: Substance P (NK1) and somatostatin (sst2A) receptor immunoreactivity in NTS-projecting rat dorsal horn neurones activated by nociceptive afferent input. *J Chem Neuroanat* 27:251-266, 2004.

98. Penn RD, Paice JA, Kroin JS: Octreotide: a potent new non-opiate analgesic for intrathecal infusion. *Pain* 49:13-19, 1992.

99. Deer TR, Penn R, Kim CK, et al: The use of continuous intrathecal infusion of octreotide in patients with chronic pain of noncancer origin: an evaluation of efficacy in a prospective double-blind fashion. *Neuromodulation* 9:284-289, 2006.

100. Hökfelt T, Brumovsky P, Shi T, et al: NPY and pain as seen from the histochemical side. *Peptides* 28:365-372, 2007.

101. Wiesenfeld-Hallin Z, Xu XJ, Hökfelt T: The role of spinal cholecystokinin in chronic pain states. *Pharmacol Toxicol* 91:398-403, 2002.

102. McCleane GJ: The cholecystokinin antagonist proglumide enhances the analgesic efficacy of morphine in humans with chronic benign pain. *Anesth Analg* 87:1117-1120, 1998.

103. Xu XJ, Hökfelt T, Wiesenfeld-Hallin Z. Galanin and spinal pain mechanisms: where do we stand in 2008? *Cell Mol Life Sci* 65:1813-1819, 2008.

104. Murck H, Held K, Ziegenbein M, et al: Intravenous administration of the neuropeptide galanin has fast antidepressant efficacy and affects the sleep EEG. *Psychoneuroendocrinology* 29:1205-1211, 2004.

105. Bauer CS, Nieto-Rostro M, Rahman W, et al: The increased trafficking of the calcium channel subunit alpha2delta-1 to presynaptic terminals in neuropathic pain is inhibited by the alpha2delta ligand pregabalin. *J Neurosci* 29:4076-4088, 2009.

106. Luo ZD, Chaplan SR, Higuera ES, et al: Upregulation of dorsal root ganglion (alpha)2(delta) calcium channel subunit and its correlation with allodynia in spinal nerve-injured rats. *J Neurosci* 21:1868-1875, 2001.

107. Basbaum AI, Bautista DM, Scherrer G, et al: Cellular and molecular mechanisms of pain. *Cell* 139:267-284, 2009.

108. Gee NS, Brown JP, Dissanayake VU, et al: The novel anticonvulsant drug, gabapentin (Neurontin), binds to the alpha2delta subunit of a calcium channel. *J Biol Chem* 271:5768-5776, 1996.

109. Hayashida K, Parker R, Eisenach JC: Oral gabapentin activates spinal cholinergic circuits to reduce hypersensitivity after peripheral nerve injury and interacts synergistically with oral donepezil. *Anesthesiology* 106:1213-1219, 2007.

110. Tanabe M, Takasu K, Kasuya N: Role of descending noradrenergic system and spinal alpha2-adrenergic receptors in the effects of gabapentin on thermal and mechanical nociception after partial nerve injury in the mouse. *Br J Pharmacol* 144:703-714, 2005.

111. Zamponi GW, Lewis RJ, Todorovic SM, et al: Role of voltage-gated calcium channels in ascending pain pathways. *Brain Res Rev* 60:84-89, 2009.

112. Malmberg AB, Yaksh TL: Effect of continuous intrathecal infusion of omega-conopeptides, N-type calcium-channel blockers, on behavior and antinociception in the formalin and hot-plate tests in rats. *Pain* 60:83-90, 1995.

113. Penn RD, Paice JA: Adverse effects associated with the intrathecal administration of ziconotide. *Pain* 85:291-296, 2000.

114. Wallace MS, Rauck R, Fisher R, et al: Intrathecal ziconotide for severe chronic pain: safety and tolerability results of an open-label, long-term trial. *Anesth Analg* 106:628-637, 2008.

115. Wood JN, Boorman JP, Okuse K, et al: Voltage-gated sodium channels and pain pathways. *J Neurobiol* 61:55-71, 2004.

116. Hains BC, Saab CY, Klein JP, et al: Altered sodium channel expression in second-order spinal sensory neurons contributes to pain after peripheral nerve injury. *J Neurosci* 24:4832-4839, 2004.

117. Lindia JA, Köhler MG, Martin WJ, et al: Relationship between sodium channel NaV1.3 expression and neuropathic pain behavior in rats. *Pain* 117:145-153, 2005.

118. Lai J, Gold MS, Kim CS, et al: Inhibition of neuropathic pain by decreased expression of the tetrodotoxin-resistant sodium channel, NaV1.8. *Pain* 95:143-152, 2002.

119. Ekberg J, Jayamanne A, Vaughan CW, et al: muO-conotoxin MrVIB selectively blocks Nav1.8 sensory neuron specific sodium channels and chronic pain behavior without motor deficits. *Proc Natl Acad Sci U S A* 103:17030-17035, 2006.

120. Amaya F, Decosterd I, Samad TA, et al: Diversity of expression of the sensory neuron-specific TTX-resistant voltage-gated sodium ion channels SNS and SNS2. *Mol Cell Neurosci* 15:331-342, 2000.

121. Caterina MJ, Schumacher MA, Tominaga M, et al: The capsaicin receptor: a heat-activated ion channel in the pain pathway. *Nature* 389:816-824, 1997.

122. Valtschanoff JG, Rustioni A, Guo A, et al: Vanilloid receptor VR1 is both presynaptic and postsynaptic in the superficial laminae of the rat dorsal horn. *J Comp Neurol* 436:225-235, 2001.

123. Kim YH, Park CK, Back SK, et al: Membrane-delimited coupling of TRPV1 and mGluR5 on presynaptic terminals of nociceptive neurons. *J Neurosci* 29:10000-10009, 2009.

124. Jeffry JA, Yu SQ, Sikand P, et al: Selective targeting of TRPV1 expressing sensory nerve terminals in the spinal cord for long lasting analgesia. *PLoS One* 4:e7021, 2009.

125. Zhou HY, Chen SR, Chen H, et al: The glutamatergic nature of TRPV1-expressing neurons in the spinal dorsal horn. *J Neurochem* 108:305-318, 2009.

126. Patwardhan AM, Scotland PE, Akopian AN, et al: Activation of TRPV1 in the spinal cord by oxidized linoleic acid metabolites contributes to inflammatory hyperalgesia. *Proc Natl Acad Sci U S A* 106:18820-18824, 2009.

127. Christoph T, Gillen C, Mika J, et al: Antinociceptive effect of antisense oligonucleotides against the vanilloid receptor VR1/TRPV1. *Neurochem Int* 50:281-290, 2007.

128. Cui M, Honore P, Zhong C, et al: TRPV1 receptors in the CNS play a key role in broad-spectrum analgesia of TRPV1 antagonists. *J Neurosci* 26:9385-9393, 2006.

129. Brown DC, Iadarola MJ, Perkowski SZ, et al: Physiologic and antinociceptive effects of intrathecal resiniferatoxin in a canine bone cancer model. *Anesthesiology* 103:1052-1059, 2005.

130. Kim YS, Son JY, Kim TH, et al: Expression of transient receptor potential ankyrin 1 (TRPA1) in the rat trigeminal sensory afferents and spinal dorsal horn. *J Comp Neurol* 518:687-698, 2010.

131. da Costa DS, Meotti FC, Andrade EL, et al: The involvement of the transient receptor potential A1 (TRPA1) in the maintenance of mechanical and cold hyperalgesia in persistent inflammation. *Pain* 148:431-437, 2010.

132. Wei H, Chapman H, Saarnilehto M, et al: Roles of cutaneous versus spinal TRPA1 channels in mechanical hypersensitivity in the diabetic or mustard oil-treated non-diabetic rat. *Neuropharmacology* 58:578-584, 2010.

133. Schmidtko A, Tegeder I, Geisslinger G: No NO, no pain? The role of nitric oxide and cGMP in spinal pain processing. *Trends Neurosci* 32:339-346, 2009.

134. Tanabe M, Nagatani Y, Saitoh K, et al: Pharmacological assessments of nitric oxide synthase isoforms and downstream diversity of NO signaling in the maintenance of thermal and mechanical hypersensitivity after peripheral nerve injury in mice. *Neuropharmacology* 56:702-708, 2009.

135. Ikeda T, Ishida Y, Naono R, et al: Effects of intrathecal administration of newer antidepressants on mechanical allodynia in rat models of neuropathic pain. *Neurosci Res* 63:42-46, 2009.

136. Jolivalt CG, Lee CA, Ramos KM, et al: Allodynia and hyperalgesia in diabetic rats are mediated by GABA and depletion of spinal potassium-chloride co-transporters. *Pain* 140:48-57, 2008.

137. Romero-Sandoval EA, Horvath RJ, DeLeo JA: Neuroimmune interactions and pain: focus on glial-modulating targets. *Curr Opin Investig Drugs* 9:726-734, 2008.

138. Watkins LR, Hutchinson MR, Rice KC, et al: The "toll" of opioid-induced glial activation: improving the clinical efficacy of opioids by targeting glia. *Trends Pharmacol Sci* 30:581-591, 2009.

139. Samad TA, Moore KA, Sapirstein A, et al: Interleukin-1beta-mediated induction of Cox-2 in the CNS contributes to inflammatory pain hypersensitivity. *Nature* 410:471-475, 2001.

140. Raghavendra V, Tanga F, DeLeo JA: Inhibition of microglial activation attenuates the development but not existing hypersensitivity in a rat model of neuropathy. *J Pharmacol Exp Ther* 306:624-630, 2003.

141. Milligan ED, Zapata V, Chacur M, et al: Evidence that exogenous and endogenous fractalkine can induce spinal nociceptive facilitation in rats. *Eur J Neurosci* 20:2294-2302, 2004.

142. Zhuang ZY, Kawasaki Y, Tan PH, et al: Role of the CX3CR1/p38 MAPK pathway in spinal microglia for the development of neuropathic pain following nerve injury-induced cleavage of fractalkine. *Brain Behav Immun* 21:642-651, 2007.

2 Pharmacological Agents and Compounding of Intrathecal Drugs

Shalini Shah, Peter S. Staats, and Sudhir Diwan

CHAPTER OVERVIEW

Chapter Synopsis: Intrathecal infusion of analgesics for pain from various sources can be very effective but faces certain challenges. Typically, intrathecal delivery is used only after more conservative treatments have failed, but studies show that this delivery may provide better analgesia and fewer side effects than maximal medication. Morphine represents the so-called gold standard of pain relief at multiple receptor subtypes in the spinal cord. However, with chronic intrathecal infusion, issues must be considered such as side effects that can arise from high central nervous system concentration and spinal metabolites. The heavy reliance on morphine as an analgesic has led to some improvements in this therapy, including development of hydromorphone, a semisynthetic morphine derivative with a fivefold higher potency and several other advantages. Fentanyl and its derivatives have even greater potency and represent the largest class of synthetic opioids. Certain local anesthetics, which act at sodium channels, can be safely and effectively used intrathecally. Among other voltage-gated channel blockers is the intriguingly efficacious calcium channel conotoxin ziconotide. Clonidine, an adrenergic receptor antagonist, has also seen increased use as a spinal anesthetic, as have γ-aminobutyric acid agonists. Special consideration must be given when attempting to provide a regimen of combined drugs for intrathecal delivery, both to the intended receptor targets and the possibly array of side effects that may arise. Finally, procedural details are particularly important when delivering drugs in this manner to prevent adverse outcomes.

Important Points:

- Intrathecal therapy should be considered after more conservative approaches have failed or patients have significant side effects with systemic analgesics.
- Intrathecal opiate therapy may have a lower side effect profile and better analgesia and probably leads to improved life expectancy in patients with cancer.
- Opioids act through several cellular mechanisms, including inhibition of presynaptic neurotransmitter release from primary afferents via presynaptic calcium channel inhibition. In addition, opioids may act at the postsynaptic level via G-protein-regulated inwardly rectifying K+ channels (GIRKs) inducing neuronal hyperpolarization.
- Morphine is currently the only opioid approved by the Food and Drug Administration (FDA) for intrathecal use and remains the gold standard of therapy. Intrathecally injected morphine is not detected in plasma until 2 hours after administration. Respiratory depression is a function of its rostral spread and redistribution from the cerebrospinal fluid (CSF).
- The role of metabolites is also an important consideration for implantable drug delivery systems, as chronic infusions of morphine do yield potent metabolites that may not be significant with intravenous administration. Morphine-3-glucoronide (M3G) plays a large role with chronic infusions.
- The potency of intrathecal M3G is approximately 10 to 45 times that of morphine and has been associated with sedation, hyperalgesia, allodynia, and myoclonus.[10] Morphine-6-glucuronide (M6G) is associated with potentially fatal renal impairment, ultimately leading to profound sedation and respiratory depression.
- Morphine at dosages of 12 mg/day or greater for longer than 28 days of infusion produces inflammatory masses consisting of multifocal immunoreactive cells, most often observed at the dura-arachnoid layer, aseptic in nature, and ultimately leading to motor weakness secondary to mass evolution and compression if not treated.
- Intrathecal infusions of hydromorphone may be a potential alternative to morphine for patients with pain refractory to morphine or with adverse effects related to morphine use and have been shown to have improved analgesic response by at least 25% in patients who were switched from morphine to hydromorphone because of poor pain relief.
- Fentanyl has shown to be stable as a monotherapy or in combination with bupivacaine, midazolam, or both at room and physiological temperatures for use in an infusion pump. Studies for the use of implantable infusions of fentanyl have shown significant reductions in Visual Analogue Scale (VAS) pain scores and reduction of toxicity in terminal cancer pain patients and in patients with nonmalignant low back pain.
- Bupivacaine is currently the most used local anesthetic in clinical practice for intrathecal infusion systems. Because the pharmacokinetic and pharmacodynamic properties of bupivacaine are well understood, they can be used to guide dosing effect.
- The addition of intrathecal bupivacaine to opioids has been shown to improve analgesia in cancer patients who have failed intrathecal opioid therapy alone. Such combinations have led to similar results in nonmalignant pain. The addition of bupivacaine to intrathecal opioids either decreased opioid side effects or enhanced analgesia in 77% of a population with chronic intrathecal infusion therapy of 1 year's duration.
- α$_2$-Adrenoceptor agonists such as clonidine decrease presynaptic calcium currents and thus decrease the release of pro-nociceptive neurotransmitters such as substance P and calcitonin gene-related peptide. In addition, α$_2$-adrenoceptor agonists increase

CHAPTER OVERVIEW—cont'd

potassium conductance and hyperpolarize dorsal horn neurons. Clinically, clonidine has been shown to be effective for the treatment of cancer pain, neuropathic pain, chronic benign pain, experimental hyperalgesia, and spasticity.
- Ziconotide is a neuron-specific calcium channel blocker used intrathecally in the management of pain. The drug works by blocking neurotransmission from primary afferents of neuronal dendrites and axon terminals. Previously, ziconotide was relegated as a last-attempt agent when trials with all other opioids, including intrathecal morphine, had failed. However, based on new literature, a recent consensus statement recommended moving ziconotide as a first-line agent to a level 1 drug with morphine and hydromorphone for chronic intrathecal drug delivery systems.

Clinical Pearls:
- The practice of blending, or "cocktailing," includes an understanding of achieving a response by different receptor site activation while minimizing risks of adverse effects such as respiratory depression and granuloma formation. Common admixtures of two opioids or opioids and local anesthetic agents are created to minimize the maximal dose of a single agent such to avoid toxicity, possible allergy to the drug, adverse drug events, and inflammatory reactions as a result of high concentrations of a single agent.
- A "compounded sterile preparation" (CSP) is defined in USP Chapter 797 as a dosage unit that (1) is prepared according to manufacturer's labeled instructions; (2) contains nonsterile ingredients or uses nonsterile components and devices that must be sterilized before administration; or (3) is biologic, diagnostic, drug, nutrient, or pharmaceutical that possesses either of the two previous characteristics and that includes, but are not limited to, baths and soaks for live organs and tissues, implants, inhalations, injections, powder for injection, irrigations, metered sprays, and ophthalmic and otic preparations.
- Powders derived from high-grade chemicals approved by the United States Pharmacopeia (USP) are combined according to the chemical formula for mixture, weighted and dissolved in sterile water, and filtered for injection. The USP-National Formulary (USP-NF) has required all sterile compounding comply with Chapter 797, which outlines the mandatory requirements to prepare sterile injectables.
- A cleanroom has a controlled level of contamination that is specified by the number of particles per cubic meter at a specified particle size and are categorized accordingly into classes. All agents prepared for intrathecal use must be prepared in a Class 100 cleanroom.
- After medications have been prepared and filtered in a laboratory, they are filtered again by the physician before delivery to the CSF. Sterile filtration requires a 0.2-μm size filter or smaller.

Clinical Pitfalls:
- The principles behind compounding agents for intrathecal use is preparing products that are not readily available for commercial use. Currently, there are no FDA suggested recommendations for mixed or blended compounds of two or more agents.
- It is well known that the stability of intrathecal agents at physiological temperature is important to the ultimate success of the analgesic therapy. Some agents are not stable at certain concentrations, certain temperatures, or when mixed in combination with other agents. Although most pharmacological agents are intended for use within 1 to 2 weeks of manufacture date, intrathecal agents are not intended for shelf life and must be administered either on the date of preparation or the beyond use date that has been established for the drug as a result of stability testing.
- All infusion admixtures of single- and mixed-entity agents are off label. There are no instructions or approved monographs yet by the FDA. Physicians who administer the medications typically give patients instructions on maintenance of the pump and how to prepare for adverse effects.

Introduction

Chronic intrathecal infusion of analgesics has been used increasingly for the management of chronic benign, neuropathic, and cancer pain in patients who have failed more conservative therapies. Originally, intrathecal morphine was used as the sole agent for patients with severe pain. It was later recognized that there were numerous receptor-specific agents that could modulate transmission, which has stimulated research on specific agents. Because many of the analgesia receptors are located in the spinal cord, application of low doses of analgesics can provide profound relief. The spinal receptor pharmacology has a provided a foundation for intrathecal drug delivery and leads to the belief that numerous agents may be able to modulate pain transmission.

Intrathecal therapy should be considered after more conservative approaches have failed or patients have significant side effects with systemic analgesics. One study that randomized patients to receive intrathecal analgesia versus maximal medical management found that intrathecal opiate therapy has a lower side effect profile and better analgesia and probably leads to improved life expectancy in patients with cancer.[1] The aim of this chapter is to expand the current knowledge concerning the diverse array of intrathecal drugs that are potentially available for clinical use for the management of chronic pain (**Table 2-1**) as well understand the principles

Table 2-1: Commonly Used Intrathecal Agents by Class

Commonly Used Intrathecal Agent by Class	Medication	FDA Approved for Intrathecal Injection
Opioids	Morphine	Approved
	Hydromorphone	Not approved
	Fentanyl	Not approved
	Sufentanil	Not approved
	Meperidine	Not approved
	Methadone	Not approved
Local anesthetics	Lidocaine	Not approved
	Bupivacaine	Not approved
	Ropivacaine	Not approved
	Tetracaine	Not approved
GABA-receptor agonists	Baclofen	Approved
	Midazolam	Not approved
Calcium channel antagonist	Ziconotide	Approved
Adrenergic agonist	Clonidine	Not approved

FDA, Food and Drug Administration; GABA, γ-aminobutyric acid.

of preparing and compounding these drugs for intrathecal drug delivery systems (IDDS).

Morphine

Morphine is considered by some the "gold standard." The discovery of opioid receptors in the intrathecal space by Yaksh and Rudy[2] marked a milestone in analgesic therapy, and further developments in intraspinal drug delivery have rapidly evolved since. Intrathecal opioids act at the substantia gelatinosa in the dorsal horn of the spinal cord at specific μ, κ, and δ receptors. Studies suggest that peripheral and spinal δ and κ opioid receptors are important when nociceptive behaviors are established. In contrast, μ opioid receptors are more important at the beginning of the injury when the sensory system has not changed.[3] Apart from specific receptor activation, opioids may also act through several cellular mechanisms, including inhibition of presynaptic neurotransmitter release from primary afferents via presynaptic calcium channel inhibition.[4,5] In addition, opioids may act at the postsynaptic level via G-protein–regulated inwardly rectifying K+ channels (GIRKs) inducing neuronal hyperpolarization.[6]

Morphine is currently the only opioid approved by the Food and Drug Administration (FDA) for intrathecal use. Intrathecal morphine is approximately 10 times more potent than the same dose administered epidurally. Because of the small volume of distribution of the cerebrospinal fluid (CSF) space, the CSF concentration of a given intrathecal dose of morphine is much higher than vascular absorption from an epidural dose. Therefore, the duration of action of an intrathecal dose is relatively long given to the fact that the rate of elimination from CSF is similar to rate of elimination from plasma. After intrathecal injection, morphine is not detected in plasma until 2 hours after administration. Respiratory depression is a function of its rostral spread and redistribution from the CSF. Elimination also occurs via systemic vascular absorption from the spinal capillary bed supplying the spinal cord. However, because duration of action is a function of redistribution from CSF to plasma, limited metabolism occurs in the spinal cord. The role of metabolites is an important consideration for implantable drug delivery systems because chronic infusions of morphine do yield potent metabolites that may not be significant with intravenous (IV) administration. Morphine-3-glucuronide (M3G) plays a large role with chronic infusions because the potency of intrathecal M3G is approximately 10 to 45 times that of morphine and has been associated with sedation, hyperalgesia, allodynia, and myoclonus.[7] Morphine-6-glucuronide (M6G) is associated with chronic nausea and vomiting and profound sedation, ultimately leading to respiratory depression in patients with compromised renal function. Intrathecal administration of morphine varies in many ways from epidural or IV pharmacokinetics, which is important for clinicians to understand, particularly for long-term chronic infusion delivery systems.

Drug-related side effects of intrathecal opioids are secondary to either the presence of direct opioid receptor activation in the CSF or of systemic absorption into the plasma. Almost all intrathecal opioid-related side effects are mediated by opioid receptors because vascular uptake, although it does occur to some degree, is clinically insignificant.[8,9] Morphine, with low lipophilicity, slowly ascends the spinal column and produces a slower onset and longer duration of action of analgesia but also a higher incidence of drug-related adverse effects. Most commonly seen are pruritus (incidence varies from 0% to 100%), nausea and vomiting (30%), urinary retention (42% to 80%), constipation (30%), dose-dependent mental status

change (10% to 14%), sexual dysfunction and loss of libido from hypothalamic-pituitary suppression, hyperalgesia (in animal models, particularly with high doses), and respiratory depression.[8-12] Respiratory depression caused by intrathecal opioids can be classified as bimodal: early (within 2 hours of drug delivery) or delayed. Early respiratory depression due to intrathecal morphine has yet to be reported. Delayed depression results from the cephalad migration of opioids and eventual respiratory center depression of the ventral medulla oblongata, and a paucity of case reports exist in the literature secondary to long-term intrathecal morphine therapy.[8] Respiratory depression can be reversed with μ-receptor antagonists such as naloxone or a mixed antagonist such as nalbuphine; however, the analgesic effect may or may not be maintained. Side effects of intrathecal infusions of opioids such as morphine are most commonly encountered at the initiation of therapy and generally resolve on an average of 3 months after the start of therapy.[13] The incidence of adverse effects secondary to long-term intrathecal opioid delivery systems decreases with effective medical management and dose reductions as therapy continues.[14]

Clinical Efficacy

The clinical efficacy of intrathecal morphine for chronic infusions has been extensively studied for chronic refractory malignant and nonmalignant pain. Strong evidence suggests that intrathecal analgesia is more effectively treated in patients with nociceptive pain disorders than neuropathic or deafferentation pain syndromes in the short term; however, the long-term effectiveness is higher in the neuropathic and deafferentation populations, although this is not always the case.[12,13] Patients who received intrathecal morphine for longer than 2 years showed an escalation of dose requirements, and the best long-term results were for mixed pain syndromes and deafferentation pain. Initially, nociceptive pain showed the best improvement (average pain reduction, 78%) in symptoms, but long-term analysis demonstrated a diminishing rate of improvement in pain control (average pain reduction at 6 months, 68%).[13] When patients with severe pain problems are selected as pump candidates, they will likely improve with the therapy, but their overall severity of pain and symptoms will remain high.[15]

In patients with refractory cancer pain, an IDDS with an infusion of morphine provides sustained pain control, significantly less drug-related toxicity, and possible better survival than medical management in short term (4 weeks) and long term (>28 days to 6 months) therapy.[1,16] On average, there is a significant decrease in toxicity (50% vs. 17%) and pain (52% vs. 39%) and increased survival (54% vs. 37%) in patients treated with IDDS over multidisciplinary medical management. Drug-related adverse effects such as fatigue and mentation are also predictably lower in IDDS-treated patients in the short term and long term as a result of decrease in systemic opioid use. Consistently, patients with refractory cancer pain achieve better analgesia and less adverse effects when managed with chronic infusions of intrathecal morphine.

Hydromorphone

Hydromorphone is a semisynthetic hydrogenated ketone derivative of morphine. Hydromorphone's potency appears to be five times greater than morphine and faster acting because of its greater lipophilic properties. Hydromorphone, similar to morphine, also binds at μ-opioid receptors, and its effects are similarly mediated via presynaptic inhibition of neurotransmitter release and hyperpolarization of postsynaptic neurons in the dorsal horn. Although hydromorphone and morphine may be similar mechanistically, inherent pharmacokinetic properties of hydromorphone may provide many advantages over morphine when delivered intrathecally. Intrathecal infusions of hydromorphone may be a potential alternative to morphine for patients with pain refractory to morphine or with adverse effects related to morphine use and has been shown to have improved analgesic response by at least 25% in patients who were switched from morphine to hydromorphone because of poor pain relief.[17,18] Also as a result of its high relative potency, an intrathecal hydromorphone dose is one-fifth of morphine at equianalgesic dose, hence decreased side effects.[18] Unlike morphine, hydromorphone has no active metabolites, which would prevent side effects such as sedation, hyperalgesia, allodynia, and myoclonus seen with M3G.

Hydromorphone as a single analgesic for intractable nonmalignant pain has been shown to be a very effective analgesic in short- and long-term monotherapy with an unchanged side effect profile.[19] Stability and compatibility in an implantable infusion system was analyzed using high-performance liquid chromatography (HPLC) and shown to be stable at physiological temperatures for at least 4 months and that current clinical practice of refilling the pump every 3 months is appropriate.[20]

Fentanyl and Sufentanil

Fentanyl and the fentanyl derivatives such as sufentanil are currently the most commonly used synthetic opioids in clinical practice. They are highly lipophilic and readily cross lipophilic barriers and with relative potency greater than 100:1 for fentanyl to morphine and 1000:1 for sufentanil to fentanyl. Intrathecal fentanyl has 10 to 20 times greater potency than systemic administration secondary to its high lipophilicity. Fentanyl has shown to be stable as a monotherapy or in combination with bupivacaine, midazolam, or both at room and physiological temperature for use in an infusion pump.[12] Studies for the use of implantable infusions of fentanyl have shown significant reduction in VAS pain scores and reduction of toxicity in terminal cancer pain patients and in non-malignant low back pain.[7,21,22] More studies, however, are needed to enhance understanding of the efficacy and side effects of chronic infusions.

Local Anesthetics

Local anesthetics such as bupivacaine, lidocaine, and ropivacaine bind to the intracellular portion of sodium channels and block sodium influx into neurons to prevent cellular depolarization. The safety of chronic infusion of local anesthetics has been questioned for certain local anesthetics, such as lidocaine and tetracaine, secondary to potential neurotoxicity. In contrast, the safety and efficacy of bupivacaine have been demonstrated for the treatment of cancer pain and nonmalignant pain. Bupivacaine is currently the most used local anesthetic in clinical practice for intrathecal infusion systems. Because the pharmacokinetic and pharmacodynamic properties of bupivacaine are well understood, they can be used to guide dosing effect.

Bupivacaine elimination is based on the total dose infused, rate of delivery, drug concentration, route of delivery, and vascularity of the site. Compared with lidocaine, the onset of action of bupivacaine is moderate, and the duration of action is significantly prolonged; however, the time to peak serum levels after intrathecal administration is not yet clearly defined.[23] Bupivacaine is metabolized via conjugation with glucuronic acid and renal excretion. Of note, the systemic absorption of bupivacaine after intrathecal administration is not affected by age.[24] Common adverse effects include paresthesias, motor block, hypotension, or

urinary retention, which can limit dose titration to analgesic effect. Tachyphylaxis can develop with chronic infusion. However, bupivacaine is an effective analgesic adjuvant when combined with opioids for chronic intrathecal infusion.

Animal studies to identify potential toxicity with bupivacaine for intrathecal use have primarily provided safe results. Neurotoxicity after chronic subarachnoid infusion in rat models shows time-dependent correlation with clinical findings at 0.5% bupivacaine concentration. The incidence of paralysis was dependent on the duration of exposure to the local anesthetic, but no abnormal histopathological differences could correlate with clinical findings.[25] Studies in dog models suggest that chronic intrathecal bupivacaine infusion through an implantable pump system may be a short-term alternative to intrathecal morphine in the control of cancer pain.[26] According to Yamashita and colleagues,[27] characteristic histopathological changes were vacuolation in the dorsal funiculus and chromatolytic damage of motor neurons in week infusions with rabbit models. The extent of vacuolation of the dorsal funiculus was in the order of lidocaine equal to tetracaine followed by bupivacaine and ultimately ropivacaine with the least changes. Large concentrations of local anesthetics administered intrathecally increased glutamate concentrations in the CSF. The therapeutic index of neurotoxicity is narrowest with lidocaine.[27]

The addition of intrathecal bupivacaine to opioids has been shown to improve analgesia in cancer patients who have failed intrathecal opioid therapy alone.[28] Such combinations have led to similar results in nonmalignant pain. The addition of bupivacaine to intrathecal opioids either decreased opioid side effects or enhanced analgesia in 77% of population with chronic intrathecal infusion therapy of 1 year's duration.[29] Although these results seem promising, all studies thus far have primarily been case reports or nonrandomized trials. One recent long-term multicenter, randomized, double-blinded clinical trial found that bupivacaine up to 8 mg/day did not provide any extra analgesic relief than opioid alone.[30] Development of tolerance to long-term infusions of opioids and local anesthetics may also be a factor.

Clonidine (α₂-Agonists)

Intraspinal clonidine has gained widespread popularity for the treatment of chronic pain. In general, α_2-adrenoceptor agonists decrease presynaptic calcium currents and thus decrease the release of pro-nociceptive neurotransmitters such as substance P and calcitonin gene-related peptide (CGRP). In addition, α_2-adrenoceptor agonists increase potassium conductance and hyperpolarize dorsal horn neurons. Clinically, clonidine has been shown to be effective for the treatment of cancer pain, neuropathic pain, chronic benign pain, experimental hyperalgesia, and spasticity.[31-33] The reported dose range for clonidine is 17 to 1500 μg/24 hr with a usual starting dosage of 75 to 150 μg/24 hr. Because α_2-adrenoceptor agonists also decrease sympathetic outflow, the ability to achieve effective analgesia with monotherapy is limited frequently by hypotension, bradycardia, and sedation. Similar to opioids, chronic infusion of these agents is associated with tolerance that often requires an increase in dose.

Midazolam (GABA-A Agonist)

γ-Aminobutyric acid-A (GABA-A) and GABA-B receptor agonists have been injected spinally for the treatment of chronic pain. In general, GABA-B agonists hyperpolarize neurons by increasing outward potassium conductance and decrease neurotransmitter release by reducing inward calcium conductance. In contrast,

GABA-A agonists likely enhance the effect of the inhibitory neurotransmitter GABA on the chlorine ionophore of the GABA-A receptor. Concerns regarding neurotoxicity in animals have limited the use of the GABA-A receptor agonist midazolam in the clinical setting. Nevertheless, several reports suggest that intrathecal midazolam mixed with morphine provides relief of intractable cancer pain, and midazolam mixed with clonidine seems to benefit patients with benign neurogenic and musculoskeletal pain.[34]

Baclofen (GABA-B Agonist)

In contrast, the GABA-B receptor agonist baclofen has a long history of safety after spinal administration and has been shown to be efficacious in the treatment of central pain secondary to spinal cord injury, neuropathic pain, and spasticity.[35] The reported dose range for baclofen is 100 to 400 µg/24 hr. Side effects such as motor weakness, lethargy, and seizures can limit the ability to achieve adequate analgesia. Compared with the widespread effectiveness of baclofen in diverse animal models of pain, the use of baclofen for the treatment of chronic pain in humans has been less rewarding.[36-38] Although baclofen has been combined with morphine for treating mixed pain syndromes, long-term studies on the stability and neurotoxicity of the drug mixture have not been performed. Detailed coverage of intrathecal baclofen is addressed in Chapters 20 and 21.

Ziconotide

Ziconotide is a neuron-specific calcium channel blocker used intrathecally in the management of pain and works by blocking neurotransmission from primary afferents of neuronal dendrites and axon terminals. It is a synthetic derivative of ω-conopeptide MVIIA, a 25-aminoacid polypeptide found in the venom of the conus magnus snail.[39] It has been shown to be more effective than placebo in cancer-related pain and nonmalignant pain. Previously, ziconotide was relegated as a last-attempt agent when trials with all other opioids, including intrathecal morphine, had failed. However, based on the literature, a recent consensus statement recommended moving ziconotide as a first-line agent with morphine and hydromorphone for chronic intrathecal delivery systems.[12] Ziconotide, as yet, is only approved for chronic infusions via implantable delivery systems and not for single injection use. It has been shown to be more efficacious for neuropathic pain, but it has shown good results for nociceptive and mixed etiologies as well.[40]

The structure of ziconotide has many implications for its use as an intrathecal agent. Primarily, the length and folding of the 25 amino acid sequence present a serious challenge for the production of clinical supplies. Therefore, the cost of the drug, on a molar basis, is likely significantly higher for ziconotide than for small-molecule agents of average structure complexity. Second, although its hydrophilicity may make it readily formulable in aqueous pharmaceutical preparations, its large size and hydrophilicity limit its tissue penetration. Thus, ziconotide is most effective when delivered directly to the compartment where its molecular target resides.[41] In the case of chronic pain therapy, this compartment is the spinal cord and CSF. After it has been delivered to its targeted area, it does not clear from that compartment by diffusion because of its low tissue permeability unlike most other analgesic compounds; these factors must be considered in preparing for its use.

The pharmacokinetics of intrathecally administered ziconotide have been studied in terms of its distribution, metabolism, and elimination in rat models. Ziconotide has a narrow therapeutic window, and adverse neurological events seems primarily to be dose dependent. In contrast to its short half-life demonstrated in serum animal models (22 to 44 min), the CSF half-life is approximately 4.5 hours, and the clearance rate is 0.26 mL/min, which is similar to the rate of CSF production (0.35 mL/min).[41] These values suggest that ziconotide clearance depends on CSF flow rather than drug metabolism, and dose regimens should be titrated accordingly.

If opioids and ziconotide both selectively block N-type voltage-gated calcium channels on presynaptic afferents, how is it possible that ziconotide is the drug of choice for patients who have failed opioid therapy? The answer lies with detailed understanding of the molecular mechanism of action of ziconotide compared with opioids. Whereas ziconotide is a direct inhibitor of neuronal voltage-gated calcium channels, opioids indirectly inhibit voltage-gated calcium channels via a G-protein coupled mechanism triggered by µ-receptor activation. However, ziconotide is a direct inhibitor of the same channels and permanently blocks the pore conductance of calcium within the neuron on all presynaptic afferents (C and A), not C fibers only. As a result, the mixture of morphine and ziconotide has uniquely additive antinociceptive properties, even in morphine-tolerant patients. The differential blockade as well as permanent impedance of calcium conductance as a result of direct channel blockade is consistent with effects of ziconotide even in patients who failed opioid therapy.[41]

The direct receptor antagonism by ziconotide also explains the lack of tolerance to the drug and is consistent with the general observation that tolerance is more likely to develop to an agonist than to an antagonist.[41] Although the mechanisms of tolerance may still need further review, it is correlated to opiate-receptor uncoupling of voltage-gated calcium channels. However, no such uncoupling mechanism is possible with a direct calcium channel antagonist such as ziconotide, which may explain the mechanism of lack of tolerance seen in several animal studies. Thus, ziconotide has unusual and unique molecular pharmacology that is responsible for three novel properties of ziconotide consistent with its observed effects: (1) efficacy in patients who have failed opiate therapy, (2) additive analgesia with opioids, and (3) a lack of tolerance to ziconotide. Therefore, ziconotide can be used effectively alone or in combination with morphine to enhance antinociceptive activity.[41]

The dose-dependent adverse effects of intrathecal administration may, however, limit ziconotide's use in a subpopulation of pain patients. The most commonly experienced side effects are neurological and vestibulopathical, presumably secondary to its calcium channel antagonism in the cerebellum. Sedation, nausea, headache, vertigo, ataxia, slurred speech, double vision, memory loss, and significant neuropsychiatric symptoms (e.g., anxiety, depression, mood instability, hallucinations) have been reported. Meningitis has also often been reported. Symptoms correlate with the rate of infusion and concentration of drug infused, and a low mean dose is associated with significant improvement in pain and better tolerated than faster titrations.[42] The starting dose of intrathecal ziconotide begin at a low of 0.5 µg/day with increases of no more than 0.5 µg/day. Filtered delivery of the drug product is mandatory to decrease the risk of infection. Patients being considered for therapy with ziconotide should be educated about the high potential for neuropsychiatric adverse effects of the drug and should provide consent that they have been advised of the risks and benefits before initiating therapy.

The large, complex 25-amino acid polypeptide structure of ziconotide causes stability issues at physiological temperatures for long-term IDDS. Ziconotide has been shown to be useful in approximately 37% of patients.[41] It presents with many adverse effects and is not easy to mix with other agents. Single-agent stability is approximately 90 to 120 days, but in combination with other agents, pump refill time is approximately 4 weeks. Ziconotide has more molecular stability at concentrations greater than 1 μg/mL, and certainly greater stability as a single agent over an admixture.[12] Interestingly, hydromorphone has greater stability (40 days at 37° C) with ziconotide than morphine (15 days) when measured by HPLC. Morphine and hydromorphone accelerate ziconotide degradation, so admixtures with lower concentrations of opioids are more stable.[12,43] Fentanyl, with higher intrinsic potency, should potentially show most stability with ziconotide; however, no studies are available. When considering adding an opioid admixture with ziconotide to ziconotide-refractory patients, compounding with low opioid doses has been shown to improve efficacy.[12]

Compounding Drugs for Intrathecal Use

Physicians need to have an understanding of the safety and efficacy before considering compounding or administering novel analgesic combinations into the intrathecal space. A clear understanding of the toxicities and risk is necessary. The principles behind compounding agents for intrathecal use include preparing products that are not readily available for commercial use. Solutions prepared from powders of single-entity salts (e.g., morphine sulfate) are compounded in sterile environments and generally prepared for same day administration, not for shelf life unless testing has been done to ensure stability for longer periods. Many of these drugs and combinations of drugs are not specifically approved for intrathecal administration. Currently, there are no FDA-suggested recommendations for mixed or blended compounds of two or more agents. There is even less literature on how to compound admixtures and the methodological regulations necessary for this purpose. Therefore, it is necessary for physicians to understand the principles of customizing blends of medications for intrathecal drug infusion systems to create an efficacious form on an individual basis as indicated for the patient. In addition, the compounding pharmacist that is consulted must have a thorough knowledge of the pharmacokinetics of each of the agents, and the facilities used to prepare these compounds must comply with the highest standards of practice.

Understanding Targeted Receptors

As with all other medication administration regimens, therapy should be targeted to activation and inhibition of specific receptors. The concept of polyanalgesia in intrathecal infusion systems is to target the specific receptors involved in the pain response (**Table 2-2**). For example, μ-receptor activation specifically inhibits nociceptive signals, and *N*-methyl-D-aspartate (NMDA) or sodium channel blockers are more efficacious for neuropathic pain. The polyanalgesic approach provides aggressive pain control while minimizing drug-related side effects of a high concentration of a single agent and may reduce pain and improve quality of life.[44]

Combination Therapy

The practice of blending, or "cocktailing," includes an understanding of achieving a response by different receptor site activation while minimizing the risks of adverse effects such as respiratory depression, sedation, and granuloma formation. Common admixtures of two opioids or opioids and local anesthetic agents are created to minimize the maximal dose of a single agent to avoid

Table 2-2: Targeted Receptors for Common Intrathecal Drug Infusions

Receptors	Desired Response	Intrathecal Medication
μ	Nociceptive pain	Morphine, fentanyl, hydromorphone, methadone, meperidine
GABA	Neuropathic pain, spasticity, anti-emesis	Baclofen, midazolam
α_2-Receptors	Neuropathic pain Sympathetic and visceral pain	Clonidine Clonidine
NMDA	Neuropathic pain	Methadone, ketamine
Sodium channel antagonists	Neuropathic pain	Local anesthetics
	Sympathetic and visceral pain	Local anesthetics
Calcium channel antagonists	Neuropathic pain, nociceptive pain	Ziconotide

GABA, γ-aminobutyric acid; *N*-methyl-D-aspartate.

toxicity, possible allergy to the drug, adverse drug events, and inflammatory reactions (granulomas) as a result of high concentrations of a single agent. Popular combinations include morphine and fentanyl; morphine and hydromorphone; morphine and clonidine; and morphine, bupivacaine, fentanyl, and clonidine. The addition of a local anesthetic, for example, has been shown to be very effective in treating phantom limb pain in which denervation of central pain fibers can contribute to peripheral nerve pain. Baclofen may be added for tremors.[45] Midazolam has been shown to be effective against persistent nausea and vomiting from opioid infusions.[46] Pitfalls to single-entity delivery systems do exist, as in the example of morphine in which granulomas can occur, causing a mass effect on the spinal cord as a result of poor placement of the catheter tip. Placing a catheter too caudal in an area that cannot tolerate a high concentration or rapid infusion rate can result in severe inflammatory granulomatous reactions. In such a situation it may be advisable to infuse an admixture of clonidine and morphine, which has extensively been shown to inhibit the formation of granulomas while achieving the same level of analgesia.[31,47] **Table 2-3** outlines current standard of polyanalgesic admixtures for first-, second-, and third-line therapies.

Preparation of Agents and Sterile Technique

A "compounded sterile preparation" (CSP) is defined in United States Pharmacopeia (USP) Chapter 797 as a dosage unit that (1) is prepared according to manufacturer's labeled instructions; (2) contains nonsterile ingredients or uses nonsterile components and devices that must be sterilized before administration; or (3) is biologic, diagnostic, drug, nutrient, or pharmaceutical agent that possesses either of the two previous characteristics and that includes, but is not limited to, baths and soaks for live organs and tissues, implants, inhalations, injections, powder for injection, irrigations, metered sprays, and ophthalmic and otic preparations.[48] Powders derived from high-grade USP-approved chemicals are combined according to the chemical formula for mixture, weighted

Table 2-3: Recommendations for Commonly Used Polyanalgesic Admixtures for Intrathecal Infusion*

First-line agents	Morphine	Hydromorphone		Ziconotide
Second-line agents	Fentanyl	Morphine or hydromorphone + ziconotide		Morphine or hydromorphone + bupivacaine or clonidine
Third-line agents	Clonidine	Morphine, fentanyl, or hydromorphone + bupivacaine or clonidine + ziconotide		
Fourth-line agents	Sufentanil	Sufentanil + bupivacaine or clonidine + ziconotide		

*Morphine and ziconotide are approved by the Food and Drug Administration for intrathecal infusions and are first-line therapies along with hydromorphone for nociceptive, neuropathic, and mixed pain syndromes. Fentanyl and clonidine are added as second-line agents for their proposed granuloma-sparing effects. Experimental drugs (fifth- and sixth-line drugs) are not included in this table because a paucity of literature exists to support their efficacy.
Adapted from 2007 Polyanalgesic Consensus Conference Algorithm for intrathecal polyanalgesic therapies. *Neuromodulation* 10:300-328, 2007.

Table 2-4: Requirements for Risk-Level Appropriate Compounding

Classification	Requirements
Low-risk compounding	Simple admixtures compounded using closed-system methods Prepared in an ISO Class 5 (Class 100) hood Located in an ISO Class 8 (Class 100,000) cleanroom with anteroom area Routine disinfection and air quality testing Review for correct identity and amounts of components before and after compounding
Medium-risk compounding	Admixtures compounded using multiple additives, small volumes, or both May involve multiple pooled sterile products for multiple patients (batched antibiotics) Preparation for use over several days Powders prepared in ISO Class 5 hood located in an ISO Class 8 cleanroom with an anteroom area
High-risk compounding	Nonsterile (bulk powders) ingredients or prepared from sterile ingredients but exposed to less than ISO Class 5 More than a 6-hour delay from compounding to sterilization Purity of components is assumed but not verified by documentation Open system transfers

ISO, International Standardization Organization.
Adapted from Kastango E: *The ASHP Discussion Guide for Compounding Sterile Preparations: Summary and Implementation of USP Chapter 797.* Washington, DC, 2004, ASHP Publishing.

and dissolved in sterile water, and filtered for injection. The USP-National Formulary (USP-NF) has required all sterile compounding comply with mandatory requirements to prepare sterile injectables (**Table 2-4**). The USP-NF defines designs of the environment, which include a cleanroom with and without gloveboxes or hoods and outlines procedures for gowning, gloving, and masking during sterilization. End-product testing for sterility, pyrogenicity, and endotoxin and potency testing is also regulated.

Microbial Contamination Risk Level

To compound level 3, or highest risk, drugs, such as sterile intrathecal agents, preparation begins with compliance of Chapter 797 regulations and risk-level determination. Appropriate risk level

(low, level 1; moderate, level 2; and high, level 3) is assigned according to the corresponding probability of contamination with microbes (organisms, spores, endotoxins), foreign chemicals, or physical matter. Risk-level classification is, in general, not prescriptive. Ultimately, assigning the appropriate risk level to a CSP requires the professional judgment of the pharmacist.

Previously, implanted intrathecally delivered medications were considered level 2 or moderate risk as were all medications delivered over several days without containing a broad-spectrum bacteriostatic substance. Current literature, however, agrees that all intrathecal medications are level 3 (high) risk because they lack bacteriostatic preservatives and include products exposed to an inadequately controlled environment even if the final preparation is sterilized before use. Preparations of a sterile solution, such as intrathecal agents, from a nonsterile powder are always at a level 3 risk.

Key High Risk-Level Requirements[49]

- CSPs are compounded from sterile commercial drugs using commercial sterile devices.
- Compounding occurs in International Standardization Organization (ISO) Class 5 (formerly known as Class 100) environment at all times.
- Compounding procedures involve only a few closed system, basic, simple aseptic transfers and manipulations.
- Routine disinfection and air quality testing to maintain ISO Class 5 occurs.
- There is adequate personnel garb for sterile preparation.
- A review for correct identity and amounts of components occurs before and after compounding.
- There is a final visual inspection of each sterile preparation.
- A semi-annual media-fill test procedure for each person who compounds is performed to validate proper aseptic technique.

Example of low-risk agents include hydration fluids produced for extemporaneous IV-piggyback use; moderate risk includes prepackaged syringes or total parenteral nutrition formulations; and high risk involves measuring raw chemicals, weighing, dissolving, and finalizing with filtered technique in a standardized cleanroom (**Table 2-5**).

A cleanroom is a controlled environment that has a low level of environmental pollutants such as dust, airborne microbes, aerosolized particles, and chemical vapors. More accurately, a cleanroom has a controlled level of contamination that is specified by the number of particles per cubic meter at a specified particle size and is categorized accordingly into classes (**Table 2-6**). All agents

Table 2-5: United States Pharmacopeia Chapter 797 Pharmacy Compounding Risk-Level Assessment

Compounding Activity	Location	Examples of Medications	USP 797 Risk Level Determination
Reconstitution of vials of powder with sterile diluent then transferred to bag of parenteral solution *one at a time*	In pharmacy using an ISO Class 5 hood in an ISO Class 8 cleanroom	Reconstitution of single-dose vials; preparation of hydration solutions	Low-risk level
Reconstitution of vials of powder with sterile diluent; resulting solution then transferred to several bags of parenteral solution	In pharmacy using an ISO Class 5 hood in an ISO Class 8 cleanroom	TPN, batch preparations (e.g., syringes), chemotherapy infusions, previously included intrathecal medications	Medium-risk level
Reconstitution of single vial of powder with sterile diluent for transfer to bag of parenteral solution	Nursing station, ambulatory care center, or at patients bedside without any engineering controls	Prepared from bulk, nonsterile components (morphine, other narcotics) or containers that are nonsterile	High-risk level

ISO, International Standardization Organization; TPN, total parenteral nutrition; USP, United States Pharmacopeia.
Adapted from Kastango E: *The ASHP Discussion Guide for Compounding Sterile Preparations: Summary and Implementation of USP Chapter 797*. Washington, DC, 2004, ASHP Publishing.

Table 2-6: International Organization for Standardization for Cleanrooms

ISO	≥0.1 µm	≥0.2 µm	≥0.3 µm	≥0.5 µm	≥5 µm	Class
ISO 3	35	7	3	1		1
ISO 4	350	75	30	10		10
ISO 5		750	300	100		100
ISO 6				1000	7	1000
ISO 7				10000	70	10,000
ISO 8				100000	700	100,000

Cleanrooms are classified according to the number and size of particles permitted per volume of air. "Class 100" or "Class 1000" denote the number of particles of size 0.5-µm or larger permitted per cubic foot of air. Intrathecal preparations require Class 100 or International Standardization Organization 5 standards at minimum.
ISO, International Standardization Organization.
Adapted from U.S. Department of Commerce FED-STD-209E standard, which was officially cancelled in 2001 but is still widely used.

prepared for intrathecal use must be prepared in at least a Class 100 cleanroom. The ambient air outside in a typical urban environment contains 35,000,000 particles per cubic meter, 0.5 µm and larger in diameter, corresponding to a Class 1,000,000 cleanroom.

The air entering a cleanroom is filtered from the outside to exclude dust, and the air inside is constantly recirculated through high-efficiency particulate air (HEPA) or ultra low particulate air (ULPA) filters to remove internally generated contaminants. Staff enter and leave through an anteroom (sometimes including an air shower stage) and wear protective clothing such as hats, face masks, gloves, boots, and coveralls. Equipment inside the cleanroom is designed to generate minimal air contamination. Cleanrooms are not sterile (i.e., free of uncontrolled microbes), and more attention is given to airborne particles. Particle levels are usually tested using a particle counter.

Class 100 of Chapter 797 is mandated protocol for a production environment of intrathecal agents. Class 100 environment, also known as ISO Class 5 (i.e., maximally 100 particles 0.5 µm and larger in diameter are allowed per cubic foot) compliance, may include a sterile hood within a sterile room or only a sterile isolator within a cleanroom.

Filtration
After medications have been prepared and filtered in laboratory, they are filtered again by the physician before delivery to the CSF.

Because intrathecal medications have no barrier, physicians rely on the assumption that the pharmacy is preparing the agent sterilely and pyrogen free; therefore, a double-filtration process is the final step. Sterile filtration requires a 0.22-µm size filter or smaller. A filter with 0.22 pore size can prevent most forms of bacteria and some very large viruses from passing through the filter because bacteria tend to range from about 0.1 to 600 µm. Many viruses are smaller than 0.1 µm, so a 0.22-µm micron filter is not nearly as effective for viruses. A high-flow 0.22-µm pore size filter was specifically designed for sterilization and bacteria-retentive applications.

Responsibility of Compounding Labs
USP Chapter 797 sets standards, guidance, and examples for compounding sterile preparations. However, it does not provide specific and comprehensive information describing how to meet those standards. Therefore, pharmacists who compound sterile preparations should exercise their professional judgment to obtain the education and training necessary to prove their competence in managing sterile compounding facilities and in sterile compounding processes and quality assurance. Each compounding laboratory writes its own policies and procedures necessary to meet Chapter 797 standards for intrathecal medications based on its individual laboratory facilities.[48]

Chapter 797 also has training and certification requirements of the laboratory personnel working with low-risk medication

Table 2-7: Solubility and pKa Coefficients for Commonly Used Intrathecal Agents

Drug	Octanol: Buffer (Oil: Water) Solubility Coefficient	pKa	Solubility at Physiological pH
Morphine	1.42	7.9	Water
Hydromorphone	0.32	8.2	Water
Fentanyl	860	8.4	Lipid
Bupivacaine	346	8.1	Lipid
Clonidine	114	8.05	Lipid
Ziconotide	1.4	Unpublished	Water

preparation. The pharmacists and technicians must meet certification and training requirements, and media tested every 6 months. It is a highly skilled field with the highest standards for disciplines involved in sterile compounding.

The FDA has long expressed concern about the quality of compounded medications. Recent deaths caused by microbial contamination of injectable steroids have prompted several state boards of pharmacy to strengthen compounding regulations. Although the American Society of Health-System Pharmacists (ASHP) published the profession's first sterile compounding standards in 1992, sterile compounding practices have potential for low compliance with voluntary standards. Enforceable standards, when they are seriously implemented, will improve compliance and greatly enhance patient safety.[49]

Stability and Solubility

It is well known that the stability of intrathecal agents at physiological temperature is important to the ultimate success of analgesic therapy. Some agents are not stable at certain concentrations, certain temperatures, or when mixed in combination with other agents. Although most pharmacological agents are intended for use within 1 to 2 weeks of manufacture date, intrathecal agents are not intended for shelf life and must be administered either on the date of preparation or the beyond use date that has been established for the drug as a result of stability testing. Furthermore, because an agent will remain within the pump chamber, it is important to test the agent for stability at 25° C and 37° C for 90 to 120 days. Refill intervals should not exceed the period of stability. Morphine, hydromorphone, clonidine, and baclofen are stable at room and body temperature for 3 months.[12,20,47,50] Bupivacaine is stable for 60 days.[23] Again, concentrations, particularly high concentrations of single agents, have the potential for decreased stability over agents with lower concentrations. Polyanalgesic therapy admixtures are injected sooner, so stability is tested for a 60- to 75-pump day run. There are currently three medications approved by the FDA for intrathecal infusions for chronic pain: morphine, baclofen, and ziconotide. Although an agent may be approved for intraspinal injection, the concentration given for chronic intrathecal delivery systems is too high than is commercially prepared and packaged. This is known as "off-label use." All infusion admixtures of single- and mixed-entity agents are off label. There are no instructions or approved monographs by the FDA. Physicians who administer the medications typically give patients instructions on maintenance of the pump and how to prepare for adverse effects. Physicians have the obligation to explain the off-label use of compounded medications and document such discussions.

There may be issues of stability when certain agents are compounded for clinical use. The definition of stability is an agent that is stable when 90% or more of the active form of the drug remains at the time point specified.[43] Stability is also a function of solubility at 25° C room temperature up to physiological temperature at 37° C. All agents indicated for intrathecal use are prepared and maintained at this temperature (**Table 2-7**). The challenge in compounding agents for IDDS is customizing admixtures as appropriate for each patient on an individual basis, so solubility and stability testing should be determined for the exact admixture before infusion. Each individual laboratory has determined its own proprietary data of stability testing for 6-month infusions of single- and multiple-agent mixtures. The clinician may readily attain these data from the compounding laboratory supplying the intrathecal medications for review before starting therapy. This is important to prevent precipitations of solution that may cause corrosive damage and ultimately lead to pump failure. For example, bupivacaine at 4% is the highest concentration one can solubilize the drug. If this concentration is exposed to temperatures below room temperature, it will crystallize out of solution.[51] This is in contrast with morphine, which may remain in solution up to 55 mg/mL. Therefore, stability is a function of temperature, concentration, and solubility coefficients. Ziconotide at a concentration less than 1 μg/cc is not very stable but appears to have molecular stability at concentrations higher than 1 μg/cc. Morphine and hydromorphone accelerate the rate of ziconotide degradation, so combinations of ziconotide with lower concentrations of the compounded opioid agents is expected to be more stable.[12]

All medications intended for intrathecal infusion systems are prepared free of preservatives. Preservatives are neurotoxic and should not be used for any agent intended for neuraxial use. Common preservatives include benzyl alcohol, mercuries, and ethylenediamine-tetraacetic acid (EDTA).

Pump Stability and Failure

Pump failure is also a concern with high concentrations of opioids. The average life expectancy of most intrathecal pump systems is 3 to 5 years. Pump failure secondary to high concentrations within the pump chamber can corrode the mechanism of the delivering system, leading to failure of the pump earlier than 3 to 5 years. In cancer pain, the clinician is far less concerned with the life of the pump than in patients with chronic nonmalignant pain. Unfortunately, because the average life expectancy of cancer patients implanted with intrathecal pumps is 18 to 24 months, the clinician may chose to be more heroic in blends with higher concentrations because the issue is quality of life rather than pump mechanism failure in these selected patients.

For patients with chronic nonmalignant pain, one major concern is how often patients can make time for follow-up appointments for pump refills. Ideally, high concentrations are favorable to lengthen time periods between pump refills; however, these are not always advisable. (The average time span between refills is 25 to 30 days, 40 cc with each refill). However, local anesthetics can be added to the opioid to create an admixture to extend the time between pump refills to average 40 to 70 days. Therefore, although the pump chamber contains high concentrations of opioids, the amount delivery is at lower concentrations, and the patient can achieve the same amount of analgesia without the need for multiple refills.

Risks of Intrathecal Therapy

There are a variety of risks of intrathecal therapy. Briefly, complication can occur with the pump and catheter or with the drugs, implantation of the device, or pump refill. This topic is covered in Chapters 4 and 14.

Insertion of the Device

At the time of insertion of the device, one needs to take great care to avoid infection and avoid damage of the spinal cord with insertion of the catheter. The pump needs to be stabilized at the correct level in the abdomen to avoid pump flipping or being placed too deeply or superficially. In this situation, the pump may flip, rotate, and dislodge the catheter, and it may not be able to be refilled (if placed too deeply), or if it is placed too superficially, it can erode through the skin wall.

If a pump malfunctions, one can have a stalled pump, leading to no drug being released, or a pump dump could result in the entire supply of the pump releasing acutely. This obviously would lead to life-threatening respiratory failure and overdose of intrathecal medications. The catheters can also kink or break, leading to no extravasation of drugs or drugs being slowly released into the subcutaneous tissue.

Pump Refill

If the pump is not accessed correctly, it is possible to inject 18 to 40 cc of medication into the subcutaneous tissue. This could lead to respiratory depression and acute overdose of medication.

Medication Problems

Problems with medications include adverse drug reactions, allergic reactions, respiratory and neurologic depression, suppression of testosterone, and possibly lead to the development of osteoporosis. Neurotoxicity of the spinal cord could occur with off-label use of drugs. In addition, if the compounding pharmacy does not use appropriate technique, it is possible to refill the pump with incorrect or unstable drugs. Suppression of natural killer (NK) cell activity has also been reported in animal models leading to a concern of increasing the chance of metastatic spread. Currently the most feared complication is the development of granuloma formation.

Granuloma Formation

Granulomas are inflammatory masses that can form inside the spinal canal with infusions of intrathecal agents. In extreme cases, they can cause spinal cord compression and paralysis. For this reason, caution needs to be used in the use of intrathecal pumps. Granulomas are most commonly seen with intrathecal opiates but have been also seen with nonopiates, including baclofen.[52]

Intrathecal morphine was the first drug to be associated with granulomatous masses from continuous intrathecal therapy. They can occur from weeks to years after initiating therapy and have been seen at low doses as well as higher doses of intrathecal therapy. They seem to be associated with high concentration and low-flow pumps.

The safety of chronic intrathecal morphine infusion has been extensively studied for potential neurotoxic effects and has been demonstrated to be dose dependent determined by the amount of morphine infused.[53] Intrathecal morphine dosages of 12 to 18 mg/day produced inflammatory masses extending from the catheter tip down the length of the catheter within the intrathecal space in a sheep model within 28 days of infusion.[53] A dose of 3 mg/day produced no neurotoxicity, and spinal histopathologic changes were equivalent to those observed in saline-treated animals.[53] Nevertheless, concentration-dependent neurotoxicity is well established, with dose-dependent allodynia usually presenting as the initial sign soon after initiation of high-dose morphine (morphine dose >9 mg/day), ultimately leading to motor weakness secondary to mass evolution and compression.[50] Morphine at dosages of 12 mg/day or greater for longer than 28 days of infusion produces inflammatory masses in all animal models studied, consisting of multifocal immunoreactive cells (macrophages, neutrophils, cytokines), most often observed between the dura and arachnoid layers, and aseptic in nature.[50,53] Human cases have been reported in patients receiving intrathecal opioids alone or in combination with other intrathecal agents or in patients receiving investigational agents not intended for long-term intrathecal use.[47,54]

Future Directions

Intrathecal therapy can be a very effective therapy for patients with chronic pain. However, a thorough understanding of the various agents used and expected doses are necessary when managing implantable pumps. Although some risks are associated with intrathecal therapy, they can relieve pain, lower side effects, and improve the quality of life in patients with intractable pain.

Acknowledgement

The authors would like to sincerely thank Stephen S. Laddy, RPh, MS, CEO MASTERPHARM, LLC, for his guidance and contribution to this chapter.

References

1. Smith TJ, Coyne PJ, Staats PS, et al: An implantable drug delivery system (IDDS) for refractory cancer pain provides sustained pain control, less drug-related toxicity, and possibly better survival compared with comprehensive medical management (CMM). *Ann Oncol* 16:825-833, 2005.
2. Yaksh TL, Rudy TA: Analgesia mediated by a direct spinal action of narcotics. *Science* 192:1357-1358, 1976.
3. Ambriz-Tututi M, Rocha-Gonzalez HI, Castaneda-Corral G, et al: Role of opioid receptors in the reduction of formalin-induced secondary allodynia and hyperalgesia in rats. *Eur J Pharmacol* 619:25-32, 2009.
4. Brescia FJ: An overview of pain and symptom management in advanced cancer. *J Pain Symptom Manage* 2(suppl):S7-S11, 1987.
5. Nallu R, Radhakrishnan R: Spinal release of acetylcholine in response to morphine. *J Pain* 8(suppl):S19, 2007.
6. Terenius L: Characteristics of the "receptor" for narcotic analgesics in synaptic plasma membrane fraction from rat brain. *Acta Pharmacol Toxicol (Copenh)* 33:377-384, 1973.
7. Bennett G, Serafini M, Burchiel K, et al: Evidence-based review of the literature on intrathecal delivery of pain medication. *J Pain Symptom Manage* 20(suppl):S12-S36, 2000.
8. Ruan X: Drug-related side effects of long term intrathecal morphine therapy. *Pain Physician* 10:357-365, 2007.
9. Chaney MA: Side effects of intrathecal and epidural opioids. *Can J Anaesth* 42:891-903, 1995.

10. Chauvin M, Samii K, Schermann JM, et al: Plasma pharmacokinetics of morphine after I.M., extradural and intrathecal administration. *Br J Anaesth* 54:843-847, 1982.

11. Porreca F, Filla A, Burks TF: Spinal cord-mediated opiate effects on gastrointestinal transit in mice. *Eur J Pharmacol* 86:135-136, 1982.

12. Deer T, Krames ES, Hassenbusch SJ, et al: Polyanalgesic Consensus Conference 2007: Recommendations for the management of pain by intrathecal (intraspinal) drug delivery: report of an interdisciplinary expert panel. *Neuromodulation* 10:300-328, 2007.

13. Kumar K, Kelly M, Pirlot T: Continuous intrathecal morphine treatment for chronic pain of nonmalignant etiology: long-term benefits and efficacy. *Surg Neurol* 55:79-86; discussion 86-78, 2001.

14. Anderson VC, Burchiel KJ: A prospective study of long-term intrathecal morphine in the management of chronic nonmalignant pain. *Neurosurgery* 44:289-300; discussion 300-281, 1999.

15. Thimineur MA, Kravitz E, Vodapally MS: Intrathecal opioid treatment for chronic non-malignant pain: a 3-year prospective study. *Pain* 109:242-249, 2004.

16. Rauck RL, Cherry D, Boyer MF, et al: Long-term intrathecal opioid therapy with a patient-activated, implanted delivery system for the treatment of refractory cancer pain. *J Pain* 4:441-447, 2003.

17. Smith HS, Deer TR, Staats PS, et al: Intrathecal drug delivery. *Pain Physician* 11(suppl):S89-S104, 2008.

18. Anderson VC, Cooke B, Burchiel KJ: Intrathecal hydromorphone for chronic nonmalignant pain: a retrospective study. *Pain Med* 2:287-297, 2001.

19. Du Pen S, Du Pen A, Hillyer J: Intrathecal hydromorphone for intractable nonmalignant pain: a retrospective study. *Pain Med* 7:10-15, 2006.

20. Hildebrand KR, Elsberry DE, Anderson VC: Stability and compatibility of hydromorphone hydrochloride in an implantable infusion system. *J Pain Symptom Manage* 22:1042-1047, 2001.

21. Aldrete JA: Extended epidural catheter infusions with analgesics for patients with noncancer pain at their homes. *Reg Anesth* 22:35-42, 1997.

22. Motsch J, Bleser W, Ismaily AJ, et al: [Continuous intrathecal opiate therapy with a portable drug pump in cancer pain]. *Anasth Intensivther Notfallmed* 23:271-275, 1988.

23. Deer TR, Serafini M, Buchser E, et al: Intrathecal bupivacaine for chronic pain: a review of current knowledge. *Neuromodulation* 5:196-207, 2002.

24. Etches RC, Gammer TL, Cornish R: Patient-controlled epidural analgesia after thoracotomy: a comparison of meperidine with and without bupivacaine. *Anesth Analg* 83:81-86, 1996.

25. Li DF, Bahar M, Cole G, et al: Neurological toxicity of the subarachnoid infusion of bupivacaine, lignocaine or 2-chloroprocaine in the rat. *Br J Anaesth* 57:424-429, 1985.

26. Kroin JS, McCarthy RJ, Penn RD, et al: The effect of chronic subarachnoid bupivacaine infusion in dogs. *Anesthesiology* 66:737-742, 1987.

27. Yamashita A, Matsumoto M, Matsumoto S, et al: A comparison of the neurotoxic effects on the spinal cord of tetracaine, lidocaine, bupivacaine, and ropivacaine administered intrathecally in rabbits. *Anesth Analg* 97:512-519, table of contents, 2003.

28. Van Dongen RT, Crul BJ, De Bock M: Long-term intrathecal infusion of morphine and morphine/bupivacaine mixtures in the treatment of cancer pain: a retrospective analysis of 51 cases. *Pain* 55:119-123, 1993.

29. Krames ES: Intrathecal infusional therapies for intractable pain: patient management guidelines. *J Pain Symptom Manage* 8:36-46, 1993.

30. Buchser E, Durrer A, Chedel D, et al: Efficacy of intrathecal bupivacaine: how important is the flow rate? *Pain Med* 5:248-252, 2004.

31. Siddall PJ, Gray M, Rutkowski S, et al: Intrathecal morphine and clonidine in the management of spinal cord injury pain: a case report. *Pain* 59:147-148, 1994.

32. Tumber PS, Fitzgibbon DR: The control of severe cancer pain by continuous intrathecal infusion and patient controlled intrathecal analgesia with morphine, bupivacaine and clonidine. *Pain* 78:217-220, 1998.

33. Eisenach JC, Hood DD, Curry R: Intrathecal, but not intravenous, clonidine reduces experimental thermal or capsaicin-induced pain and hyperalgesia in normal volunteers. *Anesth Analg* 87:591-596, 1998.

34. Borg PA, Krijnen HJ: Long-term intrathecal administration of midazolam and clonidine. *Clin J Pain* 12:63-68, 1996.

35. Middleton JW, Siddall PJ, Walker S, et al: Intrathecal clonidine and baclofen in the management of spasticity and neuropathic pain following spinal cord injury: a case study. *Arch Phys Med Rehabil* 77:824-826, 1996.

36. Herman RM, D'Luzansky SC, Ippolito R: Intrathecal baclofen suppresses central pain in patients with spinal lesions. A pilot study. *Clin J Pain* 8:338-345, 1992.

37. Zuniga RE, Schlicht CR, Abram SE: Intrathecal baclofen is analgesic in patients with chronic pain. *Anesthesiology* 92:876-880, 2000.

38. Coffey JR, Cahill D, Steers W, et al: Intrathecal baclofen for intractable spasticity of spinal origin: results of a long-term multicenter study. *J Neurosurg* 78:226-232, 1993.

39. Olivera BM, Gray WR, Zeikus R, et al: Peptide neurotoxins from fish-hunting cone snails. *Science* 230:1338-1343, 1985.

40. Staats PS, Yearwood T, Charapata SG, et al: Intrathecal ziconotide in the treatment of refractory pain in patients with cancer or AIDS: a randomized controlled trial. *JAMA* 291:63-70, 2004.

41. Miljanich GP: Ziconotide: neuronal calcium channel blocker for treating severe chronic pain. *Curr Med Chem* 11:3029-3040, 2004.

42. Rauck RL, Wallace MS, Leong MS, et al: A randomized, double-blind, placebo-controlled study of intrathecal ziconotide in adults with severe chronic pain. *J Pain Symptom Manage* 31:393-406, 2006.

43. Trissel L, editor: *Trissel's stability of compounded formulations*, ed 4, Washington, DC, 2009, APHA Publications.

44. Stearns L, Boortz-Marx R, Du Pen S, et al: Intrathecal drug delivery for the management of cancer pain: a multidisciplinary consensus of best clinical practices. *J Support Oncol* 3:399-408, 2005.

45. Weiss N, North RB, Ohara S, et al: Attenuation of cerebellar tremor with implantation of an intrathecal baclofen pump: the role of gamma-aminobutyric acidergic pathways. Case report. *J Neurosurg* 99:768-771, 2003.

46. Ho KM, Ismail H: Use of intrathecal midazolam to improve perioperative analgesia: a meta-analysis. *Anaesth Intensive Care* 36:365-373, 2008.

47. Yaksh TL, Hassenbusch S, Burchiel K, et al: Inflammatory masses associated with intrathecal drug infusion: a review of preclinical evidence and human data. *Pain Med* 3:300-312, 2002.

48. Convention USP: *Chapter 797, United States Pharmacopeia/National Formulary*, ed 1, U.S., 2009, Pharmacopeia, pp 4139.

49. Kastango E: *The ASHP discussion guide for compounding sterile preparations: summary and implementation of USP Chapter 797*, Washington, DC, 2004, ASHP Publishing.

50. Yaksh TL, Horais KA, Tozier NA, et al: Chronically infused intrathecal morphine in dogs. *Anesthesiology* 99:174-187, 2003.

51. O'Neil M, Smith A, Heckelman P, et al, editors: *Merck index*, ed 13, Hoboken, NJ, 2001, John Wiley & Sons.

52. Deer TR, Raso LJ, Coffey RJ, et al: Intrathecal baclofen and catheter tip inflammatory mass lesions (granulomas): a reevaluation of case reports and imaging findings in light of experimental, clinicopathological, and radiological evidence. *Pain Med* 9:391-395, 2008.

53. Gradert TL, Baze WB, Satterfield WC, et al: Safety of chronic intrathecal morphine infusion in a sheep model. *Anesthesiology* 99:188-198, 2003.

54. Coffey RJ, Burchiel K: Inflammatory mass lesions associated with intrathecal drug infusion catheters: report and observations on 41 patients. *Neurosurgery* 50:78-86; discussion 86-87, 2002.

3 Polyanalgesia for Implantable Drug Delivery Systems

Bryan S. Williams

CHAPTER OVERVIEW

Chapter Synopsis: Intrathecal drug delivery systems (IDDS) represent a pharmaceutical treatment option when all other drug-based approaches for chronic back pain have been exhausted. Although morphine sulfate remains the only opioid medication approved by the U.S. Food and Drug Administration for IDDS, others are routinely used as well. But "monotherapy," in which one drug (usually morphine) is used alone, may not attenuate the multifaceted nature of chronic pain. Nociceptive and neuropathic pain may respond differently to opioids than, for example, to the calcium channel blocker ziconotide. (Local anesthetics such as bupivacaine and α_2-adrenergic receptor agonists such as clonidine are also drug candidates.) This chapter examines drug combinations that may be delivered intrathecally to produce polyanalgesia. Using multiple pharmaceutical agents from different drug classes can produce both additive and synergistic effects. Additionally, monotherapy can produce significant side effects that may be avoided with lower doses of combination drug therapy.

Important Points:
- Polyanalgesia provides analgesia by interaction at different points in the pain transmission pathway, treating mixed pain states (nociceptive and neuropathic) present in many chronic pain conditions.
- Enteral adjuvants should be continued as part of a polyanalgesic or multimodal treatment regimen.

Clinical Pearls:
- Set clear expectations of analgesic response with patient.
- Initiate therapy at the lowest effective dose.
- Ensure the integrity and function of the delivery systems (connections, catheter tip placement, etc.).

Clinical Pitfalls:
- Opioid monotherapy for nonmalignant pain often leads to dose escalation, tolerance, and side effects.
- Neuropathic pain may be opioid nonresponsive, necessitating adjuvant intrathecal medication administration.

Introduction

Intrathecal drug delivery systems have become an analgesic option for patients who have failed all other treatment modalities; patients with inadequate analgesia taking high-dose enteral, parenteral, or transdermal agents; and those with unacceptable side effects. Intrathecal (IT) analgesics have been increasingly used for the treatment of patients with chronic, intractable pain (i.e., cancer-related pain). Opioid medications are a mainstay of analgesic medications, and the first application of IT morphine for clinical use for intractable cancer pain was done in 1979,[1] and the use of an implantable IT opioid (ITO) delivery device followed in 1981.[2] Morphine sulfate remains the only opioid approved by the U.S. Food and Drug Administration (FDA) for IT administration. The use of morphine as an agent for IT delivery has been and remains the most frequently used medication for initiation of IT therapy.[3] Recommendations from a consensus panel have been put forth for the rational use of IT medications. The Polyanalgesic Consensus Panel advocates monotherapy with morphine, hydromorphone, or ziconotide as first-line agents for IT delivery.[4] Monotherapy with these agents may provide adequate and prolonged analgesia, but if these medications fail to provide expected analgesia, additional IT

medications may additively or synergistically enhance analgesia. The long-term use of monotherapy with medications such as morphine has been controversial because adverse events and side effects may present (**Box 3-1**). Additionally, the multifaceted nature of many pain states lends credence to the delivery of multiple medications (polyanalgesia) with different mechanisms of analgesia. Chapter 2 discusses the agents used in IT therapy, and this chapter presents the use of polyanalgesia using the most commonly used medications for IT therapy (opioids, local anesthetics, α_2-adrenergic agonists, and calcium channel blockers). Other less used medications (ketamine, gabapentin, midazolam) have been used for delivery to the IT space for attenuation of pain, but the paucity of information regarding their safety and efficacy limits their IT use.

What Is Polyanalgesia?

Polyanalgesia utilizes different classes of medications with different receptor modulation capabilities to address pain attenuation at different points in the pain transmission pathway. The concept of polyanalgesia was created out of the lack of efficacy of long-term IT opioid therapy in nonmalignant pain states and mixed pain states (nociceptive and neuropathic) present in many chronic pain conditions treated with IT medications. For example, Grond et al[5] found that 64.1%, 5.4%, and 30.5% of study participants experienced cancer-related nociceptive, neuropathic, and mixed pain, respectively. Although the best response to spinal morphine is obtained in cases of continuous somatic or visceral pain, neuropathic pain, visceral pain from intestinal distention, incident pain on movement, as well as pain from cutaneous ulcerations have poor responses.[6] The rationale for this strategy is the achievement of sufficient analgesia because of the additive or synergistic effects of different classes of analgesics by affecting the transmission of painful stimuli at multiple sites. Polyanalgesia is achieved by combining different analgesics that act by different mechanisms (e.g., opioids, α₂-adrenergic agonist, calcium channel blockers, local anesthetics), resulting in additive or synergistic analgesia, lower total doses of analgesics, and fewer side effects. This allows for a reduction in the doses of individual drugs and thus a theoretically lower incidence of adverse effects from any particular IT medication.

Why Polyanalgesia?

Opioid medications (e.g., morphine) have long been the drugs of choice when initiating IT therapy for refractory pain states. Morphine and other opioids have been used extensively as

> **Box 3-1: Adverse Events and Side Effects of Intrathecal Opioids**
>
> - Sedation
> - Constipation
> - Pruritus
> - Peripheral edema
> - Urinary retention
> - Nausea or vomiting
> - Sweating
> - Respiratory depression
> - Tolerance
> - Hypogonadism (sexual dysfunction, osteoporosis)
> - Inflammatory granulomatous mass formation

monotherapy to treat patients with cancer-related pain, complex regional pain syndrome, failed back surgery syndrome, and other chronic pain conditions. Although the efficacy of opioids delivered to the IT space has been established,[1] controversy remains whether long-term opioid therapy for severe nonmalignant pain is effective. The issues related to long-term delivery of opioids include, but are not limited to, tolerance, side effects of high-dose opioids (e.g., sedation, pruritus, edema, nausea, urine retention), psychological dependency, and the development of catheter-related granulomatous inflammatory masses.

The delivery of opioid monotherapy for cancer-related pain has been proven beneficial in multiple studies compared with enteral delivery, including comprehensive medical management.[7,8] In comparison, support for the use of opioid monotherapy for patients with nonmalignant pain conditions is contentious. After a successful trial of ITO medications, pain scores indicate improvement, but increases in opioid dosage and changes in medication are often needed to maintain pain improvement.[9] Mercadante et al[10] demonstrated that the average opioid dose escalates quickly during titration and then stabilizes in cancer patients compared with a more gradual, linear increase in dose observed in patients without cancer. The tolerance and dose escalation witnessed in nonmalignant pain is partly attributable to the life span of use in nonmalignant pain patients (**Fig. 3-1**). In an effort to avoid continued dose escalations of opioids, adjuvant medications have been used to provide analgesia by effecting different receptors in the pain pathway. The application of adjuvant medication, and polyanalgesia, improves analgesic efficacy, and potentially reduces side effects and opioid dose escalation.

Polyanalgesic Medications

Local anesthetics have been delivered intrathecally since the late nineteenth century and when combined with ITOs the medications act synergistically, enhancing the antinociceptive effects of opioids and inhibiting wind-up of the nerve cell, thus reducing amplification and prolongation of nociceptive transmission in the spinal cord and reduction of neuronal excitability as they act by different neural mechanisms.[6] Clinically, the addition of bupivacaine has shown synergistic properties, enhancing the effect of the ITOs

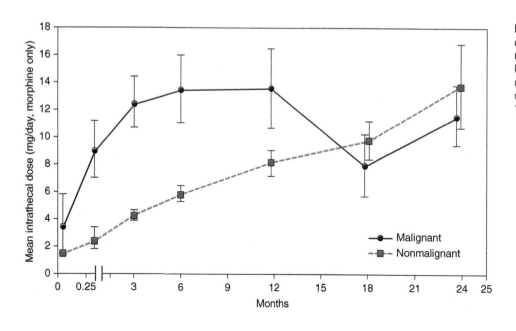

Fig. 3-1 Intrathecal morphine dose escalation in malignant and nonmalignant patients. (Modified from Paice JA, Penn RD, Shott S: Intraspinal morphine for chronic pain: a retrospective, multicenter study. *J Pain Symptom Manage* 11:71-80, 1996.)

when used in combination.[4,11] The decision to add local anesthetics (bupivacaine) may be based on the inadequate analgesia with opioid monotherapy or pain characteristics. Opioids may provide analgesia for primary nociceptive pain, but the response to neuropathic pain has proven less responsive to the opioid analgesics.[12] Additionally, local anesthetics may reduce the incidence of IT granulomatous mass formation because a lower ITO dose is required for adequate pain relief.[13] Patients who present with pain described as spontaneous or evoked, sharp, shooting, burning, lancinating, or electric pain or those with significant neural (e.g., lumbar plexus) involvement may benefit from either the addition of local anesthetics or trialing with opioid and local anesthetic combinations. In a retrospective study by van Dongen et al,[14] the authors report that the addition of IT bupivacaine to opioids resulted in satisfactory analgesia in 10 of 17 cancer patients who failed IT opioid monotherapy. The mean follow-up in this study was 112 days. In a double-blind, randomized, prospective trial comparing IT morphine monotherapy with IT morphine and bupivacaine in 20 cancer patients, the combination group developed less opioid tolerance than the morphine monotherapy group.[15] Kumar et al[13] investigated the efficacy and safety of the addition of bupivacaine in patients with chronic nonmalignant pain refractory to ITOs. The addition of bupivacaine improved the quality of life, improved their functional level, and improved pain scores. The stability of an admixture of morphine, bupivacaine, and clonidine was examined, and the medications were found to be stable at 90 days.[16] The addition of bupivacaine or other local anesthetics does warrant careful titration and monitoring because side effects such as sensorimotor weakness, hypotension, and urinary retention may surface.

Clonidine

The mechanism of action of clonidine, an α_2-adrenergic agonist, is mediated through nonopioid interactions. The usefulness of clonidine is for patients who have developed tolerance to opioids, those who are nonresponsive to opioids, those who are allergic to opioids, and those with neuropathic or mixed pain conditions. Monotherapy using clonidine is a third-line agent in the Polyanalgesic Consensus algorithm, but the addition of clonidine to opioids is a second-line therapeutic modality (Table 3-1). Polyanalgesia using clonidine and opioids has demonstrated efficacy in cancer-related pain states[17] and noncancer pain conditions.[18] Although clonidine has shown analgesic efficacy by modulating α_2-adrenoceptors in the dorsal horn of the spinal cord, monotherapy has not shown long-term efficacy, which may be related to cerebrospinal fluid (CSF) concentration. Siddall et al[19] have indicated that there is a significant correlation between CSF concentration of clonidine and pain relief. Regardless of catheter position within the IT compartment, CSF concentration can be increased by simply increasing the daily infusion rate. However, if clonidine requires a critical local or segmental concentration at its site of action, positioning of the drug delivery catheter may be a critical issue.[18]

Ziconotide

The nonopioid adjuvant medication ziconotide has analgesic effects by interruption of spinal transmission of pain information selectively and reversibly block N-type voltage-sensitive calcium channels, thus decreasing neurotransmitter release from nociceptive afferents that terminate in the dorsal horn of the spinal cord.[20] This blockade inhibits the presynaptic release of neurotransmitters (e.g., glutamate) and neuropeptides (e.g., substance P and calcitonin gene-related peptide) from sensory neurons, which results in

Table 3-1: Polyanalgesic Algorithm for Intrathecal Therapies (2007)*

Line #1	Morphine ↔ Hydromorphone ↔ Ziconotide
Line #2	Fentanyl ↔ Morphine/hydromorphone ↔ Morphine/hydromorphone + Ziconotide + Bupivacaine/clonidine
Line #3	Clonidine ↔ Morphine/hydromorphone/fentanyl/bupivacaine + Clonidine + Ziconotide
Line #4	Sufentanil ↔ Sufentanil + Bupivacaine + Clonidine + Ziconotide
Line #5	Ropivacaine ↔ Buprenorphine ↔ Midazolam ↔ Ketorolac
Line #6	Experimental agents: Gabapentin, octreotide, conpeptide, neostigmine, adenosine, XEN2174, AM336, XEN, ZGX 160

*Recommended algorithm for intrathecal polyanalgesic therapies, 2007. Line 1: Morphine and ziconotide are approved by the U.S. Food and Drug Administration for intrathecal analgesic use and are recommended for first-line therapy for nociceptive, mixed, and neuropathic pain. Hydromorphone is recommended based on clinical widespread usage and apparent safety. Line 2: Because of its apparent granuloma-sparing effect and its wide apparent use and identified safety, fentanyl has been upgraded to a line 2 agent by the consensus conference when the use of the more hydrophilic agents of line 1 result in intractable supraspinal side effects. Combinations of opioid + ziconotide or opioid + bupivacaine or clonidine are recommended for mixed and neuropathic pain and may be used interchangeably. When admixing opioids with ziconotide, attention must be made to the guidelines for admixing ziconotide with other agents. Line 3: Clonidine alone or opioids such as morphine/hydromorphone/fentanyl with bupivacaine and/or clonidine mixed with ziconotide may be used when agents in line 2 fail to provide analgesia or side effects occur when these agents are used. Line 4: Because of its proven safety in animals and humans and its apparent granuloma-sparing effects, sufentanil alone or mixed with bupivacaine and/or clonidine plus ziconotide is recommended in this line. The addition of clonidine, bupivacaine, and/or ziconotide is to be used in patients with mixed or neuropathic pain. In patients at the end of life, the panelists believed that midazolam and octreotide should be tried when all other agents in lines 1 to 4 have failed. Line 5: These agents, although not experimental, have little information about them in the literature, and use is recommended with caution and obvious informed consent regarding the paucity of information regarding the safety and efficacy of their use. Line 6: Experimental agents must only be used experimentally and with appropriate Independent Review Board-approved protocols. (Adapted with permission from Deer T, Krames ES, Hassenbusch SJ, et al: Polyanalgesic Consensus Conference 2007: recommendations for the management of pain by intrathecal (intraspinal) drug delivery: report of an interdisciplinary expert panel, *Neuromodulation* 10(4):300-328, 2007.)

antinociception.[21] In contrast to opioid monotherapy, ziconotide is effective as a monotherapy across all pain types and its potential should not be diminished by considering it as an adjuvant based on little scientific evidence. The large dose range of ziconotide should be maximally exploited in favor of combining drugs when the effects or toxicities are unknown.[21] Ziconotide has been investigated in multiple pain states with results showing favor to the analgesic effectiveness of the medication. In a controversial article, Staats et al[22] investigated the safety and efficacy of IT ziconotide in patients with pain that was refractory to conventional treatment. The randomized, double-blind, placebo-controlled study consisted of patients with AIDS-related chronic pain or cancer-related pain. The authors concluded that ziconotide was clinically and statistically significant analgesic effect of IT ziconotide in a heterogeneous, complex, and treatment-refractory patient population. Similar results have been reported with nonmalignant chronic pain states.

In a randomized, double-blind, placebo-controlled trial, in patients with severe chronic nonmalignant pain unresponsive to conventional therapy, ziconotide therapy produced a mean percent reduction in Visual Analog Scale of Pain Intensity (VASPI) score from baseline of 31.2% and 6.0% for ziconotide- and placebo-treated patients, respectively ($P \leq 0.001$).[23] Since FDA approval of ziconotide in 2004, a multitude of randomized control trials (RCT), case series, and case reports have investigated the efficacy of the medication. Many of the RCTs have focused on ziconotide as a monotherapy, partly because ziconotide is a peptide that is sensitive to oxidative degradation, so its stability when combined with other drugs is limited.[21] The concentration of ziconotide decreases in the presence of morphine and hydromorphone when stored at 37° C or 5° C in Medtronic SynchroMed II pumps.[21] An admixture of ziconotide and hydromorphone retains 80% stability for 40 days compared with only 15 days for the ziconotide and morphine combination. Morphine and hydromorphone were stable in the presence of ziconotide under all conditions. This degradation of ziconotide admixtures limits the use in polyanalgesia because the refill interval decreases with these admixtures. However, the efficacy of opioid and ziconotide admixtures has been examined. Webster et al[24] examined the safety and efficacy of adding IT morphine to patients taking IT ziconotide with suboptimal pain relief receiving stable ziconotide doses. The authors concluded that pain improved by an average of 26.3% over 4 weeks, and the additional systemic opioid consumption decreased by 49.1%. An additional multicenter, open-label study investigated the safety and efficacy of adding IT ziconotide to IT morphine in patients with suboptimal pain relief being treated with a stable IT morphine dose.[25] The average VASPI score decreased by 14.5% with the addition of ziconotide.

Guidelines

The use of IT monotherapy and admixtures (polyanalgesia) is based on the best evidence available. The Polyanalgesic Consensus Conference of 2007 set forth recommendations for IT drug delivery, but the authors concede that "In spite of these efforts, clinical research on IT analgesics that meets the 'gold standard' of evidenced-based studies has not kept pace with the growing need for innovative approaches to pain management. Rigorous supporting data on the safety and efficacy of a broad cross-section of opioid and nonopioid IT medications remains, to this day, inadequate."[4] The current algorithm for drug selection provides a set of practical clinical guidelines for optimizing the therapeutic use of analgesic medications and drug combinations in a rational and prioritized order. The medications in the current algorithm are arranged in a hierarchy based on evidence on safety, efficacy, and broad clinical parameters gleaned from previous and current consensus literature reviews, ratings of published studies, and expert opinion from three Polyanalgesic Consensus Conferences.[4]

The algorithm has been set forth from the conference initiates IT delivery with monotherapy and progresses through several medication admixtures, with decreasing clinical experience. Alternatively, IT trials should be conducted with medications that address the pain characteristic present. Patients with primary nociceptive pain may benefit from monotherapy with opioids, but patients with mixed pain states may benefit from the addition of adjuvant medications during the trial period.

The Polyanalgesic Consensus Panel[4] recommends monotherapy when initiating IT treatment. As first-line medications, morphine, hydromorphone, and ziconotide may provide adequate analgesia, but when these medications fail to provide expected analgesia, admixtures of adjuvant medications should be added. In particular, an opioid plus bupivacaine or clonidine has shown efficacy in providing analgesia in patients with chronic malignant and nonmalignant pain conditions. The addition of adjuvant medications to ziconotide has shown efficacy, but questions of admixture stability may limit its use. Other less used and clinically studied medications have been used for IT delivery, but safety and efficacy may limit their use.

Polyanalgesia or Multimodal Therapy

Medications such as selective serotonin–norepinephrine reuptake inhibitors (e.g., duloxetine), tricyclic antidepressants (e.g., amitriptyline), and antiepileptic medications (e.g., pregabalin) have shown efficacy in depressive states, alleviating neuropathic pain, and improving sleep hygiene. These medications should not be abandoned but rather continued as part of a polyanalgesic treatment plan. Patients with intractable cancer-related pain may require supplemental opioid medications as part of a treatment regimen, but their use may indicate the need for IT titration. Alternatively, the continued use of supplemental opioid medications in noncancer-related pain is controversial, but clinicians use supplemental medications for incident pain in an attempt to provide additional pain attenuation. The unpredictability of incident pain not covered by IT delivery has been a challenge, certainly in the constant-flow IT devices. The Medtronic SynchroMed II with the Patient Therapy Manager remote control now has provisions for bolus dosing after a defined interval. This advancement may provide better control of incident pain, displacing the need for supplemental opioid medications.[26]

Conclusion

Morphine remains the IT medication of choice for initiating IT therapy.[3] Although morphine is the medication of choice in many pain conditions, and is most effective in treating nociceptive pain, when treating neuropathic pain or mixed pain states, the efficacy of monotherapy using morphine remains questionable. When neuropathic pain is present or mixed pain states (nociceptive and neuropathic), opioids alone may fail to provide analgesia. Continued titration of IT opioids should prompt the clinician to investigate the integrity and proper function of the delivery system. Additionally the lack of analgesia may indicate an opioid nonresponsive or poorly responsive pain condition. In particular, neuropathic pain conditions may benefit from the addition of an adjuvant medication. Therefore the addition of adjuvant medications (bupivacaine, clonidine) should occur when titration of IT opioids fails to provide adequate analgesia, in neuropathic pain conditions, and high opioid concentration and daily delivery demands. These medications may provide a more favorable opioid dose-response curve and delay the virtually inevitable development of opioid tolerance. The medications that may prove most beneficial in neuropathic pain are opioid plus bupivacaine, clonidine, or ziconotide. This practice of polyanalgesia targeting different receptors and channels in the pain transmission pathway will continue through future IT research. Medications will be developed that provide analgesia as monotherapy and possibly reduce the need for multiple-medication IT therapy.

References

1. Wang JK, Nauss LA, Thomas JE: Pain relief by intrathecally applied morphine in man. *Anesthesiology* 50(2):149-151, 1979.
2. Onofrio BM, Yaksh TL, Arnold PG: Continuous low-dose intrathecal morphine administration in the treatment of chronic pain of malignant origin. *Mayo Clin Proc* 56(8):516-520, 1981.
3. Deer TR, Krames E, Levy RM, et al: Practice choices and challenges in the current intrathecal therapy environment: an online survey. *Pain Med* 10(2):304-309, 2009.
4. Deer T, Krames ES, Hassenbusch SJ, et al: Polyanalgesic Consensus Conference 2007: recommendations for the management of pain by intrathecal (intraspinal) drug delivery: report of an interdisciplinary expert panel. *Neuromodulation* 10(4):300-328, 2007.
5. Grond S, Radbruch L, Meuser T, et al: Assessment and treatment of neuropathic cancer pain following WHO guideline. *Pain* 79(1):15-20, 1999.
6. Mercadante S: Problems of long-term spinal opioid treatment in advanced cancer patients. *Pain* 79(1):1-13, 1999.
7. Smith TJ, Staats PS, Deer T, et al: Randomized clinical trial of an implantable drug delivery system compared with comprehensive medical management for refractory cancer pain: impact on pain, drug-related toxicity, and survival. *J Clin Oncol* 20(19):4040-4049, 2002.
8. Rauck RL, Cherry D, Boyer MF, et al: Long-term intrathecal opioid therapy with a patient-activated, implanted delivery system for the treatment of refractory cancer pain. *J Pain* 4(8):441-447, 2003.
9. Turner JA, Sears JM, Loeser JD: Programmable intrathecal opioid delivery systems for chronic noncancer pain: a systematic review of effectiveness and complications. *Clin J Pain* 23(2):180-195, 2007.
10. Mercadante S, Intravaia G, Villari P, et al: Intrathecal treatment in cancer patients unresponsive to multiple trials of systemic opioids. *Clin J Pain* 23(9):793-798, 2007.
11. Sjoberg M, Appelgren L, Einarsson S, et al: Long-term intrathecal morphine and bupivacaine in "refractory" cancer pain. I. Results from the first series of 52 patients. *Acta Anaesthesiol Scand* 35(1):30-43, 1991.
12. Krames ES: Intraspinal opioid therapy for chronic nonmalignant pain: current practice and clinical guidelines. *J Pain Symptom Manage* 11(6):333-352, 1996.
13. Kumar K, Bodani V, Bishop S, et al: Use of intrathecal bupivacaine in refractory chronic nonmalignant pain. *Pain Med* 10(5):819-828, 2009.
14. van Dongen RT, Crul BJ, De Bock M: Long-term intrathecal infusion of morphine and morphine/bupivacaine mixtures in the treatment of cancer pain: a retrospective analysis of 51 cases. *Pain* 55(1):119-123, 1993.
15. van Dongen RT, Crul BJ, van Egmond J: Intrathecal coadministration of bupivacaine diminishes morphine dose progression during long-term intrathecal infusion in cancer patients. *Clin J Pain* 15(3):166-172, 1999.
16. Classen AM, Wimbish GH, Kupiec TC: Stability of admixture containing morphine sulfate, bupivacaine hydrochloride, and clonidine hydrochloride in an implantable infusion system. *J Pain Symptom Manage* 28(6):603-611, 2004.
17. Coombs DW, Saunders RL, Fratkin JD, et al: Continuous intrathecal hydromorphone and clonidine for intractable cancer pain. *J Neurosurg* 64(6):890-894, 1986.
18. Ackerman LL, Follett KA, Rosenquist RW: Long-term outcomes during treatment of chronic pain with intrathecal clonidine or clonidine/opioid combinations. *J Pain Symptom Manage* 26(1):668-677, 2003.
19. Siddall PJ, Molloy AR, Walker S, et al: The efficacy of intrathecal morphine and clonidine in the treatment of pain after spinal cord injury. *Anesth Analg* 91(6):1493-1498, 2000.
20. Wang YX, Bowersox SS: Analgesic properties of ziconotide, a selective blocker of N-type neuronal calcium channels. *CNS Drug Rev* 6(1): 1-20, 2006.
21. Kress HG, Simpson KH, Marchettini P, et al: Intrathecal therapy: what has changed with the introduction of ziconotide. *Pain Pract* 9(5):338-347, 2009.
22. Staats PS, Yearwood T, Charapata SG, et al: Intrathecal ziconotide in the treatment of refractory pain in patients with cancer or AIDS: a randomized controlled trial. *JAMA* 291(1):63-70, 2004.
23. Wallace MS, Charapata SG, Fisher R, et al: Intrathecal ziconotide in the treatment of chronic nonmalignant pain: a randomized, double-blind, placebo-controlled clinical trial. *Neuromodulation* 9(2):75-86, 2006.
24. Webster LR, Fakata KL, Charapata S, et al: Open-label, multicenter study of combined intrathecal morphine and ziconotide: addition of morphine in patients receiving ziconotide for severe chronic pain. *Pain Med* 9(3):282-290, 2008.
25. Wallace MS, Kosek PS, Staats P, et al: Phase II, open-label, multicenter study of combined intrathecal morphine and ziconotide: addition of ziconotide in patients receiving intrathecal morphine for severe chronic pain. *Pain Med* 9(3):271-281, 2008.
26. Ilias W, le Polain B, Buchser E, et al: Patient-controlled analgesia in chronic pain patients: experience with a new device designed to be used with implanted programmable pumps. *Pain Pract* 8(3):164-170, 2008.

4 Principles of Patient Management for Intrathecal Analgesia

Shannon L. Bianchi and Michael A. Ashburn

CHAPTER OVERVIEW

Chapter Synopsis: Intrathecal infusion of analgesic drugs is an invasive, chronic treatment with facets that some find troubling. Chapter 4 outlines the specific details that need to be considered by clinicians when pursuing and maintaining treatment with an implanted intrathecal drug delivery system (ITDDS). It is important that an ITDDS be used as part of an integrated treatment plan (including physical and behavioral therapies) and that the patient have realistic expectations for outcome, which is almost never complete pain relief. Because most of our understanding of intrathecal delivery of opioids is based on systemic delivery, extreme care must be taken to achieve a proper and safe dosage in ITDDS. Likewise, drug combination therapies must be undertaken with a keen eye to the literature. Because treatment includes implantation of an infusion pump and catheter, the procedure is subject to serious adverse events, including overdose, often caused by human error. With common sense and attention to detail, the treatment can be quite effective and successful.

Important Points: Intrathecal therapy should be integrated into a multidisciplinary pain treatment approach, including, but not limited to, physical therapy and cognitive-behavioral therapy. To achieve the best possible outcome, associated disorders such as depression and sleep disturbances must be treated concurrently. The expected outcome of treatment with an ITDDS must be clear to both the patient and physician because pain relief, although significant, will likely be incomplete. Patients and families must be partners in therapy and should be educated about the risks of intrathecal treatment. Controversy remains as to whether intrathecal analgesia provides greater pain relief in the long term compared with systemic opioids in both cancer and noncancer pain. Morphine is the only opioid approved by the Food and Drug Administration (FDA) for intrathecal use and is most commonly used for primary therapy. Ziconotide, the only other medication FDA approved for intrathecal use, may be particularly useful in neuropathic or opioid-refractory chronic pain. Most patients are already opioid tolerant before beginning ITDDS, and the opioid dose selected to start intrathecal analgesia therapy should be adjusted accordingly.

Clinical Pearls: In most patients, therapy should be started using morphine. Care should be taken in selecting the initial dose; the patient's current systemic dose may serve as a guide. It is recommended that intrathecal doses be increased by 20% to 30% no more than once a week to allow sufficient time to assess for adverse effects and efficacy. If time is limited in cancer pain, doses may be increased by up to 50% every 2 to 3 days. If morphine fails, consider changing to a different opioid, such as hydromorphone, using care in selecting the dose, considering equianalgesic doses and a decrease in dose to account for incomplete opioid cross-tolerance. Bupivacaine may be added if opioids alone are not effective. Ziconotide can be considered, either as a first-line drug for neuropathic pain, or if opioids and opioids with local anesthetics fail.

Clinical Pitfalls: Medication and dose efficacy varies from patient to patient. Some clinicians advocate starting intrathecal analgesia at 10% of the patient's daily intravenous morphine dose, but this method is controversial, can be complicated when converting from multiple systemic opioids, and may result in too high of a starting intrathecal opioid dose. Although many of the side effects of intrathecal opioid therapy are similar to those of systemic opioid therapy, life-threatening respiratory depression can occur much more quickly. The addition of a local anesthetic may increase the risk of nerve injury or lesion. Lidocaine has been associated with nerve injury in some studies. Clinicians should check and recheck the drug type and concentration, injection site, and programming because programming errors or wrong drug type, concentration, or site of injection can cause fatal overdoses. Drug overdose and respiratory arrest has been reported following pump refills. These events are often attributed to errors during the refill process, most often injection of the drug subcutaneously rather than into the pump. Therefore, extreme care should be taken to ensure that refills are properly done. Serious side effects may not be apparent immediately after pump refills or dose change. Abrupt discontinuation of intrathecal opioid therapy can cause uncomfortable withdrawal symptoms, and abrupt baclofen withdrawal can be life threatening and must be recognized and treated immediately. Clinicians should consider magnetic resonance imaging or dye study if the cause of withdrawal is not readily apparent.

Introduction

An intrathecal drug delivery system (ITDDS) is implanted. The catheter is placed in the intrathecal space and verified with three-dimensional imaging that no signs or symptoms of infection exist and the wound is nicely closed. The clinician then needs to decide how to start drug therapy. With a multitude of choices available for therapy and the limited preclinical and clinical evidence of safety and efficacy for most of the available drugs, choosing the appropriate medication and determining the progression of dosing and medication addition, subtraction, or change can be daunting. However, there is hope. The recommended intrathecal trial performed before permanent implantation should provide at least an approximate starting point in the vast sea of medication type and dosing.

The goals of therapy must be clear to the physician, the patient, and the patient's family. Patients should not expect complete resolution of their pain after intrathecal analgesic therapy. Systemic long-term opioid administration is associated with only a 40% mean decrease in patient-reported pain intensity. Although the expected efficacy may be better after intrathecal therapy, pain relief, although being clinically meaningful, may not be as great as either the physician or patient hoped.[1] Outcomes associated with intrathecal analgesia appear to be better than systemic opioids in patients with cancer.[2] However, other investigators have reported that although intrathecal analgesia may initially be better than systemic opioids, long-term outcomes are similar.[3] Patients receiving intrathecal opioids for the treatment of chronic noncancer pain have worse outcomes than observed in patients with cancer-related pain and often continue to report high levels of pain and other symptoms.[4,5]

Currently, the long-term effectiveness of intrathecal analgesia relative to other therapy, such as systemic opioid administration, is not known.[6] Clearly, the decision of whether to initiate intrathecal therapy in appropriate patients must be made by judiciously weighing the known risks of the therapy against both the possible benefits and the risks of the alternative options such as high-dose oral opioid administration and then only after all other conventional therapies have failed.

The selection of medication and dose varies by physician preference and patient profiles. Although there is not uniform agreement on a standard protocol to be used in each patient, data are available in the literature to guide decision making.[7,8] This chapter provides an overview of the management of patients receiving intrathecal analgesic therapy. Information regarding the safety and efficacy of specific medications can be found in Chapters 2 and 3. In addition, information regarding the management of patients receiving intrathecal therapy for spasticity can be found in Chapter 22.

Drug Therapy

Initial Therapy
Morphine is recommended for primary therapy.[7,8] Morphine is approved by the Food and Drug Administration (FDA) for this indication and has significant data supporting its use.[4,9-11] Morphine is the most frequently used opioid for the initiation of intrathecal therapy.[12] Hydromorphone is an alternative to morphine in patients who do not experience adequate pain relief or have unacceptable adverse events after administration of morphine.[9,13] Although no commercial interest has applied for FDA approval for this indication, significant preclinical and clinical data support its use.[14-16]

Ziconotide, which is discussed in detail in Chapter 24, is FDA approved for intrathecal analgesia and may be especially useful in the treatment of patients with neuropathic pain.[17] Many clinicians initiate intrathecal analgesia using opioids and reserve the use of ziconotide for patients who do not report adequate analgesia after opioid or opioid local anesthetic therapy. As a result, ziconotide may be reserved for use as a second- or third-tier choice for intrathecal analgesic therapy, although this is based on physician preference.[8,9]

Intrathecal opioid therapy is often started in patients who have either not experienced adequate pain relief or report unacceptable adverse effects after the administration of systemic opioids. In addition, these patients have completed a successful trial of either intrathecal or epidural opioids before the decision was made to proceed with implantation of the intrathecal catheter and infusion pump. As a result, the patient may be opioid tolerant. In addition, important information regarding the patient's response to the opioid used during the trial is available to guide decision making regarding which drug and dosage should be used to start intrathecal analgesic therapy.

One of the greatest risks of intrathecal therapy is the possibility of overdose at the time of implant, or immediately following a refill.[18] Drug overdose can be due to an error in calculating the starting dose, an error in programming, or due to subcutaneous injection of the opioid rather than injection of the medication into the device. In addition, life-threatening respiratory depression has been reported after intrathecal morphine administration, which may be due to multiple causes as discussed above. Respiratory depression usually occurs after initiation of therapy in a patient who is not opioid tolerant. However, respiratory depression has also been reported in patients receiving long-term intrathecal opioid therapy, usually after a change in opioid dose.[19]

The implanting physician should be vigilant in choosing the initial opioid dose in order to lower the risk of error. The lowest effective dose should be used based on the information available from the trial completed before implantation.[9] Some investigators have used the total systemic opioid dose as a guide, estimating that the intrathecal dose of morphine is about 10% of the daily dose of intravenous (IV) morphine (**Fig. 4-1**). However, the method of converting from systemic to intrathecal opioid doses has been questioned.[20] In addition, the calculation becomes more difficult when converting from one or more opioids to a different opioid to be administered intrathecally. In this case, one may wish to decrease the calculated dose by 30% to 40% to account for incomplete opioid cross-tolerance.

Much of our understanding of the dosing of intrathecal opioids is based on our experience with systemic opioids even though the pharmacodynamic effects of intrathecal opioids for the treatment of acute pain are very different than when the same medications are administered by other systemic routes.[21] In general, the same considerations exist regarding the use of this class of medications by these different delivery routes, with some important differences as outlined below.

Patients receiving intrathecal opioids may experience the adverse effects common after systemic delivery, and the risk depends on the dose and duration of therapy. Tolerance develops to most adverse effects with the exception of constipation. Some patients also experience pedal edema that is persistent over time. Tolerance can develop over time, which may impact efficacy and may result in patients reporting less pain relief over time. The increase in daily dosing of opioids may result in improved analgesia in some patients, but this is not a uniform response. In addition, continuously increasing the opioid dose over time is not sustainable, especially because the risk of some adverse effects with chronic opioid therapy appears to rise with increases in daily dose.

Intrathecal analgesia should start with a single opioid at the lowest dose possible. This initial starting drug may be modified based on response to trialing, and in some patients, drug combinations may be necessary to obtain a positive response. This is more common in mixed or primary neuropathic pain. Initial therapy should include optimization of the dose in combination with optimizing the use of appropriate systemic medications as well as other interdisciplinary pain therapy. Care should be taken to make sure that treatment of associated disorders, such as depression and sleep disturbances, is optimized. Likewise, withdrawal of systemic opioids, if it was an initial goal of therapy, should be completed.

SUGGESTED INTRATHECAL THERAPY ALGORITHM

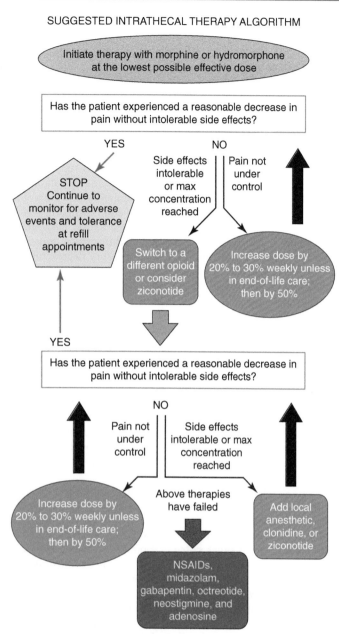

Fig. 4-1 Maximum recommended concentrations and daily dosages for common intrathecal medications. NSAID, nonsteroidal antiinflammatory drug.

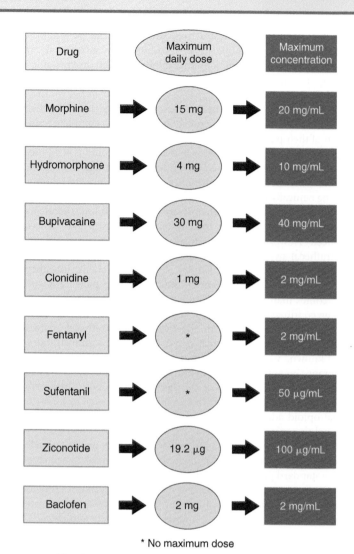

* No maximum dose

Fig. 4-2 Suggested intrathecal therapy algorithm.

Patients should be strongly encouraged to participate in cognitive-behavioral therapy and physical therapy as part of their integrated pain care when appropriate. Regardless, both the physician and the patient should not focus entirely on intrathecal drug delivery as a single-modality pain therapy with the expectation of complete resolution of pain.

When titrating the opioid dose upward, the dose may be increased based on physician experience and patient characteristics to treat inadequate analgesia.[7] Typical changes in dosing vary from 1% to 20% but may be more aggressive at end of life or after initial implant. There is a wide variability of the pace and amount of dose increases over time reported in the literature. Turner and associates[6] reported that the mean intrathecal morphine-equivalent dose increased 2.6- to 7.4-fold over a follow-up period of up to 24 months. In general, the dose should not be increased more often

than weekly to allow the patient time to experience the analgesic effects associated with the increased dose and to be able to adequately assess the presence of adverse effects associated with the increased dose. On the other hand, physicians often increase opioid doses more quickly when treating patients with cancer pain. In these patients, the dose may be increased by up to 50%, and dose changes may be completed every 2 to 3 days, depending on the opioid being used.[7] When titrating the initial opioid dose, patients, especially those who are opioid tolerant, should be carefully followed to monitor for the development of opioid-induced adverse effects.

Second-Line Therapy

There are several options for the treatment of pain not well controlled after initial therapy. Fig. 4-2 provides an overview of treatment options that can be considered. The order used when considering these options is not data driven and should be guided by the individual physician's experience with the use of the individual medications as well as the availability of the specific medications. Some options may not be available because of cost or other constraints, and other options may be contraindicated based on the patient's underlying medical condition or past experience with the medication.

If a single opioid does not provide adequate pain relief, the physician may change to a different opioid. Patients may report improved pain control after opioid rotation. Physicians may consider adjusting the daily dose of the new opioid downward by 30% to 40% to accommodate for incomplete cross-tolerance. There are several choices of agents, starting with morphine and hydromorphone. The next most common choices are fentanyl or sufentanil, although the use of these medications requires special attention because compounding of lipid-soluble opioids for intrathecal drug delivery presents special challenges (see Chapter 2). In addition, there are limited data to support the long-term safety and efficacy for these medications when used for this indication.[22]

The next option for consideration is the addition of a local anesthetic to the opioid. There is extensive experience with the epidural administration of a dilute local anesthetic with an opioid to treat patients with acute pain. In this setting, the combination appears to provide more effective pain relief than that experienced with either medication used alone. Similar experience has been reported after intrathecal delivery for the treatment of cancer-related[23] and chronic pain.[9,23] However most of the reports regarding the chronic use of local anesthetics such as bupivacaine with opioids were uncontrolled and nonrandomized case series.[24] Nerve injury and spinal cord lesions have been attributed to formulations containing local anesthetics, although they were not solo agents, and there is no evidence that these drugs caused the lesions.[25,26]

Bupivacaine is commonly used and appears to be safe and effective for this indication. However, chronic intrathecal infusion of bupivacaine has not been approved by the FDA, and there are limited data regarding the safety and efficacy of its use for this purpose in the literature. Lidocaine has also been used but should probably be avoided because intrathecal administration has been associated with neurological injury.[27] Other local anesthetics such as ropivacaine have also been used, but less data are available in the literature to guide therapy.

Patients may report initial improvement with the addition of the local anesthetic only to report decreased efficacy over time. Tachyphylaxis has been reported after chronic administration of local anesthetics. Although dose increases may initially be effective, further increases in local anesthetic dose may not be possible because patients often report numbness or weakness with higher doses of local anesthetics. Common adverse side effects include paresthesia, motor and sensory blockade, hypotension, diarrhea, and urinary retention.[9] Adverse side effects are usually dose related, and the incidence is much higher at daily doses of bupivacaine of more than 45 mg in 24 hours.[28]

Ziconotide should be considered in patients who do not experience adequate pain relief with opioid monotherapy or with opioids in combination with local anesthetics. Ziconotide can also be used as a first-line drug to treat neuropathic pain. Ziconotide may be more effective than opioids in patients with neuropathic pain but has been used for the treatment of nociceptive pain.[29-31] Ziconotide trial and dosing are discussed in detail in Chapter 24. Ziconotide may be used in combination with opioids or opioids with local anesthetics, although such use presents challenges regarding ziconotide stability (see Chapters 2 and 3). Mean pain relief after administration of ziconotide for the treatment of chronic pain is 12% 21 days after starting therapy.[32]

Clonidine, a potent α_2-agonist, has been used intrathecally, either as a single agent or in combination with other agents such as opioids. Clonidine appears to provide improved pain control compared with opioids alone, especially for the treatment of neuropathic pain.[33,34] However, no commercial interest has applied for FDA approval for intrathecal clonidine, and there are gaps in our understanding of the drug's safety and efficacy when used for this purpose. Common adverse side effects include sedation, hypotension, dry mouth, and bradycardia.[35,36] These side effects can often be avoided with slow titration and by using catheters in the lower thoracic or lumbar spine.

Several other medications from several drug classes have been evaluated for intrathecal analgesia. These include nonsteroidal antiinflammatory drugs, midazolam and other benzodiazepines, gabapentin, octreotide, neostigmine, and adenosine. There are limited data to document the safety and efficacy of these medications, and their use should probably be within the context of an institutional review board-approved clinical trial.

Therapy-Related Adverse Events

Unfortunately, adverse events associated with intrathecal analgesia do occur. There are numerous potential sources for complications, including complications related to placement of the infusion pump and catheter, failure of these devices to function properly, adverse reactions to medications, and human error. In fact, patients with noncancer pain treated with intrathecal opioid therapy experience increased mortality compared with similar patients treated with other therapies.[18] Although it has not been definitely proven, human error related to medication management, including errors during pump refill and programming, appear to be an important source of potentially serious adverse events.[37]

Medication Overdose

The causes of human error that lead to overdose are multifactorial and include placing the wrong drug or drug concentration into the pump, injecting the drug subcutaneously or intrathecally via the side port, or committing programming errors.[7] Even minor errors in programming can lead to serious complications because high concentrations of opioids are often used to avoid frequent pump refills.

It is important to note that adverse events may not occur immediately after a pump refill or reprogramming. Rather, the effects of an error or intended medication change may not present for several hours after institution of the change. In addition, both physicians and patients must be aware that intrathecal medications can certainly interact with systemically administered medications, including alcohol and recreational drugs.

Care must be taken by the medical team to ensure that extreme diligence is exercised each and every time a pump is reprogrammed or refilled. Providers should use a standardized process for patient care related to these high-risk patient care activities. For example, extreme care should be taken when initiating, reinitiating, or simply refilling the device reservoir to ensure that the injection is placed into the correct port and that the injection is not subcutaneous. The drug(s) and drug(s) concentration should be carefully reviewed and verified. Likewise, the programming should be verified. When initiating therapy in patients at increased risk for adverse events, consideration should be given to the location of therapy to ensure that proper monitoring is completed and that necessary equipment is available to care for the patient in the event of emergency.

Patients must play an active role whenever possible in their therapy, including efforts to avoid error. Education generally starts before the intrathecal analgesic trial and continues throughout therapy. When possible, patients should be aware of the medications they are receiving. In addition, patients and their immediate family members should be aware of potential adverse events and what to do if these complications occur.

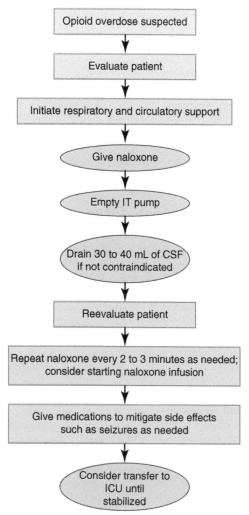

Fig. 4-3 Opioid overdose algorithm. CSF, cerebrospinal fluid; ICU, intensive care unit; IT, intrathecal.

Opioid Overdose   The diagnosis of an intrathecal opioid overdose is a clinical one. Signs of overdose include altered mental status, including confusion and sedation, and respiratory depression or arrest. Cardiac arrest and death may occur if proper medical care is not immediately initiated.

Initial medical care is supportive and includes support of oxygenation and ventilation, as well as discontinuation of opioid therapy as soon as possible. Naloxone may be administered initially via IV bolus, but then via IV infusion, because the half-life of naloxone is far shorter than the respiratory depressant effects of intrathecal opioids.

In addition to discontinuation of the intrathecal opioid infusion, the medication in the pump should be replaced with saline to avoid administration of additional opioid. Consideration should be given to aspiration of the intrathecal catheter via the side port so that all opioid is removed from the system to avoid continued dosing. During this procedure, 30 to 40 mL of cerebrospinal fluid (CSF) can be withdrawn in an attempt to lower the intrathecal concentration (**Fig. 4-3**).[38]

Ziconotide Overdose   Although ziconotide overdose is unpleasant, it does not usually cause respiratory depression or death. However, ziconotide toxicity has been associated with brief periods of apnea, unresponsiveness, delirium, and agitation. Ziconotide overdose presents as ataxia, nystagmus, dizziness, stupor, unresponsiveness, spinal myoclonus, confusion, sedation, hypotension, word-finding difficulties, garbled speech, nausea, and vomiting.[39]

Although ziconotide overdose is unlikely to be life threatening, the patient will certainly require appropriate supportive care if he or she becomes unresponsive or develops apnea. There is no antagonist for ziconotide. Therapy for overdose includes discontinuation of the intrathecal infusion. As with intrathecal opioid overdose, the medication in the pump should be replaced with saline, and consideration should be given to aspiration of the intrathecal catheter via the side port so that all medication is removed from the system to avoid continued dosing. During this procedure, 30 to 40 mL of CSF can be withdrawn in an attempt to lower the intrathecal concentration of the drug. The effects of ziconotide often diminish significantly within 24 hours because the CSF half-life is 4.6 hours, and the plasma half-life is 1.3 hours. However, the patient may report drug effects that last for weeks to months.[40]

Withdrawal Syndrome
As with systemic medications, intrathecal medications can induce increased levels of receptors and therefore tolerance. Abrupt discontinuation of intrathecal opioids can lead to a withdrawal syndrome that can be very uncomfortable but is rarely life threatening. However, abrupt discontinuation of baclofen can lead to a life-threatening withdrawal syndrome. Alternatively, ziconotide and local anesthetics can be rapidly discontinued without risk of a withdrawal syndrome.

Causes of drug withdrawal are multifactorial. Reports have been made and theories have been proposed of missed refill appointments, pump malfunctions, catheter obstruction, catheter disconnections, magnetic resonance imaging (MRI) interference, radiation therapy, and low battery output precipitating withdrawal. The first step to treatment is determining the cause. A missed refill appointment is easily remedied and easily treated. The pump should be queried, records reviewed, and the patient evaluated. However, if the cause of withdrawal is not immediately recognizable, then the condition should be treated until further testing can be initiated in the form of MRI, a dye study, or fluoroscopy, to name a few. Further descriptions of pump and catheter troubleshooting can be found in Chapter 15.

Opioid Withdrawal   After abrupt cessation of intrathecal opioid infusion, withdrawal may present with the following symptoms: malaise, severe pain, anxiety, myalgia, insomnia, dehydration, and fever. The cause of withdrawal and an immediate remedy must be determined to prevent continued withdrawal and increased pain. If intrathecal therapy cannot be resumed, systemic opioids can be started.

Baclofen Withdrawal   Because baclofen withdrawal can be life threatening, evidence of abrupt discontinuation requires immediate attention, and the development of symptoms of baclofen withdrawal is a medical emergency. Further management details are provided in Chapter 22.

Conclusion

Little evidence exists as to the best way to begin and manage intrathecal drug therapy, which can cause trepidation in even the most experienced clinicians. Fortunately, based on extensive experience coupled with the available data, consensus guidelines have been determined. Clinicians can, with care and common sense, determine the appropriate management course specific to each patient's particular needs and medical history. Most clinicians start with opioids and may eventually add local anesthetics or clonidine as needed to palliate refractory pain as much as possible. However, only morphine and nonopiate ziconotide are currently FDA approved for intrathecal use. Further research needs to be done to elucidate these medications' efficacies and to develop an evidence-based standard of care for intrathecal therapy. Regardless, ITDDS can be an effective, safe therapy for patients who have failed conventional oral medications or interventions.

On the other hand, intrathecal therapy can precipitate serious adverse events, and the clinician and patient should be aware of the risks. The patient needs to commit to being a partner in his or her own therapy by learning about the ITDDS and the signs and symptoms of overdose, withdrawal, and other complications. Finally, the patient's and clinician's expectations must be realistic and in parallel. Intrathecal medication infusion cannot provide 100% pain relief. Therefore, as with oral medications or other interventions, adjunct treatment with physical therapy, behavioral therapy, antidepressants, or sleep medications can be continued or initiated for a more complete treatment.

References

1. Noble M, Treadwell JR, Tregear SJ, et al: Long-term opioid management for chronic noncancer pain. *Cochrane Database Syst Rev* CD006605, 2010.
2. Smith TJ, Staats PS, Deer T, et al: Randomized clinical trial of an implantable drug delivery system compared with comprehensive medical management for refractory cancer pain: impact on pain, drug-related toxicity, and survival. *J Clin Oncol* 20:4040-4049, 2002.
3. Rauck RL, Cherry D, Boyer MF, et al: Long-term intrathecal opioid therapy with a patient-activated, implanted delivery system for the treatment of refractory cancer pain. *J Pain* 4:441-447, 2003.
4. Thimineur MA, Kravitz E, Vodapally MS: Intrathecal opioid treatment for chronic non-malignant pain: a 3-year prospective study. *Pain* 109:242-249, 2004.
5. Cohen SP, Dragovich A: Intrathecal analgesia. *Med Clin North Am* 91:251-270, 2007.
6. Turner JA, Sears JM, Loeser JD: Programmable intrathecal opioid delivery systems for chronic noncancer pain: a systematic review of effectiveness and complications. *Clin J Pain* 23:180-195, 2007.
7. Deer T, Krames ES, Hassenbusch SJ, et al: Polyanalgesic consensus conference 2007: recommendations for the management of pain by intrathecal (intraspinal) drug delivery: report of an interdisciplinary expert panel. *Neuromodulation* 10:300-328, 2007.
8. Hassenbusch SJ, Portenoy RK, Cousins M, et al: Polyanalgesic Consensus Conference 2003: an update on the management of pain by intraspinal drug delivery—report of an expert panel. *J Pain Symptom Manage* 27:540-563, 2004.
9. Ghafoor VL, Epshteyn M, Carlson GH, et al: Intrathecal drug therapy for long-term pain management. *Am J Health Syst Pharm* 64:2447-2461, 2007.
10. Roberts LJ, Finch PM, Goucke CR, Price LM: Outcome of intrathecal opioids in chronic non-cancer pain. *Eur J Pain* 5:353-361, 2001.
11. Follett KA, Hitchon PW, Piper J, et al: Response of intractable pain to continuous intrathecal morphine: a retrospective study. *Pain* 49:21-25, 1992.
12. Deer TR, Krames E, Levy RM, et al: Practice choices and challenges in the current intrathecal therapy environment: an online survey. *Pain Med* 10:304-309, 2009.
13. Hassenbusch SJ, Stanton-Hicks M, Covington EC, et al: Long-term intraspinal infusions of opioids in the treatment of neuropathic pain. *J Pain Symptom Manage* 10:527-543, 1995.
14. Johansen MJ, Satterfield WC, Baze WB, et al: Continuous intrathecal infusion of hydromorphone: safety in the sheep model and clinical implications. *Pain Med* 5:14-25, 2004.
15. Anderson VC, Cooke B, Burchiel KJ: Intrathecal hydromorphone for chronic nonmalignant pain: a retrospective study. *Pain Med* 2:287-297, 2001.
16. Du Pen S, Du Pen A, Hillyer J: Intrathecal hydromorphone for intractable nonmalignant pain: a retrospective study. *Pain Med* 7:10-15, 2006.
17. Rauck RL, Wallace MS, Burton AW, et al: Intrathecal ziconotide for neuropathic pain: a review. *Pain Pract* 9:327-337, 2009.
18. Coffey RJ, Owens ML, Broste SK, et al: Mortality associated with implantation and management of intrathecal opioid drug infusion systems to treat noncancer pain. *Anesthesiology* 111:881-891, 2009.
19. Scherens A, Kagel T, Zenz M, Maier C: Long-term respiratory depression induced by intrathecal morphine treatment for chronic neuropathic pain. *Anesthesiology* 105:431-433, 2006.
20. Mercadante S: Neuraxial techniques for cancer pain: an opinion about unresolved therapeutic dilemmas. *Reg Anesth Pain Med* 24:74-83, 1999.
21. Rathmell JP, Lair TR, Nauman B: The role of intrathecal drugs in the treatment of acute pain. *Anesth Analg* 101:S30-S43, 2005.
22. Waara-Wolleat KL, Hildebrand KR, Stewart GR: A review of intrathecal fentanyl and sufentanil for the treatment of chronic pain. *Pain Med* 7:251-259, 2006.
23. Sjoberg M, Nitescu P, Appelgren L, Curelaru I: Long-term intrathecal morphine and bupivacaine in patients with refractory cancer pain. Results from a morphine:bupivacaine dose regimen of 0.5:4.75 mg/ml. *Anesthesiology* 80:284-297, 1994.
24. Deer TR, Caraway DL, Kim CK, et al: Clinical experience with intrathecal bupivacaine in combination with opioid for the treatment of chronic pain related to failed back surgery syndrome and metastatic cancer pain of the spine. *Spine J* 2:274-278, 2002.
25. Wadhwa RK, Shaya MR, Nanda A: Spinal cord compression in a patient with a pain pump for failed back syndrome: a chalk-like precipitate mimicking a spinal cord neoplasm: case report. *Neurosurgery* 58:E387; discussion E387, 2006.
26. Perren F, Buchser E, Chedel D, et al: Spinal cord lesion after long-term intrathecal clonidine and bupivacaine treatment for the management of intractable pain. *Pain* 109:189-194, 2004.
27. Hodgson PS, Neal JM, Pollock JE, Liu SS: The neurotoxicity of drugs given intrathecally (spinal). *Anesth Analg* 88:797-809, 1999.
28. Dahm P, Nitescu P, Appelgren L, Curelaru I: Efficacy and technical complications of long-term continuous intraspinal infusions of opioid and/or bupivacaine in refractory nonmalignant pain: a comparison between the epidural and the intrathecal approach with externalized or implanted catheters and infusion pumps. *Clin J Pain* 14:4-16, 1998.
29. Stanton-Hicks M, Kapural L: An effective treatment of severe complex regional pain syndrome type 1 in a child using high doses of intrathecal ziconotide. *J Pain Symptom Manage* 32:509-511, 2006.
30. Lynch SS, Cheng CM, Yee JL: Intrathecal ziconotide for refractory chronic pain. *Ann Pharmacother* 40:1293-1300, 2006.
31. Rauck RL, Wallace MS, Leong MS, et al: A randomized, double-blind, placebo-controlled study of intrathecal ziconotide in adults with severe chronic pain. *J Pain Symptom Manage* 31:393-406, 2006.
32. Prialt Package Insert, approved April 18, 2007.
33. Ackerman LL, Follett KA, Rosenquist RW: Long-term outcomes during treatment of chronic pain with intrathecal clonidine or clonidine/opioid combinations. *J Pain Symptom Manage* 26:668-677, 2003.
34. Rainov NG, Heidecke V, Burkert W: Long-term intrathecal infusion of drug combinations for chronic back and leg pain. *J Pain Symptom Manage* 22:862-871, 2001.
35. Borg PA, Krijnen HJ: Long-term intrathecal administration of midazolam and clonidine. *Clin J Pain* 12:63-68, 1996.
36. Eisenach JC, DuPen S, Dubois M, et al: Epidural clonidine analgesia for intractable cancer pain. The Epidural Clonidine Study Group. *Pain* 61:391-399, 1995.

37. Rathmell JP, Miller MJ: Death after initiation of intrathecal drug therapy for chronic pain: assessing risk and designing prevention. *Anesthesiology* 111:706-708, 2009.

38. Medtronic Professional: *Emergency Procedure for Morphine Intrathecal/Epidural Overdose*, Minneapolis MN, 2009, Medtronic, Inc.

39. Smith HS, Deer TR: Safety and efficacy of intrathecal ziconotide in the management of severe chronic pain. *Ther Clin Risk Manage* 5:521-534, 2009.

40. Schmidtko A, Lotsch J, Freynhagen R, Geisslinger G: Ziconotide for treatment of severe chronic pain. *Lancet* 375:1569-1577, 2010.

5 Patient Selection for Intrathecal Infusion to Treat Chronic Pain

Allen Dennis and Miles Day

CHAPTER OVERVIEW

Chapter Synopsis: As is the case for so many treatments for chronic pain, patient selection remains one of the most important factors in a successful course of treatment with intrathecal drug infusion. Perhaps most strikingly, a patient's expectations seem to be an enormous contributing factor to success or failure. Naturally, psychosocial comorbidities (e.g., depression) contribute to the tendency to expect bad outcomes and experience more pain, which can leave this huge group of patients as contraindicated to intrathecal drug delivery systems (IDDS) therapy. On the other hand, psychological screening may reveal other psychological therapeutic avenues that could provide synergistic benefit to the patient along with IDDS. The patient's likelihood to comply with treatment requirements also contributes to success. Because the therapy is invasive in nature, it calls for a different risk-to-benefit analysis. Noncancer patients are generally considered only if they have refractory pain or severe side effects to more conventional therapies, but they should have a demonstrated opioid analgesia. When considering costs, IDDS therapy appears to become cost effective at about 2 years. IDDS is generally contraindicated in cancer patients with short life expectancies.

Important Points:
- Indications for IDDS require demonstration of pathologies consistent with chronic pain, inadequate relief from less invasive procedures, demonstrated opioid response to analgesia, and an intolerable adverse effects to systemic opioids.
- Contraindications include conditions that increase the risk of adverse events, indicate poor patient compliance with treatment plans, or diminish the analgesic potential of the intervention.
- Psychosocial comorbidities possess a dramatic influence toward patient compliance, ability to perceive analgesic effect, and overall failure of intrathecal infusion modalities.
- The cost of implanted IDDS has been shown to equal that of more conservative approaches at about 2 years of treatment. Percutaneous devices are more cost effective if the patient's life expectancy is less than 3 months.
- Primary pitfalls in the patient selection process generally involve underestimating the value of a successful intrathecal analgesic trial or impact of poorly controlled psychosocial comorbidities.

Clinical Pearls:
- Clinical judgment is greatly improved by a greater fund of knowledge of the clinical situation. Before utilization of implantable systems to treat chronic pain, it behooves the physician to have sufficient encounter time with the patient to both rule out less invasive therapies as viable options and to establish patient compliance and responsiveness to analgesics. Patients who display a high degree of compliance with treatment plans and respond to systemic analgesics are more likely to display beneficial results from IDDS. These tendencies are best demonstrated by time and repeated patient–doctor encounters.
- Analgesic response to systemic opioids provides evidence that intrathecal delivery of opioids will provide beneficial treatment of chronic pain.[1-7,23] Documentation of analgesia from both systemic and intrathecal opioid trials aids the decision to place permanent IDDS. It is also beneficial to observe an improved side effect profile from the intrathecal route compared with systemic dosing.[23] A display of efficacy and diminished adverse effects over time helps rule out a placebo effect from intrathecal pharmacology. In addition, patients who require rapid escalation of systemic opioids are likely to require similar escalations from the intrathecal route.

Clinical Pitfalls:
- As previously stated, intrathecal infusion therapies possess a significant level of risk compared with other interventional pain therapies.[21,22] In addition, intrathecal infusions require a high degree of patient compliance.[1-7] These factors contribute to a significant level of commitment and energy of the practitioner toward ongoing intrathecal infusion therapy. Therefore, efforts to discover issues that may increase patient risk, interfere with patient compliance, or decrease the probable efficacy of intrathecal therapies must not be ignored. Progression to implantation of IDDS without sufficient time and interaction with a patient to judge the appropriateness of intrathecal therapies can have disastrous consequences.[7,21]
- Underestimating coexisting psychological comorbidities during the selection process risks both an insufficient response to intrathecal infusions and serious complications to therapy.[1-7,24-26] Certainly, implantation of IDDS in patients with untreated major psychopathologies places the patient at high risk of serious complications for either noncompliance or self-harm. Furthermore, poorly controlled minor psychopathologies can interfere with perception of analgesia.[1-7,24-26] As with anatomic and physiologic pathologies, minor psychiatric pathologies may develop into more serious conditions.

■ Many psychiatric comorbidities develop in conjunction with the chronic pain state; however, treatment of the pain generator poorly treats the psychiatric condition.[24-26] Posttraumatic stress disorder is a prime example of a psychopathology whose symptomatology persists long after the initiating physical stressor has resolved. In a similar fashion, depression, anxiety, and other mood disorders that are exacerbated in the presence of chronic pain likely will persist despite optimization of the pain generator.[24-26] Treatment of chronic pain with IDDS in patients with poorly optimized psychopathologies is likely to provide suboptimal results.[1-7,24-26] Intrathecal opioids are poor replacements for selective neurotransmitter reuptake inhibitors, mood stabilizers, and antipsychotic medications.

■ The pain physician may be tempted to progress toward implantation of IDDS in patients devoid of psychosocial contraindications despite a history of poor response to pharmacologic agents used in intrathecal therapies. Likelihood of successful intrathecal therapies is a balance between indicators of efficacy of therapy and absence of complicating conditions.[23] Ignoring a poor response to systemic opioids or an indeterminate intrathecal opioid trial can expose the patient to the increased risks of intrathecal infusions with little analgesic response.[23] In addition, disregard of complications from an intrathecal infusion trial, such as urinary retention, sedation, pruritus, headache, and altered mental status, places the patient at risk of chronic suffering from those adverse effects.

Introduction

The utilization of intrathecal analgesics has been a significant development in the treatment of patients with chronic and cancer pain.[1,2] As with most interventions, proper patient selection greatly affects the achieved efficacy. Skilled technique and an increased diversity of pharmacologic agents remain poor substitutes for improper patient selection for intrathecal infusion therapy.[2,3] Multiple factors must be considered before implantation of an intrathecal infusion device, including the benefits of less invasive interventions, the patient's functional and psychological status, the ability of the patient to be compliant to the treatment regimen, the type of pain, potential contraindications of pump implantation, and the cost of therapy.[1-7] Treatment of chronic nonmalignant pain with intrathecal therapies is more controversial than cancer pain and carries additional patient selection concerns.[1,7]

Indications

Intrathecal drug delivery systems (IDDS) are reserved for treatment of chronic pain refractory to other procedures or conservative therapy.[4] Generally, pain lasting more than 3 or 4 months that is refractory to accepted medical management or pain secondary to malignant conditions projected to last more than 3 months is thought of as chronic.[4] As a fairly invasive therapy, use of IDDS necessitates consideration of several inclusion criteria (**Box 5-1**) before trial or implantation.

The most common indication for implantation of IDDS is chronic pain requiring high-dose opioids resulting in intolerable opioid side effects.[5] A history of dose-dependent opioid side effect profiles is helpful when planning a trial of intrathecal opioids.[2,4-6] To predict successful analgesia with intrathecal opioids, analgesia with systemic opioids despite side effects should be demonstrated.[2,4-6] In general, intrathecal opioids provide for better side effect profiles and improved analgesia in both cancer pain and certain forms of chronic pain; however, the ineffectiveness of

high-dose opioids is a poor prognostic indicator for the efficacy of intrathecal opioid therapy.[1,2,5,6]

Opioid side effects include sedation, nausea, headache, constipation, rash, and itching, as well as other various complaints. Attempts to treat the patient's side effect profile and trial alternative systemic opioids should be made before judging the patient to be intolerant of systemic opioids.[5] Additionally, analgesia with lower doses of opioids combined with adjuvant medications such as nonsteroidal antiinflammatory drugs and neuromodulatory medications should also be attempted before intrathecal opioid trials.[4] The presence of a dose-dependent analgesic response to opioids when side effects become intolerable and adjuvant medications fail to reduce the opioid requirements are good indicators of the potential benefit of intrathecal opioid therapies.[2,4-6] Numerous studies have displayed improved analgesic affect, decreased opioid side effects, and improved quality of life with intrathecal morphine, hydromorphone, and combined morphine-bupivacaine intrathecal infusions compared with systemic opioids for the treatment of cancer and nonmalignant chronic pain.[8-20]

Although IDDS use for treatment of cancer and chronic nonmalignant pain had gained positive evidence, it is also accepted as a higher risk and more labor intensive therapy for both the practitioner and patient.[1,21,22] To further justify the risk-to-benefit ratio for chronic intrathecal analgesic infusion, failure or contraindication of less invasive therapies should be demonstrated.[1-7] Less invasive therapies include systemic medication, physical therapy, nerve blocks and neurolysis, and methods of neuromodulation.[1,3-7] Additionally, IDDS should not be considered if definitive treatment of the pain generating pathology is possible.[6] Furthermore, the presence of an identifiable pathology consistent with the patient's pain complaint should be described.[2-4,6]

Several references[4,6,10,11,20,23] suggest that certain pain types and pathologies respond better to intrathecal therapies; therefore pain type should be considered during patient selection. Nociceptive pain is generally considered to be opioid responsive.[5] Hassenbusch et al[10] reported an average 39% pain reduction in 11 of 18 patients with neuropathic pain enrolled in a prospective intrathecal morphine infusion study. However, more than half of the patients who reporting improved analgesia required daily morphine doses in excess of current intrathecal dosing recommendations.[1,10] Kumar et al[11] studied 16 patients with severe nonmalignant pain and reported better analgesia in patients with deafferentation and mixed pain. Kumar et al[11] also described early high-level analgesia that weaned with time in patients with nociceptive pain. Paice et al[20] evaluated 363 patients with either malignant or

---

Box 5-1: Inclusion Criteria for Patient Selection for Intrathecal Analgesic Therapies

■ Identifiable pathology generating chronic pain
■ Measurable opioid responsiveness
■ Failure of systemic opioid therapy secondary to high-dose requirements or intolerable side effects
■ Pain that is refractory to less invasive therapies
■ Definitive medical or surgical therapy is not indicated
■ No presence of contraindications for device implantation

nonmalignant pain and reported greater relief in patients with somatic pain and that patients with neuropathic pain required higher doses of opioid at 6 months, suggesting decreased opioid responsiveness to intrathecal opioids. Dominguez et al[23] performed a retrospective analysis of 86 patients undergoing intrathecal opioid infusion and evaluated for potential predictors of escalating dose requirements. A trend of increasing dose requirements was seen in patients with pain of cervical and visceral origin; however, these results were not statistically significant. Based on the current level of evidence for differential response of intrathecal opioid infusion toward varying types of pain, it remains difficult to stratify the importance of neuropathic versus nociceptive pain type for patient selection for IDDS. However, the evidence for the use of IDDS is strong for short-term improvement of cancer pain and moderate for long-term improvement in cancer pain; it is less supportive for use in chronic nonmalignant pain states.[1]

Contraindications

Potential complications of IDDS systems have been well documented.[1,21,22] To reduce the risk of both immediate and long-term complications during placement as well as to maintain the proposed efficacy of IDDS, evaluation for the coexistence of several conditions has been proposed (**Box 5-2**) during the patient selection period.[1-7]

Anatomically, an intrathecal infusion catheter courses through the epidural space and dwells within the subarachnoid layer. Infection or hemorrhage in these regions can produce devastating consequences, including paralysis and death.[22] Evaluation for conditions that predispose the patient to infection of implanted equipment or neuraxial hemorrhage during IDDS placement must be made during the selection process.[1-6,22] The presence of systemic infection, uncontrolled coagulopathy, and aplastic anemia are absolute contraindications to IDDS trial and placement.[2,6,7] It is also advisable to evaluate the patient for signs of infection before percutaneous maintenance of the IDDS. Inadequate body habitus and poor wound healing are considered relative contraindications for IDDS placement because tissue breakdown around the IDDS is a substantial infectious risk.[2,6,7] Hypersensitivity reactions to either infusion medications or pump and catheter material can also result in severe patient sequelae and should be considered as absolute contraindication to IDDS trial and placement.[2,6,7]

Withdrawal from intrathecal infusions can cause multiple adverse consequences ranging from severe patient discomfort to death.[22] Substance abuse in the presence of intrathecal infusions can lead to respiratory depression or arrest, hypotension, functional impairment, and death.[21] Secondary to these concerns, intrathecal infusions should only be considered in patients who have displayed a history of compliance with their respective treatments.[2,6,7] Patients and their caregivers must be able to understand and recognize the signs of intrathecal drug withdrawal and overdose.

A history of intravenous drug abuse may also be considered a contraindication to IDDS use.[2-7] Attempts by the patient to access the IDDS can result is infection, mechanical failure, and withdrawal. Furthermore, the presence of an underlying addiction can impair the analgesic efficacy of the intrathecal infusion stategy.[2] Multiple other psychiatric conditions are indicative of poor outcome with therapies for chronic pain.[24-26] The presence of certain psychiatric comorbidities should be considered contraindications to intrathecal therapies.[2-7] Further details of the psychological screen are discussed later in this chapter.

Obtaining a successful outcome with either the intrathecal trial or long-term intrathecal infusion is highly dependent on the patient's ability to judge pain relief.[7] Numerous physical conditions can impair the patient's ability to measure analgesia (**Box 5-3**) and should be corrected if possible before trialing of intrathecal therapies.[7] Uncorrectable causes of altered patient pain and analgesia perception may be considered contraindications to IDDS implantation.[7]

Psychological Screening

Coexisting psychiatric and behavioral comorbidities can negatively affect the long-term efficacy of intrathecal infusion modalities.[2-7,24-26]

Box 5-2: Contraindications for Intrathecal Analgesic Therapies

- Absolute contraindications
  - Infection
  - Aplastic anemia
  - Ongoing intravenous drug use
  - Allergy to materials present in the implantable device
  - Allergy to pharmacologic agents to be infused
  - History of poor compliance
  - Coagulopathy
  - Major psychopathology
  - Life expectancy less than 3 months
- Relative contraindications
  - Poor healing
  - Insufficient body mass to support implanted device
  - Poor familial or social support
  - Recovering intravenous drug use
  - Poor access to health care
  - Age before epiphysis fusion

Box 5-3: Conditions That Interfere with Analgesic Perception

- Metabolic conditions
  - Hypercalcemia
  - Hyponatremia
  - Hypoxia
  - Hypercarbia
  - Azotemia
  - Paraneoplastic syndrome
  - Metastatic tumor
  - Abscess
- Pharmacologic conditions
  - Narcotics
  - Tranquilizers
  - Barbiturates
  - Phenothiazine reactions
  - Cimetidine
  - Drug-induced organic brain syndrome
- Neurologic conditions
  - Encephalopathy (metabolic, hepatic, or infectious)
  - Increase intracranial pressure
  - Cerebral infarction or hemorrhage
  - Neurodegenerative disorders
  - Alzheimer disease or other forms of dementia
- Psychosocial conditions
  - Chemical dependence
  - Use of pain as a controlling or attention-seeking device
  - Use of pain to punish persons within their support group
  - Mood disorders
  - Anxiety, high magnitude of distress, or catastrophizing
  - Major psychopathology
  - Risk for self-harm

These conditions may inhibit the patient's ability to assess analgesia as well as interfere with patient compliance. Thus, a thorough psychiatric evaluation plays a significant role in the patient selection process.[2-7,24-26] Currently, there is little evidence in the literature supporting any one method of psychiatric evaluation before trial of intrathecal infusions as superior to other screening modalities.[24] It is argued that obtaining patient psychosocial information from multiple settings and methods provides superior evaluation compared with any single screening tool alone.[24-26] Psychosocial evaluation strategies may include review of patient complaints, pain inventories, intelligence testing, psychometric testing, behavioral observation, and clinical interview with a mental health practitioner.[3,6,24-26]

Major psychopathology, mood disorders, suicidal depression, severe personality disorders, dementia, anxiety, catastrophization, history of addiction, and high level of distress represent psychiatric comorbidities that are commonly accepted to negatively affect outcomes of implantable pain therapies.[2-7,24-26] Patients with these conditions tend to have a decreased ability to judge the degree of analgesia obtained to maintain compliance with the treatment strategy and may possess mental and emotional reliance on their pain state.[7] Consideration of permanent device implantation should be approached with caution if evidence exists that the patient has borderline, antisocial, or multiple personality disorders or is using pain as an attention-seeking method or means to punish persons within their support systems.[7]

The goal of the psychological assessment is to both identify comorbidities that could cause increased risk of IDDS complications as well as shed light of the markers for adequate coping skills, social support, and sufficient insight of condition and treatment to provide the best opportunity for the patient to experience optimum treatment outcomes.[2-7,24-26]

Psychological screening of patients with cancer pain is generally accepted not to be a steadfast requirement before intrathecal analgesic trial as with nonmalignant pain treatment.[3] However, the prevalence of psychosocial comorbidities of terminal patients should not be ignored.[3,6] Psychological screening in this population can both identify when counseling and other psychiatric therapies may provide synergistic benefit to pain treatments as well as identify home care needs for the patient and their personal support systems.[5,6,24-26]

Financial Considerations

Implantation and management of IDDS carries a significant financial cost.[27-32] The financial burdens of modern medical technologies and therapies has introduced the necessity of cost-to-benefit analysis of proposed treatment plans.[27,28] Various economic analysis models have been used to predict the financial burden of IDDS for both cancer and nonmalignant chronic pain treatment.[27] Understanding the goals and limitations of these methods is necessary to draw conclusions for chronic economic analysis of IDDS for treatment of chronic pain and how it pertains to patient selection for these therapies.[27]

Cost-minimization models compare the cost of two of more therapies that are judged to have equivalent outcomes.[27] Studies relying on cost minimization may fail to account for superior outcomes of one therapy above another. Cost-effective analysis attempts to compare the cost of two therapies to achieve similar outcomes.[27] To accomplish this, a monetary value is assumed per unit of outcome. Outcome measures tend to be subjective and difficult to standardize when treating chronic pain. Cost-to-benefit analysis strives to define both the cost and benefits of a therapy in terms of financial units and is beneficial for assigning society cost of particular therapies and determination of standards of care.[27]

Cost-minimization analysis of intrathecal opioids compared with equipotent opioids via alternate routes of administration for treatment of cancer pain was published by Hassenbusch et al[28] in 1997. Data from this study suggest the financial break-even point between intrathecal opioid infusion compared with systemic opioids occurs between 18 and 30 months of treatment. When compared with tunneled epidural catheter infusion for treatment of malignant pain, IDDS become more cost effective at 3 months.[28-30] Based on this finding, IDDS are recommended for treatment of cancer pain if the patient's life expectancy is longer than 3 months.

Cost-effective analysis of intrathecal analgesic therapy for the treatment of nonmalignant back pain is more difficult to perform because of numerous variables in therapy over an extended patient course.[27] de Lissovoy et al[31] used a computer projection model and prevalence of complications of IDDS to predict the cost of intrathecal therapies and conventional therapies for failed back surgery syndrome over a 5-year period. The break-even point was predicted at 22 months.[31] Kumar et al[32] reported the costs of treatment of 67 patients with failed back surgery syndrome over a 5-year period.[28] Of these patients, 23 underwent implantation of IDDS. The break-even point was seen on average at 28 months.[32]

Based on these studies, a financial benefit for intrathecal analgesic infusion over conventional therapies should not be expected for at least 2 years and is subject to numerous variables, including IDDS complications and required escalation of therapy.[31] Thus, financial considerations for patient selection for IDDS for treatment of nonmalignant pain are difficult to justify.

Recommendations

Patients with cancer pain refractory to less invasive therapies and high-dose opioids or those that have intolerable side effects to systemic opioids may be considered for intrathecal analgesic therapies. If a patient's life expectancy is less than 3 months, tunneled catheter systems are more cost effective, and IDDS are generally considered contraindicated in this population. Intrathecal opioids are more effective in patients with proven opioid responsive pain. Although psychologic screening is not seen as a requirement before IDDS implantation for cancer pain, it may discover psychosocial comorbidities that may interfere with optimal intrathecal analgesic effectiveness. Absence of contraindications to implantation of a neuraxial device is mandatory for patient selection for intrathecal analgesics.

Treatment of nonmalignant pain with IDDS requires more stringent patient selection. Psychological clearance and optimization of psychosocial and physiologic conditions that interfere with analgesic perception is mandatory before intrathecal opioid trial or device implantation. Patient compliance history should also be strongly considered in the patient selection process. Evidence of opioid responsive pain is a positive indicator for intrathecal opioids. Although some evidence for a cost-to-benefit analysis of intrathecal therapies exist over conventional therapies after 23 to 28 months, financial considerations should not play a predominant role in the selection of nonmalignant pain patients for IDDS.

References

1. Smith SS, Deer TR, Staats PS, et al: Intrathecal drug delivery. *Pain Physician* 11(suppl):S89-S104, 2008.
2. Krames ES, Olson K: Clinical realities and economic considerations: patient selection in intrathecal therapy. *J Pain Symptom Manage* 3(suppl):S3-S13, 1997.

3. Deer TR: Intrathecal drug delivery: overview of the proper use of infusion agents. In Benzon HT, editor: *Raj's practical management of pain*, ed 2, Philadelphia, 2008, Mosby Elsevier, pp 945-954.

4. Oakly J, Staats PS: The use of implanted drug delivery systems. In Raj PP, editor: *Practical management of pain*, ed 3, St. Louis, 2000, Mosby Elsevier, pp 768-778.

5. Du Pen SL, Du Pen AR: Neuraxial drug delivery. In Warfield CA, Bajwa ZH, editors: *Principles and practice of pain medicine*, ed 2, New York, 2004, McGraw-Hill, pp 720-739.

6. White C, Rajagopal A: Intraspinal therapy. In De Loon-Casasola OA, editor: *Cancer pain: pharmacological, interventional and palliative care approaches*, ed 1, Philadelphia, 2006, Saunders Elsevier, pp 417-427.

7. Waldman SD: Implantable drug delivery systems: practical considerations. In Waldman SD, editor: *Pain management*, ed 1, Philadelphia, 2007, Saunders Elsevier, pp 1382-1387.

8. Smith TJ, Staats PS, Deer TR, et al: Drug Delivery Systems Study Group. Randomized clinical trial of an implantable drug delivery system compared with comprehensive medical management for refractory cancer pain: impact on pain, drug-related toxicity, and survival. *J Clin Oncol* 20:4040-4049, 2002.

9. Rauck RL, Cherry D, Boyer MF, et al: Long-term intrathecal opioid therapy with a patient-activated, implanted delivery system for the treatment of refractory cancer pain. *J Pain* 4:441-447, 2003.

10. Hassenbusch SJ, Stanton-Hicks M, Covington EC, et al: Long-term intraspinal infusions of opioids in the treatment of neuropathic pain. *J Pain Symptom Manage* 10:527-543, 1995.

11. Kumar K, Kelly M, Pirlot T: Continuous intrathecal morphine treatment for chronic pain of nonmalignant etiology: long-term benefits and efficacy. *Surg Neurol* 55:79-86, 2001.

12. Thimineur MA, Kravitz K, Vodapally MS: Continuous intrathecal opioid treatment for chronic non-malignant pain: a 3-year prospective study. *Pain* 109:242-249, 2004.

13. Anderson VC, Cooke B, Burchiel KJ: Intrathecal hydromorphone for chronic nonmalignant pain: a retrospective study. *Pain Med* 2:287-297, 2001.

14. van Dongen RT, Crul BJ, De Bock M: Long-term intrathecal infusion of morphine and morphine/bupivacaine mixtures in the treatment of cancer pain: a retrospective analysis of 51 cases. *Pain* 55:119-123, 1993.

15. van Dongen RT, Crul BJ, van Egmond J: Intrathecal coadministration of bupivacaine diminishes morphine dose progression during long-term intrathecal infusion in cancer patients. *Clin J Pain* 15:166-172, 1999.

16. Krames ES: Intrathecal infusion therapies for intractable pain: patient management guidelines. *J Pain Symptom Manage* 8:36-46, 1993.

17. Mironer EY, Haasis JC, Chappel I, et al: Efficacy and safety of intrathecal opioid/bupivacaine mixture in chronic nonmalignant pain: a double-blind, randomized, cross-over, multicenter study by the National Forum of Independent Pain Clinicians (NFIPC). *Neuromodulation* 5:208-213, 2002.

18. Angel IF, Gould HJ, Carey ME: Intrathecal morphine pump as a treatment option in chronic pain of nonmalignant origin. *Surg Neurol* 49:92-99, 1998.

19. Anderson VC, Burchiel KJ: A prospective study of long-term intrathecal morphine in the management of chronic nonmalignant pain. *Neurosurgery* 44:289-300, 1999.

20. Paice JA, Penn RD, Shott S: Intraspinal morphine for chronic pain: a retrospective, multicenter study. *J Pain Symptom Manage* 11:71-80, 1996.

21. Coffey RJ, Owens ML, Broste SK, et al: Mortality associated with implantation and management of intrathecal opioid drug infusion systems to treat noncancer pain. *Anesthesiology* 111:881-891, 2009.

22. Staats PS: Complications of intrathecal therapy. *Pain Med* 9:102-107, 2008.

23. Dominguez E, Sahinler B, Bassam D, et al: Predictive value of intrathecal narcotic trials for long-term therapy with implantable drug administration systems in chronic non-cancer pain. *Pain Pract* 2:315-325, 2002.

24. Doyles DM, Dinoff BL: Psychological aspects of interventional therapy. *Anesthesiol Clin North Am* 21:767-783, 2003.

25. Follett KA, Doyles DM: *Selection of candidates for intrathecal drug administration system to treat chronic pain: considerations in pre-implant trials*, Minneapolis, MN, 2002, Medtronic.

26. Doyles DM, Brown J: MMPI Profile as an outcome "predictor" in the treatment of non-cancer pain patients utilizing intrathecal opioid therapy. *Neuromodulation* 4:93-97, 2001.

27. Hassenbusch SJ, Paice JA, Patt RB, et al: Clinical realities and economic considerations: economics of intrathecal therapy. *J Pain Symptom Manage* 14(suppl):S36-S48, 1997.

28. Hassenbusch SJ: Cost modeling for alternative routes of administration of opioids for cancer pain. *Oncology* 13:63-67, 1999.

29. Krames ES: Practical issues when using neuraxial infusion. *Oncology* 13:37-44, 1999.

30. Bedder MD, Burchiel K, Larson SA: Cost analysis of two implantable narcotic delivery systems. *J Pain Symptom Manage* 6:368-373, 1991.

31. de Lissovoy G, Brown RE, Halpern M, et al: Cost-effectiveness of long-term intrathecal morphine therapy for pain associated with failed back surgery syndrome. *Clin Ther* 19:96-112, 1997.

32. Kumar K, Hunter G, Demeria DD: Treatment of chronic pain by using intrathecal drug therapy compared with conventional pain therapies: a cost-effectiveness analysis. *J Neurosurg* 97:803-810, 2002.

6 Patient Preparation

Tarun Jolly and Eric Royster

CHAPTER OVERVIEW

Chapter Synopsis: This chapter includes the many aspects of intrathecal drug delivery systems (IDDS) that should be considered by both the clinician and patient before undertaking a therapeutic course. Patient education and responsibility appear to be crucial to IDDS success. The benefits of intrathecal drug therapy can be grouped into three categories. "Medication benefits" include reduced side effects, increased pain relief, and a lower systemic exposure to medication. The greatest of the so-called "patient benefits" lies in delivery. Many patients would gladly give up the task of taking several timed doses of oral medication every day. Finally, "device benefits" make accessible drugs not orally available, such as the calcium channel conotoxin ziconotide. As an invasive surgical procedure, IDDS should be undertaken only with a thorough understanding by the patient of the risks and benefits that might occur. These risks include overdose, side effects, device malfunctions, infection, paralysis, and even death. Even preparation for IDDS treatment may be grueling; opioid withdrawal may occur from presurgery tapering off. Device implantation site and maintenance (including regular refill of the pump) rank as important factors in successful treatment as well. Optimal programming of drug delivery also typically requires several weeks after implantation. With proper expectations of outcome and preparation, treatment with IDDS can be effective for chronic pain.

Important Points:
- Benefits of intrathecal drug delivery can be categorized as medication benefits, patient benefits, and device benefits, and range from decreased systemic side effects to the use of novel agents.
- Complications from IDDS can vary from surgical risks to potential harm from the medications themselves.
- Pretrial patient preparation includes evaluating a variety of trialing methodology with careful consideration of both insurance requirements as well as full patient assessment as to efficacy. Pretrial preparation should also include assessment of a patient's opioid requirements and adjustments necessary.
- Posttrial and pre-implant evaluation involves setting a patient's expectations, determining the size of the pump as well as the location, and having a discussion about the informed consent.
- The post-implant period primarily involves discussing the nature of refills as well as titrations with the patient. Emergency contact information should be given to the patient at this time.

Clinical Pearls:
- It is the physician's responsibility to ensure that the patient has reasonable expectations regarding the goals and outcomes of therapy.
- Benefits of IDDS may include decreased side effects, increased pain relief, and improved function through decreased systemic exposure to a medication.
- For assessment of pain relief, a single epidural or intrathecal bolus is often sufficient to obtain adequate data. For assessment of functional status, an indwelling temporary catheter is probably more effective.
- If it is the physician's intent to wean the patient from chronic narcotics before the trial, sufficient time should be provided to allow this to occur smoothly. Reduction in systemic opioids has been associated with reduction in pain complaints, possibly by relief of opioid-induced hyperalgesia.

Clinical Pitfalls:
- Secondary gain, history of psychosis, and issues of drug abuse or dependence are of particular concern.
- Before proceeding with IDDS, a patient must be aware of all risks associated with surgery, side effects of chronic drug administration, mechanical problems, and possible operator error.
- With proper patient selection and reasonable patient expectations, trials proceed to implant at least 80% of the time. A number much larger or smaller than this may require reexamination of trialing protocols.
- Patients should be aware that there is typically a titration phase after full implantation of the pump and catheter system. Patients should understand that when they leave the hospital after the operation, their pain may not be under maximum control and they may require oral narcotics for postoperative pain.

Introduction

After it has been determined that a patient is an acceptable candidate for intrathecal drug therapy, the process of adequately educating and preparing the patient for trial and implantation becomes extremely important. A frank and open relationship between the physician and the patient is crucial. Education, in terms of risks and benefits of intrathecal drug delivery systems (IDDS), should be undertaken in detail. It is the physician's responsibility to ensure that the patient has reasonable expectations regarding the goals and outcomes of therapy. Next, the patient should be appropriately screened from a psychological and behavioral perspective. Secondary gain, history of psychosis, and issues of drug abuse or dependence are of particular concern. Many patients who are candidates for this type of therapy have been suffering and perhaps undertreated for many years. This brings with it a spectrum of possible psychological issues. Psychological assessment of the patient for IDDS is discussed in Chapter

7. Before considering this invasive form of treatment, both the physician and patient must be fully aware of the benefits and potential complications of the procedures, pretrial and posttrial considerations, surgical preparation, and what to expect in the postoperative course. Frequently asked patient questions have been included at the end of each subsection.

Benefits

Benefits of intrathecal drug therapy for the appropriate patient are numerous and fall into the general categories of medication benefits, patient benefits, and device benefits (**Table 6-1**). The delivery of medications directly to the intrathecal space offers many distinct benefits. They may include decreased side effects, increased pain relief, and improved function through decreased systemic exposure to a medication. These advantages become apparent through a significant reduction in the daily dosage of medication compared with the oral route. From a patient's perspective, IDDS also presents unique benefits. Most patients in consideration for this type of therapy require daily use of medications. The psychological and financial burden that comes with remembering to take several pills at timed intervals throughout the day can be heavy. As a result, many patients are very enthusiastic about the opportunity to do away with this in consideration of a therapy that may only require refill and thought a few times a year. The final benefit of IDDS is intrinsic to the pump itself. Many medications such as local anesthetics and ziconotide are not available as oral preparations. Additionally, the multiple programming options allow for optimal drug delivery to the patient specific to his or her pattern of pain. Although many questions still need to be answered, the available literature seems to support the usage of intrathecal drug delivery for chronic moderate to severe pain uncontrolled by less invasive means.[1] **Box 6-1** answers some questions that patients frequently ask about benefits.

Complications

Drawbacks of intrathecal drug therapy include several broad categories. Before proceeding with IDDS, a patient must be aware of all risks associated with surgery, side effects of chronic drug administration, mechanical problems, and possible operator error (**Table 6-2**).

Patient consideration of surgical risks is a must before proceeding with this procedure. Although the surgical risks are expansive, examples include infection, hemorrhage, possible life-threatening meningitis, or even spinal cord injury (**Tables 6-3** and **6-4**). Permanent implantation of an indwelling catheter and pump also carries inherent risks (**Table 6-5**).

Further drawbacks of IDDS include the side effects and limitations of the medications. All medications currently in clinical use carry the risk of significant side effects, but some of the common side effects associated with opioid use include lethargy, fatigue, and sweating (**Table 6-6**).[2] Currently, only morphine, baclofen, and ziconotide are approved by the Food and Drug Administration for use.

Although pump device malfunctions are uncommon, they can occur. The *Medtronic Neuromodulation 2009 Product Performance Report Executive Summary*, which looked at more than 1800 devices, showed a 0.8% malfunction rate over 4 years.[3] Catheter problems occur with greater frequency and will occur even with the most experienced operator. Catheter problems could include occlusion, migration, and rupture. In a multicenter study, catheter

Table 6-1: Potential Benefits of Intrathecal Infusion Therapy

Category	Example
Medication	Reduced side effects, increased pain relief, decreased systemic exposure to medication
Patient	Independence from oral medication
Device	Ability to deliver medications not available orally, multiple programming options

Box 6-1: Frequently Asked Patient Questions About Benefits

- **What are the programming options for delivery of medication with the pump?** Several programming options exist. Your physician will work with you to determine the best options for you. Options include continuous infusion, flexible infusion doses, and patient-controlled doses.
- **What sort of conditions have been treated successfully with this system?** Many painful conditions, including various types of cancer pain, spine pain, spasticity, and nerve pain, have been successfully treated.
- **Will I be able to stop my other medications for pain?** Many patients are able to stop their long-acting medications and typically reduce much of their short-acting medications after permanent implantation.

Table 6-2: Categories of General Complication Considerations

Category	Example
Surgical	Infection
Drug related	Side effects, overdose, inadequate dosing
Mechanical	Catheter migration
Operator error	Improper programming

Table 6-3: Surgical Complications and Approximate Frequency

Complication	Frequency
Wound infection	12%
Meningitis	2%
Pump or catheter malpositioning	17%
CSF leak or postdural puncture headache	Unknown

CSF, cerebrospinal fluid.
From Follett KA, Boortz-Marx RL, Drake JM, et al: Prevention and management of intrathecal drug delivery and spinal cord stimulation system infections, *Anesthesiology* 100(6):1582-1594, 2004.

Table 6-4: Sample Data of Postoperative Wound Infections as Evaluated by Follett et al[4]

Patients implanted (*n*)	700
Overall infection rate (%)	2.5-9; 5 overall
Pump pocket infections (%)	57-80
Lumbar site infections (%)	13-33
Meningitis (%)	10-14.3
Devices explanted (%)	57-80

From Follett KA, Boortz-Marx RL, Drake JM, et al: Prevention and management of intrathecal drug delivery and spinal cord stimulation system infections, *Anesthesiology* 100(6):1582-1594, 2004.

Table 6-5: Potential Complications of Implanted Catheter and Pump Systems

Infection	Peripheral edema
Catheter migration	Endocrine disturbances
Neuraxial hemorrhage	Other hemorrhage
Persistent CSF leak	Seroma formation
Postdural puncture headache	Pump migration
Opioid overdose	Drug bolus in catheter access port
Persistent medication side effects	Pedal edema with opioids
Catheter kink, disruption, separation	CSF-oma formation
Catheter tip granuloma	Spinal cord injury
Drug infusion errors, programming	Drug infusion errors, compounding

CSF, cerebrospinal fluid.

Table 6-6: Possible Side Effects of Intrathecal Morphine

Lethargy	Sweating	Constipation
Urinary retention	Fatigue	Nausea or vomiting
Pruritus	Dysphoria	Malaise
Cold sweats	Anxiety	Diarrhea
Headaches	Dry mouth	Sleep disturbances
Nightmares	Loss of appetite	Decreased libido
Dizziness	Respiratory depression	Pedal edema
Hyperalgesia	Catheter-tip granuloma	Myoclonus

complications among providers with similar experience ranged from 5% to 56% at 2 years.[4] The most frequent complications were catheter migration from the intrathecal space (5.1%), catheter occlusion or kinking (4%), and catheter sheering or puncture (3%). Across an aggregate of three clinical trials, there was a cumulative 2-year complication rate of 20%, with 80% of catheters remaining intact and functioning properly.[4] Patients should be made aware that although every effort will be made to avoid catheter problems, they may occur at any point during the therapy. Typically, these require a fairly simple operation to revise the catheter and restore therapy.

The final category for patient consideration of complications includes operator error. Care must be taken by the programmer of the intrathecal device to ensure that all data are input as intended for delivery. Common errors include incorrect data entry at the time of implant (e.g., catheter length removed), incorrect units (e.g., milligrams instead of micrograms), or rate errors (e.g., micrograms per day instead of micrograms per hour). These mistakes can be innocuous to life threatening depending on the patient and medication. This further substantiates the case for close postoperative observation of patients after implantation. Depending on the error, a patient will likely present with overdose of the medication or increased pain because of inadequate drug delivery. **Box 6-2** answers some frequently asked questions about complications.

Box 6-2: Frequently Asked Questions About Complications:

- **What are the risks of the trial?** Risks of the trial may depend partly on the method used but include procedure-related risks such as bleeding and infection and medication risks such as overdose, nausea, itching, and sedation. Although less common, more serious complications may occur such as spinal cord injury, paralysis, or even death.
- **How will I know if there is a problem with my drug delivery system?** The first sign of a problem with your system is most likely to be an increase in your typical pain.
- **What does it mean when my pump alarms?** Your pump is equipped with several alarms to indicate possible malfunction, a low battery, or a low medication volume. If your pump alarms, contact your physician immediately for evaluation.
- **What are signs of overdose of medications?** Typically, you may notice increased sedation, aching, nausea, or urinary retention.

Pretrial Preparation

Many methods of trialing for efficacy in intrathecal drug delivery exist (see Chapter 9). Each method has its own inherent risks and benefits, and none has been shown to be necessarily better than the other. For assessment of pain relief, a single epidural or intrathecal bolus is often sufficient to obtain adequate data. For assessment of functional status, an indwelling temporary catheter is probably more effective. Also, certain insurance requirements may dictate whether a trial is performed through a temporary indwelling catheter or via a single bolus technique. Many patients may be candidates for outpatient trials of either an opioid or ziconotide, depending on their domestic situation and the distance they live from the trialing center and other medical institutions. In general, if a patient or the physician has concerns about the patient's candidacy for an outpatient trial, an inpatient trial or a single-shot trial with several hours of monitoring should be performed. Older patients, patients with moderate to severe systemic disease, and patients with little systemic opioid tolerance are a particular risk for sedation and should probably be monitored as inpatients.

The patient should be fully aware of the method the physician intends to use, the risks and benefits, and the indices by which a successful trial will be evaluated. The length of the trial and hospitalization are just as important for the patient's planning. Furthermore, the practitioner should take time to explain what will occur at the conclusion of the trial (e.g., whether the patient will be placed back on his or her home medications, how long the patient will wait before full implantation, and other practical concerns).

In general, all of the possible risks already discussed regarding ongoing IDDS apply to the trial as well. Any intrathecal trial, either single shot or continuous, carries the risk of infection, spinal cord injury, neuraxial hemorrhage, and potentially life-threatening meningitis. Bleeding into the epidural space or the intrathecal space may also occur and potentially could require surgical intervention. Postdural puncture headaches are also possible, and the patient should be prepared for this before the intrathecal trial approach is planned. The patient should understand that this is a normal physiologic response, and is quite treatable if the headache persists. The most common adverse reactions will be related to pharmacologic effect of an opioid. However, the patient should be prepared for other possible side effects of ziconotide if it is used for IDDS. Respiratory depression is not found with ziconotide, but a patient may be exposed to hallucinations, changes in mood or consciousness, and cognitive impairment. For an outpatient trial with ziconotide, the patient must be able to report to the clinic daily or semi-daily for titration. This requires a significant amount of psychosocial support.

Another pretrial consideration is the possibility of changes to a patient's chronic opioid regimen before a trial. If this is to be undertaken, the patient should be counseled and fully understand the rationale behind this. If it is the physician's intent to wean the patient from chronic narcotics before the trial, sufficient time should be provided to allow this to occur smoothly. This requires a very close relationship and trust between the physician and the patient because the idea of weaning from the patient's long-term narcotics may provoke anxiety. Furthermore, steps must be taken to avoid unnecessary suffering and withdrawal symptoms. If systemic opioids are to be discontinued, they should be stopped well before the trial. Reduction in systemic opioids has been associated with reduction in pain complaints, possibly by relief of opioid-induced hyperalgesia.[5]

The patient may also experience a subjective increase in chronic pain after a trial as pain returns to baseline. The patient may perceive this as a worsening of the condition or complication, and this may be accompanied by considerable anxiety. The patient should be prepared for this as well and provided support and encouragement if this is the case.

In the case of intrathecal or epidural trialing with opioids, the patient should be aware that over- or underdose can initially occur. The patient should be aware that there is no absolute way to predict the amount of medication he or she will require for the trial but that he or she will be monitored closely and given adequate support during the trial. Side effects of opioids may also occur with intrathecal delivery at any dose, including but not limited to nausea, pruritus, and obtundation. It is important for the physician to adequately educate the patient on this because the patient may be otherwise overly concerned with the appearance of any side effects during the trial period. Typically these side effects will attenuate with time, and it is extremely rare for patients to have ongoing side effects with intrathecal infusion.

A final consideration may be patients' inquiries with regards to medications to be used for the trial. Depending on the nature of the patient's chronic pain, several agents are available and are further discussed in Chapters 2 and 3. A common issue that patients require counseling for, though, is that of medication "allergies." Often, patients' report allergies to opioid medications that are actually systemic side effects. They should be instructed that side effects caused by systemic opioids are not a contraindication to intrathecal opioids. However, in the case of severe reactions or true allergy, precipitating medications should obviously be avoided. It is best to share with the patient your initial impression but leave the discussion open to changes in potential intraspinal drugs. This will allow the patient to participate in crafting the most appropriate therapy for the trial and contribute to his or her confidence in success. Box 6-3 answers some questions that patients frequently ask about pretrial preparation.

Posttrial Evaluation

After the trial, the patient may have many new questions regarding full implantation (**Box 6-4**). It is best to reiterate the discussions and education that have already taken place and provide the patient with any further information that they may need to make a final decision about moving to full implantation. Educational materials and discussions with the device representative may also be helpful to the patient at this stage. The patient may begin to ask very practical questions such as general support from the technical

---

Box 6-3: Frequently Asked Patient Questions About Pretrial Preparation

- **What is the chance of success of the trial?** With proper patient selection and reasonable patient expectations, trials proceed to implant at least 80% of the time.
- **How long will I have to miss work?** For a single-shot trial, you will probably be able to return to work the following day. In the case of inpatient catheter trial, you will most likely miss 2 to 3 days of work. After permanent implantation, you may expect to return to work after approximately 1 week.
- **Do I have to stay in the hospital for my trial?** Catheter trials typically require a hospital stay of 1 to 2 days, but single-shot bolus trials typically do not require an overnight stay in the hospital.

Box 6-4: Frequently Asked Patient Questions About Posttrial Evaluation

- **Will the trial provide me with long-term pain relief?** Pain relief from the trial will be short lived after either a bolus or a continuous infusion. You may expect your pain to return to previous levels after the trial and plan to resume your home medications.
- **Will I still take my home medications after the trial?** You will most likely require your home medications after the trial. However, in the case of permanent implantation, your physician may make certain changes before your surgery.

---

side, traveling issues, and any other restrictions that may be required with the pump system.

Pre-Implant Preparation

In preparing the patient for permanent implant, several considerations must be addressed. First, the patient's expectations for pain relief should be discussed. In general, the patient should go willingly into full implantation after a trial, expecting that his or her pain relief will be equal to or sometimes less than the pain relief received during the trial period; this will allow the patient's expectations to be reasonable. Both the patient and practitioner should be mindful that although a trial may verify a patient's response to a specific intrathecal medication, no trialing method can truly predict the course of long-term therapy.

Second, preoperative management of the patient's pain medications should be evaluated. The practitioner should consider tapering off the patient from long-acting opioids before full implantation because the pump will provide a continuous infusion, replacing long-acting medications. Typically, a tapering of long-acting medications can be started immediately after a successful trial, assuming 2 to 4 weeks before permanent implantation. Breakthrough medications are generally left unchanged, but in either case, no escalation of the patient's opioids should occur at this time. If the patient continues to require significant medications for breakthrough pain, the practitioner may consider use of a patient-controlled device. For the appropriate candidate, this can provide an additional amount of control for the patient and may help to wean the patient off oral narcotics entirely.

Next, consideration of the size of the pump to be implanted as well as location is important. Several factors may influence this decision. In general, placing the largest pump that the patient's body habitus will accommodate is in the patient's best interest. The

SynchroMed II 40-mL pump is essentially the same circumference as the 20-mL pump but is somewhat deeper. For most patients, the 40-mL pump will provide the most flexibility and a refill frequency that is most advantageous. However, for patients who are particularly small, who have abdominal anatomic issues, who are particularly worried about cosmetics, or who have very small requirements of medication based on a trial, the 20-mL SynchroMed 2 pump may be sufficient. The most common locations for permanent implant are the right and left lower quadrants of the abdomen. The abdomen is regarded as the optimal site of patient pump implantation by most practitioners. Implantation can be done, nonetheless, in a patient's buttocks or even the back if anatomy excludes the abdomen as a site or a patient's body habitus can accommodate implantation elsewhere. Inspection of these sites must be performed preoperatively, and any possible issues must be addressed at that time. Previous surgeries, feeding tubes, and scar tissue may also influence the site of implantation.

Also, this is the time to begin discussing the initial programming scheme and medications that will be used in the patient's therapy. Although different programming modalities can be used interchangeably at any time during the course of the patient's maintenance, it is best to prepare the patient for the baseline program the practitioner plans to set. An example may include a discussion of whether the patient will expect a continuous infusion throughout the day or intermittent boluses during set times of increased pain. Chapter 11 provides more details regarding programming options.

Finally, the patient should receive a full informed consent regarding the risks and benefits of surgery. Commonly, this operation is performed under general anesthesia, and all of the inherent risks of general anesthesia apply. For patients with moderate to severe systemic disease, clearance from an internist or anesthesiologist may be advisable.

The pump may be placed under local anesthesia and intravenous sedation, which may be preferable for patients with severe systemic disease. Patients need to stop anticoagulants preoperatively to avoid the risk of bleeding, and this may require consultation with an internist or the prescribing physician. For patients with cancer or spasticity, nutrition may be an important consideration. Patients with poor nutrition may be at increased risk for poor wound healing and infection. In these types of patients, a tunneled percutaneous catheter may be a better approach. Follett et al,[6] in a multicenter study of 700 implanted patients, found an overall infection rate of 5%, with the pump pocket site being the most commonly involved, and the vast majority of cases requiring complete removal of the system.

Frequently Asked Patient Questions About Pre-Implant Preparation

1. **If the trial is successful, how long will it take to get to full implantation?** In some cases, your surgeon may place your permanent device immediately after the trial. In other cases, your surgeon may choose to wait 1 to 2 weeks to further evaluate the success of the trial.
2. **Is it a major surgery?** Implantation of the permanent pump and catheter does routinely require general anesthesia; however, the recovery time is usually short, and the patient can return to work in 1 week.
3. **Where can the pump be placed in my body?** Possible sites for implantation of the pump include the abdomen, the buttocks, or the back. The abdomen is the most common site for implantation.

Post-Implant Considerations

Patients should be aware that there is typically a titration phase after full implantation of the pump and catheter systems. Patients should understand that they may not leave the hospital after the operation with their pain under maximum control and may require oral narcotics for postoperative pain. After the initial surgery, several visits may be required over several weeks to months to obtain maximum benefit from the system.

It is important that the patient understands what maintenance of the intrathecal infusion will require. Most notably, this will require a refill of the pump and a brief clinic visit, requiring no less than two visits per year. It must be impressed upon patients that if they allow the pump to run dry or ignore device warnings, they may run significant risks to their health because withdrawal with opioids, especially baclofen, can be quite severe and possibly life threatening. Furthermore, patients must have access to emergency contact numbers and back-up plans in the case of natural disasters (e.g., hurricane evacuations). Typically, the company providing the infusion system will have support numbers that patients can call to contact a physician who can maintain their pump in the case of an emergency.

Frequently Asked Patient Questions About Post-Implant Complications

1. **How often will I require refill of my pump medication?** Typically, your doctor will plan your therapy so that you are required to have a refill no more than three or four times a year, with twice a year being the minimum.
2. **Where may I go to get the pump refilled if my doctor is unavailable?** Most major cities have providers qualified to refill and maintain your pump. You should have your manufacturer's contact information in the case of an emergency so they may assist you with finding a provider.
3. **What does the pump refill process entail?** The refill process is a quick and simple procedure that takes place in the physician's clinic. No anesthesia is required, and the procedure takes less than 5 minutes. The physician or an assistant will access the pump in a sterile manner with a needle, remove the old medication, and replace it with your new medication.
4. **What are some of the postoperative concerns and considerations?** Immediately after your surgery, the major concerns are infection and pain from the surgery itself. Also, your surgeon may have you wear an abdominal binder to prevent fluid accumulation in the back or pocket site.
5. **Will I leave the hospital after surgery with my chronic pain under control?** Typically, after implantation, there is a process of titration of your medication that may take several weeks.
6. **How often will I have to be reprogrammed?** Initially, during the first 4 to 8 weeks of therapy, you may require frequent reprogramming of your device to obtain maximal pain control. However, after that, your need for reprogramming may be minimal and occur only during pump refills.

General Frequently Asked Patient Questions

1. **How long will the pump last?** The average pump life is 6 to 7 years. It can then be replaced with a simple outpatient procedure.
2. **Can I still have a magnetic resonance imaging (MRI) scan if I need one?** Yes, the Medtronic SynchroMed 2 pump is

approved for MRI. It is approved for use in up to a 3-Tesla MRI. However, you will need to have your practitioner verify that the pump is functioning correctly after your scan.

3. **Can I SCUBA dive?** Yes, up to 33 feet or 10 meters. Pressures higher than that may affect your pump's function.

4. **How will this affect my traveling through airports?** Your pump may set off metal detectors at airports or other places. You will need to keep your patient identification card to show to any security personnel.

5. **Will this affect my sex life?** Talk to your physician about any change in your libido because this may occur with long-term infusions of opioids. Usually, this is easily treatable with hormone replacement.

6. **Can I take a hot shower or sit in a hot tub?** Yes, but you'll need to make sure that the pump is not exposed to temperatures of greater than 102° F.

7. **Will a microwave oven, cell phone, or radio interfere with my pump?** No.

8. **Will this affect any of my activities?** In general, patients are able to carry out any activity they choose; however, activities that involve significant bending or twisting of the spine may predispose you to catheter migration issues.

References

1. Smith HS, Deer TR, Staats PS, et al: Intrathecal drug delivery. *Pain Physician* 11(suppl):S89-S104, 2008.
2. Kumar K, Kelly M, Pirlot T: Continuous intrathecal morphine treatment for chronic pain of nonmalignant etiology: long-term benefits and efficacy. *Surg Neurol* 55:79-86, 2001.
3. Medtronic: 2009 Product Performance Report. Online at http://professional.medtronic.com/product-performance/intrathecal-drug-delivery-systems/.
4. Follet KA, Burchiel K, Deer T, et al: Prevention of intrathecal drug delivery catheter-related complications. *Neuromodulation* 6(1):32-41, 2003.
5. Doleys DM, Dolce JJ, Doleys AL, et al: Evaluation, narcotics and behavioral treatment influences on pain ratings in chronic pain patients. *Arch Phys Med Rehabil* 456-457, 1986.
6. Follett KA, Boortz-Marx RL, Drake JM, et al: Prevention and management of intrathecal drug delivery and spinal cord stimulation system infections. *Anesthesiology* 100(6):1582-1594, 2004.

CHAPTER

7 Psychological Considerations in Intrathecal Drug Delivery

Daniel M. Doleys

CHAPTER OVERVIEW

Chapter Synopsis: Psychological factors play perhaps the biggest role in the successful treatment of chronic pain with intrathecal drug delivery systems (IDDS). In noncancer patients, psychological assessment is carried out in most but not all cases. Overmedicalization of pain produces a tendency to expect to be "rescued" by the IDDS treatment and can result in falsely high expectations. It is important that both the patient and clinician understand pain as a multifactorial syndrome that can be partly controlled by the patient. Likewise, an appreciation of chronic pain as a dangerous disease can improve patient outcomes. Psychological evaluation can identify not only psychological disease but also other barriers to success, such as poor understanding of pain or unrealistic expectations of outcome. Cancer patients present a different set of challenges in terms of assessing psychosocial problems that can affect their pain. Mood disturbances are present in a large proportion of cancer patients, and tools should be used to distinguish depressed mood that may come naturally with cancer diagnosis and treatment from disorders that can have a more deleterious effect on pain outcomes. In any case, this population is even more susceptible to the complex interactions of expectation and pain relief. Additionally, cancer pain is erratic and unpredictable in nature, and its course may be variably interpreted by the patient. An appreciation of the interdependent nature of psychological and physical factors on a patient's pain can increase the chances for successful treatment.

Important Points: Pain, whether in the cancer or noncancer setting, is a complex and dynamic phenomenon. A psychological and behavioral assessment, including standardized tests and questionnaires along with a clinical interview, can be beneficial in patient selection and long-term management. Such an assessment may be optional for patients with cancer-related pain and a very limited life expectancy wherein immediate comfort is the primary goal. Inclusion of a significant other, delineating the positive and negative aspects of the patient's psychosocial status, and outlining the potential benefits of adjunctive psychological and behavioral therapies should be considered as part of the evaluation process. Patients with chronic pain and their circumstances change over time. A periodic post-internalization psychosocial evaluation update and modification of the therapeutic algorithm can enhance long-term outcomes.

Clinical Pearls:
- Always treat pain, especially chronic noncancer pain, as a multifactorial and multidimensional problem.
- Pain relief is not always associated with increased functioning.
- Ongoing monitoring of the patient's psychological and behavioral status is as important as monitoring IT medications.

Clinical Pitfalls:
- Approaching pain as if it were a chemical (opioid) deficiency
- Overlooking the synergistic effect(s) of combining behavioral and functional restoration therapy with IDDS
- Overreliance on the trial as the sole or best predictor of success

---

Introduction

Psychological considerations as they relate to spinal cord stimulation (SCS) therapy for chronic pain have been discussed in a companion volume, "Neurostimulation for the Treatment of Chronic Pain" (volume 1 of this series).[1] The present chapter deals with the use of intrathecal drug delivery systems (IDDS). Although IDDS in the treatment of spasticity is covered in this volume, this chapter focuses on the treatment of both chronic noncancer and cancer-related pain.

There are some different psychological issues at play for IDDS compared with SCS. First, the Centers for Medicare and Medicaid Services does not mandate a pre-implant psychological evaluation for IDDS as it does for SCS. Second, SCS produces a consistent paresthesia not found with IDDS that may affect patient acceptance and satisfaction. Third, many of the issues that surround the use of oral opioids, including dependence, tolerance, altered cognitive function, and opioid-induced hyperalgesia, apply to intrathecal therapy (IT) as well. Next is the issue of the prevalence of patient expectations and sense of entitlement regarding dosage adjustments and oral breakthrough pain medicine as a means of achieving 24-hour relief. Related to this is the necessity of frequent post-implant office visits for IDDS management. Also, there is a much wider array of trialing options with IDDS, the interpretation of which remains an issue. Furthermore, one is more likely to encounter IDDS in the treatment of cancer-related pain than SCS. Finally, the physician's post-implantation management strategy is likely to have a more significant influence on the long-term outcome of IDDS.

Both IDDS and SCS have the same psychological concerns as they relate to the treatment of chronic pain. These include the practitioner's understanding of the nature of chronic pain and the dynamic interplay between physiological and psychological variables. Unfortunately, we live in a highly medicalized society that has come to depend on technology and pharmaceuticals, as witnessed by the various media commercials and advertisements. The emphasis on personal responsibility, empowerment of patients in their own care, and medical intervention as but a tool has gradually eroded away. Some, if not a great percentage of it, is tied into insurance reimbursement policies. Patients "naturally" gravitate to treatment or intervention that is financially covered by their insurance companies. At the other extreme is the apparent irresistible urge to spend billions of dollars on a "promise" of a cure despite the lack of any credible scientific evidence or scrutiny. This latter trend is perhaps the greatest testimony one can give for the utter psychological power of persuasion (i.e., advertising). Thus, we have to alert ourselves to the psychology of society, the practitioner, and patient alike.

Unfortunately, IDDS is often considered to be a therapy of "last resort." It is reserved for those who have failed all other less invasive treatments, including physical therapy, medication management, behavioral and psychological therapies, and so on, and for whom no pain-concordant, surgically correctable lesion could be found. It is falsely assumed that chronic pain itself is benign and, unlike diseases such as diabetes, poses no real threat to the individual. Furthermore, this approach ignores the negative impact of requiring repeated treatment failure in order to have access to a potentially effective treatment. Because of their "minimally invasive nature," some[2] have argued for placing neuromodulation in a more fundamental position in the therapeutic algorithm. Although this argument can be made based on the type of pain, quality of life (QoL) issues, seriousness of the physical pathology, and clinical experience, the degree to which neuromodulation, including IDDS, can be considered "minimally invasive" is relative to the comparison procedure and the experience and skill of the implanter.

Learning to appreciate pain as a disease and IT opioids as akin to insulin in the treatment of the diabetic patient may add some clarity to the therapy. No one would presume that the effect of insulin therapy on a patient with diabetes is unrelated to other factors such as diet, weight, and exercise. Insulin is often used as a means to an end. By aggressively addressing comorbid factors such as obesity, some otherwise insulin-dependent diabetics can live with no or minimal insulin replacement therapy. Furthermore, it would be foolhardy to require the patient with a blood glucose level of 500 mg/dL or a hemoglobin A1c of 9%, to fail diet, weight control, and exercise therapy before considering more aggressive insulin therapy. In like fashion, IT therapy in responsive patients, especially in the setting of disabling chronic pain wherein restoration of function is considered critical, should not be relegated to the last rung of the therapeutic ladder. It makes little sense to perform irreversible procedures such as surgery before procedures that are reversible. Indeed, in the past 2 years, we have had three of our IDDS patients faded off the IDDS with little or no reliance on other oral medications as a result of psychological or behavioral and physical rehabilitation efforts and continue to report adequate pain control and, perhaps more importantly, a very satisfactory QoL.

Although many of us involved in the day-to-day care of chronic pain patients manifesting pathology-concordant pain, disability or dysfunction, and reduced QoL recognize the past and potential benefit of IDDS, external reviews, such as that by the Emergency Care Research Institute prepared for the Washington State Heath Care Authority (available at http://www.hta.hca.wa.gov), do not embrace the therapy very strongly. This, of course, is in large part because of the relatively poor methodological quality of the published research, at least from their standpoint and that of their reviewers. Indeed, Dr. John Loeser noted that the issue is more about the absence of meaningful outcome assessment rather then the presence of data that are not supportive.

Evaluation of Noncancer Pain Patients

When performing a psychological evaluation, it is important to consider several basic assumptions of pain management. Persistent pain, regardless of its associated physical pathology (e.g., malignant tumor, degenerative disc disease, osteoarthritis), is multidimensional and therefore influenced by psychosocial factors. These psychosocial factors can influence the outcomes of pain relief–oriented therapies; in addition, co-utilization of behavioral or psychological therapies along with somatic therapies can enhance pain relief. Finally, the prominence and priority of psychosocial factors can vary according to the type and degree of pain and pain-related pathology. Much of the material discussed herein comes from two recent consensus papers headed by Drs. Timothy Deer and Howard Smith on IT therapy for cancer and noncancer chronic pain.[3]

Insurance companies vary as to their policies regarding performing a psychological evaluation before the IDDS trial or implantation. However, it has become a common practice—and arguably a "standard of care"—to obtain a psychological evaluation or consultation. The recommendation for such appears in guidelines on the subject. A meaningful psychological evaluation should do more that simply report the outcome of one or more tests. With an estimated 75% of chronic pain patients identified as having psychological factors relevant to their pain experience,[4] a focused pretrial psychological evaluation seems warranted and potentially beneficial.

There is a continued emphasis on outcome prediction as the goal of the evaluation. The predictive validity of any one or more tests has yet to be demonstrated. Philosophically, the emphasis on "predictability" distorts our contemporary understanding of pain and pain mechanisms as possessing the property of extreme plasticity. Likewise, although some psychological states and patient characteristics may impose constraints on the degree of change possible, there would be little reason to perform psychological pain-related therapies if change were not possible. Prediction models tend to emphasize a more linear and deterministic approach, especially for patients falling below some artificial or statistically derived "cut-off score."

Presuming the existence of "predictors" of outcome also assumes a standard set of outcomes or goals for each patient. In fact, the goals are likely to vary for cancer versus noncancer pain and for pain versus spasticity. The specific condition (e.g., severe complex regional pain syndrome [CRPS] I or II vs. failed back surgery syndrome or multilevel degenerative disc disease) may influence the therapeutic goals. The outcome goal(s) for a 38-year-old man with a mild radiculopathy after modified microdiscectomy who is otherwise in good health with 15 years of formal education possessing "transferable" skills and aspirations of returning to work may be quite different than for a 78-year-old woman with multiple-level compression fractures. The identification of a fixed set of psychosocial predictors is most likely to occur when examining a highly constrained and homogenous group of patients.[5] To date, it also appears more likely that one will identify characteristics associated with "poor outcomes" than with "good outcomes."[6,7]

Despite the potential limited prognostic value, the evaluation process can serve several other functions. First, it can be used to facilitate the development of an individualized treatment plan. Second, it provides an opportunity to properly prepare and educate the patient and significant other for the trial, possible internalization, and long-term treatment.[8] Third, psychological interventions designed to mitigate the impact of maladaptive psychological issues (e.g., poor coping, limited acceptance) can be implemented and lead to a patient with a more favorable prognosis. Using the psychological evaluation process as a means of addressing potentially modifiable problems may enhance the overall efficacy of IT therapy and prevent an overemphasis on the development of absolute exclusionary criteria.[9]

The psychological evaluation should include an assessment of the patient's ability (1) to be educated as to expectations for and benefit of IDDS; (2) to prepare for, commit to, and subjectively assess long-term therapeutic impact; and (3) to participate in and gain benefit from concomitant behavioral or cognitive therapy designed to improve functional activities and maximize QoL.[8] Psychological states such as depression and anxiety capable of enhancing the patient's experience of pain and impairing his or her ability to effectively cope but modifiable with psychological or behavioral therapies should be attended to. In their recent review of the IT literature from 1990 to 2005, Raffaeli et al[10] concluded that the psychological evaluation should explore (1) patient expectations, (2) quality and "meaning" of the patient's pain, (3) psychological disease, and (4) barriers to patient and family compliance with treatment.

Suicidal depression, psychotic conditions such as schizophrenia, and active drug abuse or addiction have routinely been considered as contraindications for IDDS.[11] In a recent review of the literature concerning pretreatment psychological variables as predictors of outcome with surgery and SCS, Celestin et al[6] reported a positive relationship between somatization, depression, anxiety, and poor coping and poor outcomes in 92% of 25 studies reviewed. Although suggestive of a possible correlation between psychological status and pain-related treatment outcomes, the authors note that clinical research has yet to reveal a specific set of variables associated with positive or negative outcomes. The relationship between psychological variables and treatment outcomes may be obscured by (1) variability in the methodological quality of the research, (2) the number of potential psychosocial variables, (3) the types and locations of pain, (4) other medical comorbidities, and (5) changes in the patient's circumstances (e.g., new injury, loss of a job, death in the family).

In general, psychological variables should be considered as relative versus absolute contraindications. Therefore, a patient should not be included or excluded solely on the basis of any single psychological test. For example, contrary to their expectations, Doleys and Brown[12] found that patients with mildly abnormal Minnesota Multiphasic Personality Inventory-2 (MMPI[13]) personality profiles reported a higher percentage of improvement in pain after 4 years of IDDS compared with those with more "normal" MMPI profiles.

There are a number of different strategies or approaches to the psychological evaluation. The evaluation should include a clinical interview as well as psychological test(s) or questionnaires. If at all possible, a significant other should be included given their tendencies to view treatment outcomes far differently, and often not as effectively, as does the patient.[14,15] Information on events that increase and decrease the pain (i.e., pain-modifying events) should be elicited. Patients need to be informed that mood- or stress-related pain is more properly addressed with psychological than IT

therapy. Functionally-oriented questions may uncover maladaptive behavioral tendencies, including activity avoidance and anticipatory pain. In such cases, desensitization and functional restoration therapies may be indicated along with IT. The degree to which the patient continues to carry out commitments and activities of daily living gives some measure of conscientiousness and willingness to engage in activity despite pain. Conscientiousness and activity engagement may represent two positive indicators.

The clinical interview, psychological test(s) or questionnaire(s), a review of records, behavioral observations, and consultation with other health care providers and significant others can provide valuable insights into the patient's perception of his or her condition, general coping strategies, expectations of therapy, overall psychological status, and "readiness for change." Clarification of a patient's goals, priorities, and expectations is fundamental. The functional pain level (FPL; the level of pain at which the patient believes he or she can be more productive) can be useful. A patient reporting a low FPL (e.g., 0 to 2 of 10) may require some "expectation management." The more vague or ambiguous the patient, the greater the need to identify appropriate and measurable functional goals and consider a functionally-oriented trial.[16,17] Patient anxieties about an object "in the spine," continuity of care if the patient or the physician relocates geographically, options and alternative therapies, and device malfunction should also be assessed.

A variety of psychological tests and questionnaires are available for use during the evaluation. Test selection should included consideration of the instrument's sensitivity and specificity. The time required to complete the evaluation and expense to the patient should not be overlooked. Interpretation and meaning of the testing data should be done in the context of information gathered through a clinical interview. Preference should be given to scale-based instruments whose validity and reliability are supported by suitable research and those that provide a mechanism for assessing dissimilation, malingering, or symptom exaggeration or magnification (see Doleys and Doherty[18] for a more detailed discussion). In addition, the evaluation of the pain patient should incorporate a number of dimensions, including pain intensity (e.g., McGill Pain Questionnaire[19]); mood, personality, and overall psychological functioning (e.g., MMPI,[13] Symptom Checklist 90-R,[20] State Trait Anxiety Inventory[21]); pain beliefs, coping, and acceptance (e.g., Multidimensional Pain Inventory,[22] Chronic Illness Problem Inventory,[23] Coping Strategies Questionnaire,[24] Chronic Pain Acceptance Questionnaire[25]); level of functioning (e.g., Oswestry Disability Questionnaire,[26] Sickness Index Profile[27]); and cognitive functioning (e.g., Mini Mental Status Exam).[28] Schocket et al[29] describe a protocol that encompasses a number of different tests and questionnaires. Points are assigned to patient characteristics such as degree of depression, personality disorder, active workers' compensation claim, and so on. Patients are grouped according to their cumulative points as (1) acceptable to proceed, (2) requires postsurgical psychological intervention, (3) requires presurgical psychological intervention, (4) noninvasive therapy recommended, or (5) recommend no treatment.

Williams and Epstein[30] reported the presence of psychiatric disorders, including personality disorders; depression; substance abuse; secondary gain, including litigation and workers' compensation; and motivation for receiving an implantable device, to be the psychological factors most frequently evaluated. The clinician must be weary of cognitive impairment even at the mild level. This is most common among patients with dementia, traumatic brain injury, or Alzheimer's disease. However, it can also be found in those with limited education, history of drug abuse, high levels of medication, and even prolonged pain.[31] The presence of cognitive dysfunction can compromise patients' ability to comprehend the goals, expectations, and rationale for IT and negatively affect their response to treatment. These patients are more prone toward a positive short- versus long-term response. Other areas to explore during the evaluation include any untreated or undertreated major affective disorder, alcohol or drug problems, and type and degree of social support.[32] It may be beneficial for the physician to create a letter requesting a psychological evaluation of areas of interest or concern (e.g., addiction, major affective disorders, expectations) as opposed to asking for "clearance." *Psychological clearance* is an extremely vague term that can be influenced by available clinical resources, the evaluator's experience and attitudes toward IT, relationship with the physician, and economic concerns.

The elimination of chronic pain is rarely achieved with any therapy. Therefore, long-term outcomes are partly related to the patient's ability and willingness to cope with his or her "residual pain." Belief systems and coping strategies can exert a positive or negative influence on outcomes. The beliefs associated with more favorable results include (1) understanding pain as a multifactorial experience that can be affected by one's attitudes and behaviors, (2) a belief in the effectiveness of exercising coping skills and acceptance, and (3) active involvement in treatment-related decisions.[33] By contrast, viewing pain only in the context of its physical characteristics or medical cause and thus minimizing the role of psychosocial factors can result in an overreliance on medical-based therapies, a sense of helplessness, and less positive outcomes. Coping strategies can be divided into control-based, such as cognitive coping, and acceptance-based methods. Several studies in both experimental and controlled clinical settings have found acceptance-based strategies to be superior to control-based methods with regard to increasing pain threshold, pain tolerance, and associated functioning.[34-36] Assessing and modifying these belief systems and coping strategies can easily be incorporated into the evaluation process.

There may be distinct advantages to conceptualizing the pre-implant trial as an "*n* of 1," or a single-subject design. Individualized trialing goals regarding functioning, medication reduction, pain relief, and so on are developed with the patient and support person. These trialing goals become the criteria for proceeding to implant. Cepeda et al[37] illustrated this approach in a case study that focused on a patient undergoing a pre-implant trial of SCS. The investigators systematically compared the effects of SCS with transcutaneous electrical nerve stimulation across a 5-day period. In this instance, the two treatments produced similar results; therefore the device was not implanted. By thoroughly evaluating patient response in varying clinical scenarios, this approach may help to prevent "false-positive" outcomes (e.g., a positive trial followed by a poor long-term outcome). Admittedly, time constraints, clinical setting, and insurance coverage will have their influence. However, an "*n* of 1" philosophy is more consistent with how most individuals wish to be approached.

There may be situations in which the severity of the clinical condition takes precedence over the usual psychological considerations. For example, patients with CRPS manifesting a very dystrophic, swollen, and hyperalgetic extremity may require a deviation from the widespread practice of advancing from conservative to invasive pain management.[2] Although a psychological evaluation is still warranted, the criteria for proceeding may need to be more flexible and weighed against the consequences of delaying or forgoing a potentially beneficial therapy. On the other end of the continuum, it is also important to remain vigilant over patients lacking any significant maladaptive or pathological psychological conditions because the future can be very unpredictable. Brief but regular post-implant office visits for the purpose of reinforcing and supporting positive changes may pay big dividends.

IDDS may have a role in treating addicted patients with significant pain-concordant pathology.[38] The removal of overt cues and physiological effects of the drug that stimulate and maintain addictive behavior has some advantages. The addicted patient, however, should have demonstrated a significant period of abstinence, active involvement in a recovery program, and a commitment to rely only on the IT medication for the pharmacological component of treatment. Even under these conditions, treatment of an addicted patient is not without its problems and should be carried out with caution and in conjunction with an addictionologist. Although rare, patients have been known to attempt to penetrate the pump or catheter to gain access to the drug. The author encountered one such patient in treating an anesthesiologist from another state with an undiagnosed addiction to fentanyl. The addiction was discovered when he was found accessing his pump, filed with fentanyl, apparently with relative ease, which had been implanted for the treatment of what appeared to be a legitimate pain problem. After the addiction was identified and properly treated, the IDDS system was removed and the patient was managed well with minimal nonopioid substances and aggressive nonpharmacological therapy. It is also important to be vigilant to a situation in which the patient is the "mule" and provides the means for others to secure drugs for use or sale. One must never underestimate the ingenuity and persistence of some drug-addicted patients.

The incidence of personality disorders, especially in the addicted population, is significant. Such patients can be demanding, manipulative, passive-aggressive, and generally noncompliant. If cross-addicted, there is no assurance that addressing the pain problem may not result in the patient's turning to alcohol, illicit drugs, benzodiazepines, and so on. A very experienced implanter in the Midwest describes a case wherein the patient, who turned out to have borderline personality disorder, became overwrought with her situation and "cut her pump out" with a knife at home. Fortunately, she survived. The implanter notes it was one of the few times he did not listen to his "gut instincts." Although hard to define, gut instincts, especially in an experienced clinician, should play a role in the decision process.

Finally, the patient's drug-taking behavior should be assessed. There continues to be a substantial debate over the use of oral opioids, particularly during the trial and after implantation. Some have patients discontinue their opioids weeks before the trial (referred to as an "uncontaminated trial") and give little if any post-implantation. At the other end of the continuum are those who do not alter the patient's opioid intake but use it as a baseline against which to assess the effectiveness of the trial and long-term treatment. Issues of physical or psychological dependence and chemical coping become relevant. Some patients may be conditioned to the perceived or real effects of their oral medications and experience increased pain, despite significant IT dosages, without them. Although yet to be proven, chronic use of opioids after implant may negatively impact the analgesic effect of IT opioids. This may explain the loss or lack of pain relief and thus decreased functioning and poor outcomes even with high IT levels. Providing feedback to the physician and patient as to the potential negative impact of certain drug-taking patterns and alternative ways of managing breakthrough pain can be an important part of the psychological evaluation.

Summary

The following is a recapitulation of the consensus recommendation put forth a panel of experienced clinicians headed by Drs.

Timothy Deer and Howard Smith. A pretrial or pre-implantation psychological evaluation for patients with chronic noncancer pain being considered for IT should be carried out. The evaluation should highlight characteristics that may positively or negatively impact a trial or long-term therapy. The potential influence of identified psychological factors should be outlined to the patient and significant other. In addition to identifying relevant psychological conditions and behavioral patterns, the consistency among the patient's complaints, the psychological exam, and the clinical findings should be given careful consideration. Patients should be considered with great caution if they are manifesting one or more of the following conditions: (1) untreated significant addiction, (2) active psychosis with delusional or hallucinatory components, (3) major uncontrolled depression or anxiety, (4) active suicidal or homicidal behavior, (5) serious cognitive deficits, or (6) severe sleep disturbances. Patients exhibiting the following attributes can be viewed as more appropriate candidates from a psychological perspective: (1) generally stable psychologically; (2) cautious, effectively defensive, and generally optimistic regarding outcome; (3) moderate levels of self-confidence and self-efficacy; (4) realistic concerns regarding "illness" and proposed therapy; (5) mild depression appropriate to the situation; (6) ability to cope with flare-ups, complications, and side effects appropriately; (7) appropriately educated regarding procedure and device; (8) supportive and educated family or support person; (9) history of compliance and cooperativeness with previous treatment; (10) behavioral or psychological evaluation consistent with patient's complaints and reported psychosocial status; (11) comprehends instruction(s) and other information; (12) patient or significant other has appropriate expectation(s); (13) conscientiousness and activity engagement despite pain; and (14) patient able or willing to "tolerate" medication adjustments with the drug delivery system.

The psychological evaluation should also assess the need for any pretrial, pre-implantation, or post-implantation targeted psychological or behavioral interventions determined to be potentially beneficial in obtaining or sustaining a positive outcome. A multidisciplinary approach to patient selection should be undertaken wherever possible to account for the multifactorial nature of pain and to avoid isolation of the psychological components. The psychological consultant should have some level of participation in the pre-implant trial or follow-up to evaluate the utility of the assessment and help determine whether the therapeutic goals have been achieved.

Evaluation of Patients with Cancer-Related Pain

A pre-implantation psychological evaluation is reportedly carried out in approximately 11% of cases with cancer-related pain compared with 89% for noncancer pain.[39] Cancer poses a different situation than noncancer pathology. The origin of the cancer is often unknown; tumor progression and spreading are uncertain and erratic. The disease can be arrested, but this is not always predictable. Although about 62% of adults with cancer are disease free 5 years after diagnosis,[40] recurrence rates vary and can be heralded by a reemergence of pain. By virtue of it ambiguity, patients with cancer often continually monitor and can become preoccupied with physical sensations, especially pain, and are given to mis- or overinterpretation. This somatic vigilance and search for the meaning of physical sensations can be a great source of stress and anxiety.[41,42]

Patients with cancer-related pain are faced with treatment options and decisions different from those with noncancer pain. It is not difficult to imagine the emotional impact considering the potential loss of bodily functions, disfigurement, loss of autonomy and independence, abandonment and isolation, becoming a burden, and financial matters. Few concerns generate more distress than the fear of uncontrolled pain and other related end-of-life issues. Caregiver reactions, as well, may inflame or moderate those of the patient.

Approximately 50% of all types of cancer are associated with pain. It is estimated that 30% of women with metastatic breast disease report phantom breast pain after mastectomy.[43] Cancer-related pain has many unique features, including the need for patients to understand that their condition is potentially fatal. Pain is often seen as an inevitable consequence of the disease or its treatment, a sign of disease progression, and a prelude to death. Ahles et al[44] reported that 61% of patients were afraid that pain or changes in pain signified a progression of their disease. Patients tend to ascribe various meanings to their pain, often interpreting it as a challenge, punishment, or enemy. Those interpreting their disease as a punishment are likely to manifest higher levels of pain and depression.[45] Spiega and Bloom[46] noted that mood and interpretation of pain predicted patient's reported pain intensity in 86 metastatic breast cancer patients, finding that some only experienced pain *after* they were informed of their diagnosis. Anxiety, depression, expectations, cognitive appraisals, self-efficacy, and perceived control have been found to influence the reports and experience of physiological processes, fatigue, sleep, appetite nausea, and pain, and should all be assessed as part of the psychological evaluation.

In their review of the literature Zaza and Baine[47] reported that nearly 73% of patients reported an association between pain and psychological distress and that increased pain was associated with greater mood disturbance.[48] Also, the presence of a precancer psychiatric disorder was associated with increased cancer-related distress. It is estimated that between 14% and 38% of women with breast cancer develop a psychiatric disorder after the diagnosis of cancer or at the time of a recurrence.[49,50] The association of pain with anxiety and depression is especially pronounced in terminally ill patients[51] and those with pancreatic cancer.[52] A reduction in depression has been accompanied by reduced pain. Depressed mood is often a natural reaction and should be distinguished from the presence of a depressive illness. The latter may be preexisting and exacerbated by the cancer or related pain. In fact, cancer-related pain has been reported to reactivate prior emotional trauma.[53] Severe forms of depression complicate the management of pain; can influence patients' motivation and therefore compliance; and stimulate death wishes, suicidality, and the desire for euthanasia.[54] Importantly, this degree of depression is not always acknowledged by the patient. In one study, 58% of patients did not divulge certain symptoms to health care professionals, and 52% omitted complaints involving psychosocial problems.[55]

Depression in cancer patients can include social withdrawal, failure to respond to "good news" or humorous situations, persistent tearfulness, feeling like a burden to others, failure to respond to pain-relieving therapies, and a tendency to perceive cancer as a punishment.[56,57] The Hospital Anxiety and Depression Scales (HADS)[58] has been a useful and efficient instrument for detecting depression in cancer patients. Monroe[54] outlined a variety of interview questions that can aid in uncovering mood disturbances. Cancer-related pain can lead to maladaptive coping, feelings of hopelessness and helplessness, and anhedonia, resulting in withdrawal from day-to-day activities. The Brief Pain Inventory,[59] Karnofsky Index,[60] and Short-Form Health Survey[61,62] have been useful in assessing the levels of functioning and perceived pain-interference levels among cancer pain patients.

Anxiety often coexists with depression. Anxiety disorders among cancer patients include posttraumatic stress disorder (PTSD), acute-stress response, generalized anxiety disorder, obsessive-compulsive disorder, pain disorder, and phobias. When present, anxiety is known to lower the pain threshold and interfere with disclosure and problem resolution. Anxiety disorders occur in about 7% to 18% of the general population, 20% to 40% of chronic pain patients, and 13% to 16% of cancer patients, with 4% of cancer patients having a preexisting anxiety disorder. Asmundson et al[63] and Keogh[64] demonstrated that those with an anxiety sensitivity, or fear as a consequence of feeling the physical manifestations of anxiety, often misinterpret innocuous body sensation as threatening or indicative of disease progression. Anxiety tends to peak at specific points, including initial diagnosis, initiation of cancer treatment, cancer recurrence, failure of treatment, and perception of dying.[65] The presence of PTSD at all stages in cancers of mixed etiology is 3% to 19%.[52,66]

Levels of anxiety and depression will likely vary over the course of the disease and its treatment. Instruments such as the HADS,[58] STAI,[67] and Hamilton Rating Scale for Anxiety[68] have each been used to assess levels of anxiety and can be used repeatedly over time. Changes in the levels of anxiety may well affect the patient's pain level and tolerance. Having strategies in place to identify and address these changes without excessive manipulation of the IT medicine may reduce the development of tolerance or opioid-induced hyperalgesia.

The experience of pain is also influenced by the patient's appraisal of the meaning of his or her disease and pain, level of acceptance, and type of coping. Coping has been defined as the individual's effort to mange demands that are perceived as likely to exceed his or her resources.[69] Denial, rationalization, anger, avoidance, intellectualization, prayer, distraction, and catastrophizing represent common coping strategies used by patients. Adaptive coping is characterized by (1) addressing problems, (2) appropriate sense of optimism and hope, (3) revising plans, (4) willingness to use the assistance of others, and (5) open communication.[70] Acceptance is defined as "… a disengagement from struggling with pain, a realistic approach to pain and pain-related circumstances, and an engagement in positive every-day activities" (McCracken and Eccleston).[71(p198)] Acceptance does not mean giving up or giving in. Rather, it is a realistic appraisal of appropriate expectations and goals. Whereas increased pain intensity, pain interference, and anxiety have each been associated with higher levels of castastrophizing,[72-74] self-efficacy and perceived control over pain are associated with reduced pain intensity.[75,76] Inventories such as the Coping Strategies Questionnaire[75,76] and Chronic Pain Acceptance Questionnaire (CPAQ) can be of value in assessing type of coping and level of acceptance.[77]

Pain reduction is often accompanied by improvement in emotional distress. However, pain may also function as a distraction from other issues. Cahana[78] for example, reported on two patients with cancer-related pain treated by IT therapy. Both patients demonstrated a reduction of 50% or greater in pain intensity, increase in cognitive function, and increased daily activity. Unfortunately, the "side effects" of what would otherwise be considered successful treatment included an unexpected increase in depression, anxiety, conjugal conflicts, interpersonal disputes (e.g., regarding previous marital stressors, ex-spouses, children, in-laws), and the "emotional burden" of cancer and death along with decreased "well-being." Although difficult to uncover, the psychological evaluation needs to attend to the possibility of such "hidden" issues and educate the patient and family as to their possible emergence.

There are many barriers to effective treatment of cancer-related pain. Some are patient related and others caregiver related. For this reason there may be cases in which the psychological evaluation would be incomplete without incorporating the caregiver. Patient-related barriers include fear of addiction, pharmacological tolerance, treatment side effects, interpreting pain as sign of disease progression, fear of distracting the physician from treating the disease, fear of injections, fatalism, and the belief that "good" patients do not complain.[79,80] Patients harbor the fear their reported pain will be interpreted as psychological. They may also hesitate to fully disclose their residual pain for fear of disappointing their treating physicians. These and other fears are more common among the older and less educated patients and those from the lower socioeconomic strata. Caregiver-related barriers include end-of-life issues, side effects, addiction, fear of injections, and that increased pain equates to increased disease.

Summary

Whereas pre-implantation psychological evaluations with noncancer pain patients tends to focus on *trait-related* characteristics, such as personality and degree of disability, that of the cancer-related pain patient may need to address *state-related* characteristics. The rapid changing status of the disease and the impact of various treatments, such as chemotherapy and surgery, can impact the patient's emotional status and adjustment almost on a day-to-day basis. By virtue of the uncertain course of the disease (i.e., cure, disease progression, improvement followed by recurrence), and unclear longevity of IT therapy, brief psychological evaluations may need to occur periodically to reevaluate the potential benefits of adjunctive behavioral/psychological therapies.[68] Indeed, Jensen[81] has outlined a neuropsychological model of pain in which he illustrates the pairing up of certain psychological interventions based on the presence of specific maladaptive cognitive and behavioral patterns.

For the purpose of discussing the role of a psychological evaluation in cancer-related pain, the consensus panel mentioned above recommended that it may be useful to conceptualize this pain in three different categories and to proceed with evaluation or therapy based on the status of the patient's disease. Category 1 consists of those patients whose life expectancy is significantly compromised by their disease and the goal of therapy is palliation. A pretrial or internalization psychological evaluation should be considered optional. It should be done at the discretion of the physician with a focus on identifying cancer- or pain-related psychological factors potentially amenable to psychological intervention that may facilitate patient adjustment and analgesia rather than to clear the patient psychologically for IT therapy. Category 2 involves patients whose disease process has been arrested but wherein there is a significant probability of recurrence. A pretrial or internalization psychological evaluation is encouraged, with an emphasis on periodic psychological consultation or intervention to assist with changes in disease process or recurrence and coping. Finally, category 3 consists of patients whose cancer has been eradicated by surgery or other therapies but who have residual chronic pain secondary to the medical treatment or anatomical or physiological disease-related damage. Patients in this category should undergo a pretrial or internalization psychological evaluation, approached in much the same way as those with chronic noncancer pain. Whenever possible, the primary caregiver should be included to assess the type and degree of support.

References

1. Deer T, Levy R, Hayek S, editors: *Neurostimulation for the treatment of chronic pain*, Philadelphia, 2012, Saunders. Deer T, editor. Interventional and Neuromodulatory Techniques for Pain Management Series, Volume 1.

2. Prager J, Jacobs M: Evaluation of patients for implantable pain modalities: medical and behavioral assessment. *Clin J Pain* 17:206-214, 2001.

3. Deer T, Smith H, Cousins M, et al: Consensus guidelines for the selection and implantation of patients with noncancer pain for intrathecal drug delivery. *Pain Physician* 13(3):E175-E213, 2010.

4. Doleys DM, Olson K, editors: *Psychological assessment and intervention in implantable pain therapies: monograph*, Minneapolis, 1997, Medtronic Neurological, pp 1-20.

5. Howell DC: *Statistical methods in psychology*, ed 4, Belmont, CA, 1997, Wadsworth Publishing Company, p 724.

6. Celestin J, Edwards RR, Jamison RN: Pretreatment psychosocial variables as predictors of outcomes following lumbar surgery and spinal cord stimulation: a systematic review and literature synthesis. *Pain Med* 10(4):639-653, 2009.

7. Doleys DM, Klapow J, Hammer M: Psychological evaluation in spinal cord stimulation. *Pain Rev* 4:186-204, 1997.

8. Doleys DM: Preparing patients for implantable technology. In Turk DC, Gatchel RJ, editors: *Psychological approaches to pain management*, New York, 2002, The Guilford Press, pp 334-348.

9. Doleys DM, Dinoff BL: Psychological aspects of interventional therapy. *Anesthesiol Clin North Am* 21:767-783, 2003.

10. Raffaeli W, Andruccioli J, Righetti D, et al: Intraspinal therapy for the treatment of chronic pain: a review of the literature between 1990 and 2005 and suggested protocol for its rational and safe use. *Neuromodulation* 9(4):290-308, 2006.

11. Nelson DV, Kennington M, Novy DM, Squitieri P: Psychological selection criteria for implantable spinal cord stimulators. *Pain Forum* 5:93-103, 1996.

12. Doleys DM, Brown J: MMPI profiles as an outcome 'predictor' in the treatment of non-cancer pain patients utilizing intraspinal opioid therapy. *Neuromodulation* 4:93-97, 2001.

13. Keller LS, Butcher JN: *Use of the MMPI-2 with chronic pain patients*, Minneapolis, 1991, University of Minnesota Press.

14. Doleys DM, Coleton M, Tutak U: Use of intraspinal infusion therapy for non-cancer pain patients: follow-up and comparison of worker's compensation versus non-worker's compensation patients. *Neuromodulation* 1:149-159, 1998.

15. Willis KD, Doleys DM: The effects of long term intraspinal infusion therapy with non-cancer pain patients: evaluation of patient, significant-other and clinic staff appraisals. *Neuromodulation* 2:241-253, 1999.

16. Doleys DM, Kraus TJ: Trialing for intrathecal therapy: comments and considerations. *Pract Pain Manage* 7:48-49, 2007.

17. Follett KA, Doleys DM: *Selection of candidates for intrathecal drug administration to treat chronic pain: considerations in pre-implantation trials*, Minneapolis, 2004, Medtronic, pp 1-19.

18. Doleys DM, Doherty DC: Psychological and behavioral assessment. In Raj PP, editor: *Practical management of pain*, ed 3, St. Louis, 2000, Mosby, pp 408-426.

19. Melzack R: The McGill Pain Questionnaire: major properties and scoring methods. *Pain* 1:277299, 1975.

20. Derogatis LR: *Symptom-Checklist-90-R: Scoring and Procedures Manual I for the Revised Version*, Eagan, NM, 1977, Pearson Assessments.

21. Spielberger C: *The State-Trait Anxiety Inventory*, New York, 1970, Academic Press.

22. Kerns RD, Turk DC, Rudy TE: The West Haven-Yale Multidimensional Pain Inventory (WHYMPI). *Pain* 23(4):345-356, 1983

23. Kames LD, Naliboff BD, Heinrich RL, Schag CC: The Chronic Illness Problem Inventory: problem-oriented psychosocial assessment of patients with chronic illness. *Int J Psychiatry Med* 14(1):65-75, 1984.

24. Rosenstiel AK, Keefe FJ: The use of coping strategies in chronic low back pain patients: relationship to patient characteristics and current adjustment. *Pain* 17:33-44, 1983.

25. McCracken LM, Vowles KE, Eccleston C: Acceptance of chronic pain: component analysis and a revised assessment method. *Pain* 107:159-166, 2004.

26. Fairbank JC, Davies JB, Couper J, O'Brien JP: The Oswestry Low Back Pain Disability Questionnaire. *Physiotherapy* 66(8):271-273, 1980.

27. Bergner M, Bobbitt RA, Carter WB, Gibson BS: The Sickness Impact Profile: development and final revision of a health status measure. *Med Care* 19:787-805, 1981.

28. Folstein MF, Folstein SE, McHugh PR: Mini-Mental Sate: a practical method for grading the cognitive state of patients for the clinician. *J Psychiatr Res* 12:189-198, 1975.

29. Schocket KG, Gatchel RJ, Stowell AW, et al: A demonstration of a presurgical behavioral medicine evaluation for categorizing patients for implantable therapies: a preliminary study. *Neuromodulation* 11:237-248, 2008

30. Williams DA, Epstein SA: Psychological assessment prior to surgery for implantable pain-management devices. In Burchiel K, editor: *Surgical management of pain*, New York, 2002, Thieme Medical, pp 135-144.

31. Apkarian AV, Scholz J: Shared mechanisms between chronic pain and neurodegenerative disease. *Drug Discovery Today: Disease Mechanism* 3:319-326, 2006.

32. Doleys DM: Psychological considerations in spine surgery. In Follett KA, editor: *Neurosurgical pain management*, Iowa City, IA, 2004, Elsevier Saunders, pp 38-45.

33. Doleys DM: Psychologic evaluation for patients undergoing neuro-augmentative procedures. *Neurosurg Clin North Am* 14:409-417, 2003.

34. Gutierrez O, Luciano C, Rodriguez M, Fink BC: Comparison between an acceptance-based and a cognitive-control based protocol for coping with pain. *Behav Ther* 35:767-783, 2004.

35. Hayes SC, Bissett RT, Korn Z, et al: The impact of acceptance versus control rationales on pain tolerance. *Psychol Rec* 49:33-47, 1999.

36. McCracken LM, Eccleston C: Coping or acceptance: what to do about chronic pain? *Pain* 105:197-204, 2003.

37. Cepeda MS, Acevedo JC, Alvarez H, et al: An N-of-1 trial as an aide to decision making prior to implanting a permanent spinal cord stimulator. *Pain Med* 9:235-239, 2008.

38. Doleys DM, Kraus TJ: Psychological and addiction issues in intraspinal therapy. *Semin Pain Med* 2:46-51, 2004.

39. Ahmed SU, Martin NM, Chang Y: Patient selection and trial methods for intraspinal drug delivery for chronic pain: a national survey. *Neuromodulation* 8:112-120, 2005.

40. American Cancer Society: *Cancer facts and figures 2003*, accessed from http://www.camcer.org/docroot/STT/stt_O_asp?sitearea=STT&level=1.

41. Turk DC, Monarch ES, Williams AD: Cancer patients with pain: considerations for assessing the whole person. *Hematol Oncol Clin North Am* 16:511-525, 2002.

42. Turk DC, Fernandez E: On the putative uniqueness of cancer apian: do psychological principles apply? *Behav Res Therapy* 28:1-13, 1990.

43. Kronner K, Krebs B, Skov J, Jorgensen HS: Immediate and long term phantom breast syndrome after mastectomy: incidence, clinical characteristic relationship to pre-mastectomy breast pain. *Pain* 36:327-335, 1989.

44. Ahles TA, Blanchard EB, Ruckdeschel JC: The multidimensional nature of cancer-related pain. *Pain* 17:277-288, 1983.

45. Barkwell DP: Ascribed meaning: a critical factor in coping and pain attenuation in patients with cancer-related pain. *J Palliative Care* 7:5-14, 1991.

46. Spiega LD, Bloom JR: Group therapy and hypnosis reduced metastatic breast carcinoma pain. *Psychosom Med* 45:333-339, 1982.

47. Zaza C, Baine N: Cancer pain and psychological factors: a critical review of the literature. *J Pain Symptom Manage* 24:526-542, 2002.

48. Glover J, Dibble SL, Dodd MJ, Miaskowski C: Mood states of oncological outpatients: does pain make a difference? *J Pain Symptom Manage* 10:120-128, 1995.

49. Derogatis LR, Morow GR, Fetting J: The prevalence of psychiatric disorders among cancer patients. *JAMA* 249:751-757, 1983.

50. Massie MJ, Holland JC: The cancer patient with pain: psychiatric complications and their management. *J Pain Symptom Manage* 7: 99-109, 1992.
51. Kane RL, Berstein L, Wales J, Rothenber R: Hospice effectiveness in controlling pain. *JAMA* 253:2683-2686, 1985.
52. Kelsen DP, Portenoy RK, Thaler HT, et al: Pain and depression in patients with newly diagnosed pancreas cancer. *J Clin Oncol* 13: 748-755, 1995.
53. Steinman RH: The cancer patient with anxiety and chronic pain. *Pain Clin Updates* 27:1-5, 2009.
54. Monroe B: Psychological evaluation of patient and family. In Sykes N, Fallon MT, Patt RB, editors: *Clinical pain management: cancer pain*, New York, 2003, Oxford University Press, pp 73-85.
55. Rathbone GV, Horsley S, Goacher J: A self evaluated assessment suitable for seriously ill hospice patients. *Palliative Med* 8:29-34, 1994.
56. Endicott J: Measurement of depression in patients with cancer. *Cancer* 53(suppl):2243-2249, 1984.
57. Casey P: Depression in the dying: disorder or distress? *Prog Palliative Care* 2:1-3, 1994.
58. Moorey S, Greer S, Watson M, et al: The factor structure and factor stability of the Hospital Anxiety and Depression Scale with cancer. *Br J Psychiatry* 158:255-259, 1991.
59. Daunt RJ, Cleeland CS, Flannery RC: Development of the Wisconsin Brief Pain Questionnaire to assess pain in cancer and other diseases. *Pain* 197-210, 1983.
60. Karnofsky DA, Abelmann WH, Craver LF, et al: The use of the nitrogen mustards in the palliative treatment of carcinoma. *Cancer* 1: 634-656, 1948.
61. Ware JE, Kosinki M, Keller SD: *SF-36 physical and mental health summary scales: a user's manual*, Boston, 1994, The Health Institute.
62. Ware JE, Sherboune CD: The MOS 36-item short-form survey (SF-36). *Med Care* 30:473-481, 1992.
63. Asmundson GJG, Coons MJ, Taylor S, Katz J: PTSD and the experience of pain: research and clinical implications of shared vulnerability and mutual maintenance models. *Can J Psychiatry* 47:930-937, 2002.
64. Keogh E, Cochrane M: Anxiety sensitivity, coping biases and the experience of pain. *J Pain* 3:320-329, 2002.
65. Miller K, Massie MJ: Depression and anxiety. *Cancer J* 12(5): 388-397, 2006.
66. Gold J: Pain and posttraumatic stress in adults treated for cancer. *J Pain* 6(suppl):S78, 2005.
67. Van Knippenberg FC, Duivenvoorden HJ, Bonke B, Passchier J: Shortening the State-Trait Anxiety Inventory. *J Clin Epidemiol* 43:995-1000, 1990.
68. Hamilton M: The assessment of anxiety states by rating. *Br J Med Psychology* 32:50-55, 1959.
69. Lazarus RS, Folkman S: *Stress, appraisal, and coping*. New York, 1984, Springer Press.
70. Keefe FJ, Abernethy AP, Campbell LC: Psychological approaches to understanding and treating disease-related pain. *Annu Rev Psychol* 56:601-630, 2005.
71. McCracken LM, Eccleston C: Coping or acceptance: what to do about chronic pain. *Pain* 105:197-204, 2003.
72. Bishop SR, Warr D: Coping, catastrophizing and chronic pain in breast cancer. *J Behav Med* 26:265-281, 2003.
73. Lin CC: Comparison of the effects of perceived self-efficacy on coping with chronic cancer pain and coping with chronic low back pain. *Clin J Pain* 14:303-310, 1998.
74. Wilkie DJ, Keefe FJ: Coping strategies of patients with lung cancer-related pain. *Clin J Pain* 7:292-299, 1991.
75. Jacobson PB, Butler RW: Relation of cognitive coping and catastrophizing to acute pain and analgesic use following breast cancer surgery. *J Behav Med* 19:17-19, 1996.
76. Rosenstiel AK, Keefe FJ: The use of coping strategies in chronic low back pain patients: relationship to patient characteristics and current adjustment. *Pain* 17:33-44, 1983.
77. McCracken LM, Vowles KE, Eccleston C: Acceptance of chronic pain: component analysis and a revised assessment method. *Pain* 107: 159-166, 2004.
78. Cahana A: Is optimal pain relief always optimal? *APS Bull* 12(3), 2002.
79. Ward SE, Goldberg N, Miller-McCauley V, et al: Patient-related barriers to management of cancer pain. *Pain* 52:319-324, 1993.
80. Ward SE, Carlson-Dakes K, Hughes SH, et al: The impact of quality of life on patient-related barriers to pain management. *Res Nurs Health* 21(5):405-413, 1998.
81. Jensen M: A neuropsychological model of pain: research and clinical implications. *J Pain* 11(1):2-12, 2010.

8 Intrathecal Drug Delivery: Medical Necessity, Documentation, Coding, and Billing

David Schultz

CHAPTER OVERVIEW

Chapter Synopsis: With any treatment for chronic pain, both the patient and clinician must proceed with an eye to how payment for procedures will be rendered and how cost will be affected by insurance coverage. This chapter covers some of the challenges for clinicians to recover the therapy's cost, including showing medical necessity for the treatment and providing documentation, using proper coding technique, and ensuring billing compliance. Each step of the process is regulated by standard legal or corporate language and requires the physician's full attention. Other issues affect the procedure, including a required trial before implantation to show opioid sensitivity and the need for ongoing pump refilling and maintenance.

Important Point: Documentation of a detailed history and physical examination to demonstrate medical necessity are of greatest importance in getting appropriate reimbursement.

Clinical Pearl: Detailed documentation of indications for the procedure and the use of appropriate billing codes will lead to a successive medical practice.

Clinical Pitfall: Most denials of payment are due to lack of documentation for surgical interventional procedures.

Introduction

In 1979, Dr. Josef Wang at the Mayo Clinic in Rochester, Minnesota, administered intrathecal (IT) morphine by single-bolus injection to a number of patients with intractable cancer pain and demonstrated that spinal morphine exerted a powerful analgesic effect by binding directly to spinal cord pain receptors.[1] This first successful use of IT morphine opened up a realm of possibilities for spinal pain relief and was followed by widespread interest in IT drug delivery systems (IDDS) within the physician pain management community as well as within the medical device industry. The first programmable, fully implantable IT infusion pump was invented by Medtronic in 1981, and Medtronic's SynchroMed pump is now at the center of a worldwide IT drug delivery industry that currently involves more than 185,000 implanted patients with an experience involving more than 365,000 implanted devices over the past quarter century.[2]

Despite its medical efficacy, interventional pain clinics may choose not to offer this therapy because of perceived economic risks involved in implanting and managing pumps. Likewise, hospital operating room directors and surgery center administrators may balk at allowing surgeons to perform pump implants in their facilities because of the high cost of the implantable hardware and the possibility of inadequate reimbursement.[3] The present reality within the current U.S. health care system is that even the most beneficial medical treatment will not be widely available if it is not also a financially viable business for the physicians and facilities that deliver it. It is simply a fundamental economic principle that

a business, including a medical business, cannot survive over the long term unless it is able to meet its financial obligations. It follows that the providers of medical care, at least in the private sector, cannot subsidize that care over time and expect their medical practices to remain economically viable. This is especially true of IDDS, where there is a high upfront cost at therapy initiation related to the implanted hardware as well as recurring costs related to pump medication refills, pump maintenance, and ongoing management of patients with IDDS.

The purpose of this chapter is to provide implanting physicians and medical practice business managers with the information necessary to determine whether an economically viable IDDS program can be created given specific medical practice circumstances. To make sense of the current payment system and reimbursement potential for IDDS, it is important to start with a basic understanding of reimbursement principles within the U.S. health care system.

Medical Necessity and the U.S. Health Care Payment System

Medical necessity is a concept invented by government and adopted by others to help payers determine what is a legitimate treatment or service that should be reimbursed and also what is inappropriate and unnecessary care that should not be reimbursed. The principle itself is understandable. Many physicians believe that determination of the medical necessity for any particular service is part of the individual physician–patient relationship. Physicians may perceive that payer medical policy can be used improperly to both interfere with that relationship and to deny genuinely appropriate medical care as a cost-saving measure.

Regardless of perspective, medical necessity is the law. The Social Security Act, the enabling legislation for Medicare, explicitly states that no Medicare payment shall be made for items or services that "are not reasonable and necessary for the diagnosis or treatment of illness or injury or to improve the functioning of a malformed body member."[4] Virtually all private payers have similar language in their provider and member contracts. Based on this guiding precept, the Centers for Medicare and Medicaid Services (CMS), which administers Medicare, develops National Coverage Determinations (NCDs) for many treatments and services. These decisions are the outcome of a process involving technology assessment and analysis of the clinical research and scientific evidence for the treatment's benefits and risks. The results of each stage of the process are open to the public via CMS' website, and opportunities are provided for input on proposed decisions before they are finalized. Reconsiderations of prior decisions are also undertaken as new evidence becomes available.

Opioid Drugs for Treatment of Chronic Intractable Pain

An implantable infusion pump is covered when used to administer opioid drugs (e.g., morphine) intrathecally or epidurally for treatment of severe chronic intractable pain of malignant or non-malignant origin in patients who have a life expectancy of at least 3 months and who have proven unresponsive to less invasive medical therapy as determined by the following criteria: The patient's history must indicate that he or she would not respond adequately to noninvasive methods of pain control, such as systemic opioids (including attempts to eliminate physical and behavioral abnormalities that may cause an exaggerated reaction to pain), and a preliminary trial of intraspinal opioid drug administration must be undertaken with a temporary IT or epidural catheter to substantiate adequately acceptable pain relief and degree of side effects (including effects on the activities of daily living) and patient acceptance.[5]

The NCD is a general statement of medical necessity criteria for Medicare coverage. It then forms the basis for more specific Local Coverage Determinations (LCDs) developed by each Medicare carrier or contractor. While maintaining consistency with the NCD, LCDs establish more specific requirements for providers in each carrier's region.

LCDs typically identify:

- The specific Current Procedural Terminology (CPT) codes for the treatment (**Box 8-1**)
- The International Classification of Diseases (ICD-9-CM) diagnosis codes that are held to support medical necessity (**Box 8-1**)
- Documentation requirements to establish that the service was rendered

---

Box 8-1: Common Codes for Intrathecal Drug Delivery

ICD-9-CM Diagnosis Codes

338.29	Other chronic pain
338.3	Neoplasm-related pain (cancer pain)
338.4	Chronic pain syndrome
996.2	Mechanical complication of nervous system device, implant and graft
996.63	Infection and inflammatory reaction due to nervous system device, implant or graft
996.75	Other complications due to nervous system device, implant and graft
V53.09	Fitting and adjustment of devices related to nervous system

CPT Procedure Codes

62311	Injection, single (not via indwelling catheter), not including neurolytic substances, with or without contrasts (for either localization or epidurography), of diagnostic or therapeutic substance(s) (including anesthetic, antispasmodic, opioid, steroid, other solution), epidural or subarachnoid; lumbar, sacral (caudal)
62319	Injection, including catheter placement, continuous infusion or intermittent bolus, not including neurolytic substances, with or without contrast (for either localization or epidurography), of diagnostic or therapeutic substance(s) (including anesthetic, antispasmodic, opioid, steroid, other solution), epidural or subarachnoid; lumbar, sacral (caudal)
62350	Implantation, revision or repositioning of tunneled intrathecal or epidural catheter, for long-term medication administration via an external pump or implantable reservoir/infusion pump; without laminectomy
62351	Implantation, revision, or repositioning of tunneled intrathecal or epidural catheter, for long-term medication administration via an external pump or implantable reservoir/infusion pump; with laminectomy

62355	Removal of previously implanted intrathecal or epidural catheter
62362	Implantation or replacement of device for intrathecal or epidural drug infusion; programmable pump, including preparation of pump, with or without programming
62365	Removal of subcutaneous reservoir or pump, previously implanted for intrathecal or epidural infusion
62367	Electronic analysis of programmable, implanted pump for intrathecal or epidural drug infusion (includes evaluation of reservoir status, alarm status, drug prescription status); without reprogramming
62368	Electronic analysis of programmable, implanted pump for intrathecal or epidural drug infusion (includes evaluation of reservoir status, alarm status, drug prescription status); with reprogramming
61070	Puncture of reservoir for injection procedure
75809	Shuntogram for investigation of previously placed indwelling nonvascular shunt (indwelling infusion pump)
76000	Fluoroscopy
77003	Fluoroscopic guidance and localization of needle or catheter tip for spine or paraspinous diagnostic or therapeutic injection procedures (epidural, subarachnoid)
95990	Refilling and maintenance of implantable pump or reservoir for drug delivery, spinal (intrathecal, epidural) or brain (intraventricular)
95991	Refilling and maintenance of implantable pump or reservoir for drug delivery, spinal (intrathecal, epidural) or brain (intraventricular), administered by physician

HCPCS II Codes

A4220	Refill kit for implantable infusion pump
J2275	Injection, morphine sulfate (preservative-free sterile solution), per 10 mg
J2278	Injection, Ziconotide, 1 mcg
J3490	Unclassified drugs

CPT, Current Procedural Terminology; *HCPCS*, Healthcare Common Procedure Coding System; *ICD*, International Classification of Diseases.

- Utilization guidelines (e.g., site of service for drug trial, frequency of pump refill)

An individual Medicare intermediary may also explain reimbursement policy by other forms of written communication. WPS Medicare, a Midwestern CMS intermediary, has published guidelines for the states of Illinois, Michigan, Wisconsin, and Minnesota in its 2006 Medicare Part B Communique newsletter pertaining to the maintenance and filling of implanted IT infusion pumps. The WPS policy includes the following declarations and provisions:

1. Infusion pumps may typically be filled on a monthly basis.
2. Drugs used to fill IT infusion pumps are often prescribed off label by the managing physician and compounded for the patient by a compounding pharmacy.
3. The following seven pain drugs are considered covered and reimbursable by WPS when used in an IT infusion pump:
   a. Bupivacaine
   b. Clonidine
   c. Fentanyl
   d. Hydromorphone
   e. Morphine
   f. Sufentanil
   g. Ziconotide
4. These drugs or drug combinations should be billed using the J3490 (unclassified drugs) Healthcare Common Procedure Coding System (HCPCS).
5. The invoice for the drug purchase should be submitted with any paper claim or immediately available on request for electronic submissions.
6. The CPT code for electronic analysis or electronic analysis with reprogramming can be billed in addition to the refill CPT code.
7. The refill kit is bundled into the refill CPT code and cannot be billed separately.
8. An evaluation and management service is allowed, if performed at the time of the pump refill for a significant, separately identifiable reason. The applicable, appropriate E/M code should be billed with a −25 modifier.

With some variability, private payers go through a similar process in developing their medical necessity criteria, generally referred to as medical policy, clinical policy, or medical coverage policy. Although individualized for each payer, these policies are frequently informed by the criteria established in Medicare LCDs. Reflecting the trend toward use of evidence-based medicine to determine medical necessity, medical policies for private payers often cite the clinical research studies on which their decisions are based.

In the past, medical necessity criteria for Medicare have been difficult to ascertain. With modern electronic improvements, physicians who wish to know the specific criteria for any treatment can find all LCDs online via CMS' website. In recent years, other payers have also put their medical policies online. Currently, sophisticated electronic systems within the payer organizations enable the specific medical necessity criteria to be loaded into tables within claims processing software. Each bill submitted is then automatically adjudicated against these encoded criteria to determine whether the bill is covered. On a practical basis, this means that the data elements on each bill must match the data elements on the tables for the service to be covered and paid.

For example, the ICD-9-CM diagnosis code submitted on the bill must find a match on the payer's table of ICD-9-CM diagnosis codes that support medical necessity. If there is no code match, the claim will be denied as not medically necessary regardless of its clinical merit. Although this may reflect coding issues on the physician bill, it may also be attributable to omissions in the list of ICD-9-CM diagnosis codes contained within the payer's medical policy. With medical policy online, physicians can review for omitted codes and can petition the payer, usually through its medical director, to update the code list.

Another practical means of ensuring medical necessity is prior authorization. Particularly because IDDS is relatively expensive, many payers require prior authorization before the IDDS can be implanted. Medicare and many other government plans do not have a prior authorization system in place and use postprocedure audits to verify medical necessity. Even those payers with prior authorization systems perform postprocedure audits to ensure the authorization was valid. These audits rely almost entirely on the documentation in the medical record.

Documentation

Current standards dictate that treatment must not only be medically necessary, but it must also be documented in such a way that medical necessity is evident. To this end, the medical necessity language used by the payer may provide the language for the physician to use in documentation. For example, all LCDs state that IT infusion pumps are covered for "severe chronic intractable pain." To ensure that medical necessity is met, physicians must determine that the patient is experiencing "severe chronic intractable pain" and then, to ensure that medical necessity is apparent, may document this exact phrase as the indication for the pump in office notes and on the operative report. Although the primary purpose of medical record documentation is to support clinical care, physicians must also bear in mind that documentation is used for a variety of other legitimate purposes, including reimbursement and auditing by the payer.

Coding and Reimbursement

Physicians use CPT codes to communicate their services to payers. This is not just by convention but also by statute. The Health Insurance Portability and Accountability Act (HIPAA) mandates CPT as the standard code set for physician services nationwide.[6] CPT codes then form the basis for the Resource Based Relative Value Scale (RBRVS), which is the prospective payment system Medicare uses to reimburse physicians. Each CPT code is assigned a point value, which represents its worth. Each point is called a Relative Value Unit (RVU), and there are three components to the RVUs for each code: physician work, practice expense, and malpractice. The American Medical Association's (AMA's) Relative Value Updating Committee (RUC) determines the point value of each CPT code through the use of physician surveys, although CMS makes the final determination. Each year, CMS sets a flat dollar amount called the conversion factor to represent what each point is worth. The payment to the implanting physician is essentially the product of the total RVUs for the code multiplied by the conversion factor. The RVUs for each code and the conversion factor are standard nationwide. However, payment is also adjusted by a Geographic Practice Cost Index, designed to reflect variations in physician expenses among localities. The result is that, in 2010, Medicare paid a physician in Manhattan more than $100 more for implanting an infusion pump than it paid a physician in Tulsa, Oklahoma.

Hospitals also use CPT codes to bill outpatient services. Similar to RBRVS for physicians, CPT codes are the basis for Ambulatory Payment Classifications (APCs), Medicare's prospective payment system for hospital outpatient department (HOPD) reimbursement. Although some services are bundled and not paid separately, codes for significant procedures and services are assigned to specific APCs based on similarities in clinical nature as well as hospital resource use. Each APC has a relative weight reflecting its worth. The weight is then multiplied by a standard conversion factor to determine the hospital payment for each procedure. Ambulatory surgery centers (ASCs), which also use CPT codes for their services, are paid by Medicare under a prospective payment system that is based on hospital outpatient APCs but using a lower conversion factor that is a percentage of the HOPD payment.

All providers, physicians, hospitals, and ASCs currently use ICD-9-CM diagnosis codes to document the reason for the service provided. This is also mandated by HIPAA. Use of specific CPT codes and ICD-9-CM diagnosis codes is governed by various coding guidelines. Particularly when an outside audit is involved, physicians must be able to point to the guidelines they followed in making their code choices. The most defensible coding guidelines to follow are those in writing from an impeccable source. For CPT, the most credible guidelines are issued by the AMA, for example, in its monthly coding publication *CPT Assistant*. Medical specialty societies also usually have coding publications as well as coding answer services available to members.

For ICD-9-CM diagnosis coding, HIPAA mandates that the *ICD-9-CM Official Guidelines for Coding and Reporting* be followed. Among many other guidelines, this reference sets requirements for assignment and sequencing of diagnosis codes for pain-related disorders. The organizations that develop the annual *ICD-9-CM Official Guidelines*, which include CMS and the Centers for Disease Control and Prevention, also publish *Coding Clinic*, a quarterly journal of updated guidelines that are considered definitive.

The National Correct Coding Initiative (NCCI) also functions as a de facto coding standard for physicians, hospitals, and ASCs. NCCI is a set of more than 110,000 CPT coding edits that is updated quarterly. Although developed for Medicare, health care payers throughout the country have almost universally adopted NCCI edits. The edits are primarily designed to indicate which CPT codes are considered components of others and therefore cannot be assigned, billed, or paid separately. Overrides are permitted for some NCCI edits, but this must be approached with care. In general, overrides are appropriate only when the component code represents a procedure performed at a different anatomical site or at different patient encounters. NCCI's definition of different anatomical sites includes different organs or different lesions in the same organ but does not include treatment of contiguous structures of the same organ.[7] The NCCI edits are backed by a multichapter policy manual, updated annually, that articulates the rationale for many edits. The NCCI policy manual and the complete set of edits are available via the CMS website. The edits are also usually built into coding software and electronic "scrubbers" at billing clearinghouses.

Other sources for coding guidance, such as reimbursement consultants, are useful but not definitive, and consultant suggestions cannot be cited as justification for a coding practice judged to be improper by an outside auditor. Ultimately, the physician—and only the physician—bears responsibility for the choice of codes submitted to the payer.

Because the hardware associated with IDDS is expensive, the facility in which these devices are implanted will be understandably concerned about reimbursement. The programmable infusion pump, spinal catheter, and associated system components such as the tunneling device may cost the facility in the range of $10,000

to $15,000, and this cost must be paid by the facility in advance, independent of any reimbursement. So the facility is at significant financial risk if the device is not adequately reimbursed, and neither the technology vendor nor the implanting physician shares this risk. Therefore, to maintain a sustainable implant program, the implanting physician needs to be cognizant of the financial issues faced by the facility. Under a prospective payment system for Medicare or contracted rates for private payers, it is common for a hospital operating room to make money on certain surgeries and to lose money on others. For IDDS, the hospital administrator is interested in net revenues created by the implant service from an overall perspective. If a physician performs IDDS trials at the hospital and uses various hospital services such as imaging and laboratory services, the hospital may be able to make a net profit on the implant business even if it loses money on a specific surgical implant procedure. The implanting physician should facilitate discussions and cooperation between the administration and the technology vendor so the implant program can survive and prosper rather than generating net financial losses for the facility.

Billing Compliance

Medical necessity, documentation, and coding requirements create an environment in which physicians must always be mindful of compliance. Noncompliance with these requirements has genuine consequences, both economic and legal. Some are minor, but others can be life changing. Health care facilities and medical practices often have advisory reviewers in place to actively assist physicians in avoiding compliance issues. These include documentation improvement specialists at hospitals whose queries and educational in-services are designed to ensure that the documentation in medical records meet coding and payer requirements.

However, most reviewers are present specifically to detect and exploit any compliance issues. External reviewers include auditors from private payers who review records for sufficient documentation to support medical necessity and to validate the codes on which either physician or hospital payment is based. These reviewers are in a position to deny or retract payments to physicians and facilities. In fact, that is their purpose.

Government reviewers include Recovery Audit Contractors (RACs). RACs are private contractors working for CMS whose stated mission is to find Medicare overpayments. For motivation, RACs are paid on a contingency basis. The scope of RAC audits includes reviewing for services that are not medically necessary and for incorrect codes based on misapplication of coding guidelines. It also includes identifying evaluation and management (E&M) services that were paid separately but should have been included within the global period of a procedure.

For Medicare and virtually all other payers, the physician payment for a procedure encompasses multiple other services. This includes preoperative visits on the day of a minor procedure and the day before a major procedure, medical treatment of any surgical complications during the postoperative period, and follow-up visits for surgical issues during the postoperative period.[8] The postoperative period is defined individually for each CPT surgery code and is usually 0, 10, or 90 days. Physicians may not bill separately for any services related specifically to the procedure during the defined global period. However, some services are separately billable even within the global period. These include visits for unrelated diagnoses or for treatment of the underlying condition apart from the normal recovery from the surgery or procedure, as well as staged procedures and treatment of complications that require a return to the operating room. External auditors closely review all services billed during the global period of a procedure to ensure that they meet requirements for separately payable services.

Physicians should be aware that first-line auditors are rarely physicians. Instead, depending on the nature of the audit, they are typically nurses or professional coders. In practical terms, this means that documentation must be intelligible not only to other physicians but to nurses and coders as well.

Reviewing for fraud is the purview of the Office of the Inspector General (OIG), which can impose severe penalties, both civil and criminal. For example, for coding abuses, providers can be subject to penalties of up to $10,000 "for each item" plus a penalty of three times the specific overpayment. Miscoding is a felony and carries a maximum penalty of $25,000 and 5 years in prison. It is not necessary for the government to prove intent but only to establish a "pattern or practice" of miscoding.[9] Issues in medical necessity, documentation, and coding and billing compliance specific to the initial evaluation, trialing, surgical implantation, and ongoing management of IDDS patients are reviewed in the following sections.

Initial Evaluation

Medical Necessity

Because the NCD states that implantable infusion pumps are covered for "severe chronic intractable pain," the initial evaluation must focus on establishing that the patient has reached this state. The NCD does not specify what constitutes "chronic," although the medical policies for some payers define it as arising from a long-term pathological process as opposed to an immediate insult and as persisting for 6 months or more for pain of nonmalignant origin.[10,11] To substantiate intractability, the NCD also requires that the patient be demonstrably unresponsive to prior, less invasive medical therapy. Because IDDS is costly, the NCD requires the patient to have a life expectancy of at least 3 months.

Documentation

Documentation of the diagnosis and history (**Boxes 8-2** and **8-3**) are crucial to establishing medical necessity.

Box 8-2: Essential Elements of Diagnosis
"Severe chronic intractable pain"
Underlying cause of pain such as CRPS, malignancy (primary and secondary sites)
CRPS, Complex regional pain syndrome

Box 8-3: Essential Elements of History
Duration of pain
Severity of pain, such as patient's descriptive terms, scale of 1 to 10
A catalogue of all prior pain control measures, particularly systemic opioids
Need to escalate dosages
Attempts to address any physical and behavioral issues, which may heighten perception of pain, such as biofeedback
Details of the patient's response to the prior interventions, including side effects
Life expectancy (in patients whose underlying condition could draw this into question)

Documentation is also key to the E&M level assigned for the visit. Among the three components of history, physical examination, and medical decision making, medical decision making is the most difficult to convey in the documentation but is often the key to establishing higher E&M levels. Physicians should be sure to clearly document those elements that lead to higher levels for medical decision making (**Box 8-4**).

The initial evaluation may involve a significant amount of counseling. From a coding perspective, counseling includes discussion with the patient or family on the prognosis, the different management options available, and the risks and benefits of the options. If this counseling takes up more than 50% of the total time that the physician spends face to face with the patient during the visit, then time becomes the sole determinant of E&M level. For example, the typical time established for code 99214, a midlevel office visit with an established patient, is 25 minutes face to face. If the physician spends 13 or more minutes counseling the patient and documents this clearly, code 99214 can be billed regardless of the level of history, examination, and medical decision making. To code by time on the basis of counseling, the documentation must include certain elements (**Box 8-5**). Note that the documentation must describe the specific risks and benefits reviewed rather than simply refer to a generic discussion.

Coding

At one time, the main issue in coding the initial evaluation service was selecting the level of E&M code and ensuring that the documentation supported the level selected. Usually a mid- to high-level code can be justified. Depending on the payer, a code could be assigned either for a consultation or an outpatient office visit for a new or established patient. The distinction between a consultation or office visit depends on whether a transfer of care has taken place. However, for Medicare, this is a moot point. Beginning in January 2010, Medicare stopped accepting any CPT consultation codes for physician billing. This was based on an OIG study showing that consultation codes, which had higher RVUs than office visit codes, were often assigned incorrectly. To put an end to the coding issues and the payment differential, Medicare began requiring physicians to use regular office visit codes for outpatient consultations. Other payers may still accept consultation codes, although Medicare practice often becomes the standard over time.

Box 8-4: Elements Leading to Medical Decision Making
Interaction of multiple diagnoses
Whether the patient's condition is worsening
Personal review of image or discussion with performing physician
Review and summary of prior medical records
Use of controlled substances
Selection of surgical option

Box 8-5: Counseling Elements to Include in Documentation
Total time of visit (number of minutes)
Total time of counseling (number of minutes)
Who was counseled (e.g., patient, parent, spouse)
Nature of counseling (each option discussed)
Specific benefits and risks discussed for each option

Billing Compliance

For the initial evaluation, one of the primary compliance issues is the scrutiny drawn by high E&M levels. However, physicians may also draw scrutiny by billing all visits with midrange E&M codes because this can be interpreted as an attempt to avoid scrutiny. The best rule is to bill whatever level is supported by the service and the documentation.

Trialing

Medical Necessity

A trial is an essential component of medical necessity that must take place before the patient can proceed to permanent implantation. The NCD requires a "preliminary trial" of intraspinal opioids with a "temporary" catheter to substantiate an "adequately acceptable" level of pain relief. Virtually all other payers have the same requirement for a temporary trial. Although the NCD does not specify the length or setting of the trial and does not specifically require a continuous infusion through the catheter, the medical policies for some payers are more specific, requiring, for example, that the trial last at least 1 week.[12,13]

Meeting inpatient level of severity for the trial can be challenging, particularly because many payers use proprietary admission criteria. Often, though, inpatient admission can be justified on the basis of opioid use with the need for dosage adjustments and intensive monitoring. Conversely, some payer medical policies actually require an inpatient trial. A recent study published in *Anesthesiology* in October 2009 identified a significant increase in mortality immediately after IDDS implant or revision and may set a new standard for hospital admission for at least 24 hours after initiating therapy.[14]

The NCD also does not quantify what constitutes an acceptable level of pain relief during the trial for permanent pump implantation to be considered medically necessary. Some payer policies define this as at least a 50% reduction in pain.[14] In addition, some payers have a separate requirement for a comprehensive psychological evaluation performed by a psychologist or psychiatrist knowledgeable about pain to determine that the pain is not psychogenic and that the patient is an appropriate IDDS candidate.

Documentation

The documentation during the trial stage of IDDS must accomplish three things: support medical necessity, enable diagnosis and procedure coding, and record the trial results. To help meet medical necessity requirements, elements of the initial evaluation can be integrated into the trialing documentation. This is important because when faced with an outside review, the documentation for each phase must stand on its own. Pain should be documented as a distinct clinical element, and its underlying cause should be explained. As clinically appropriate, physicians should explicitly characterize the pain as severe, chronic, and intractable and must also indicate whether it is of malignant or nonmalignant origin. The pain must then be directly linked to a specific underlying diagnosis.

Procedure documentation should make clear whether the trial consisted of sequential single injections or continuous infusion via an IT or epidural catheter. Use of fluoroscopy to insert the needle or catheter should be clearly recorded. If the trial catheter was tunneled, the tunneling should be explicitly noted in the procedure report along with a statement explaining why tunneling was clinically appropriate and the difficulty it added to the procedure in terms of effort, intensity, time, and technical difficulty.

Meticulous documentation should be kept for the visits during which the patient's response is assessed. This includes a complete history and physical examination as well as highly detailed notes on the physician's medical decision making related to the patient's responses. Finally, the trial documentation must summarize its results. The trial summary should include:

- The degree of pain relief, as a percentage, as well as how it was quantified
- Any observed side effects and their impact on the patient
- Patient tolerance of the trial and willingness to proceed to permanent implantation

Coding

For diagnosis coding, ICD-9-CM contains a set of codes specifically for chronic pain as a distinct disorder. One of these chronic pain codes, typically 338.29 or 338.3, is used as the principal diagnosis "when pain control or pain management is the reason for the admission/encounter," as is the case with IDDS trialing.[15] The underlying cause of the pain is then reported as a secondary diagnosis.

For a trialing procedure with continuous infusion or intermittent bolus through an intraspinal catheter, CPT offers codes 62318 for cervical or thoracic spinal catheter or 62319 for lumbar spinal catheter. There is also CPT code 62311 for single-shot lumbar subarachnoid or epidural injection without catheter placement, although single injections without a catheter may not meet the catheter criteria outlined in the NCD. Fluoroscopy can be used when performing spinal injections or placing spinal catheters. NCCI edits bundle the general fluoroscopy codes 76000 and 76001 into the spinal injection codes. However, NCCI policy allows fluoroscopy to be coded with spinal procedures when "there is a specific CPT manual instruction indicating that it is separately reportable."[16] In the case of spinal injections, CPT manual instructions state that fluoroscopic guidance and localization is reported with 77003. NCCI edits do not bundle this specific fluoroscopy code 77003 with spinal injection codes 62311, 62318, and 62319.

Code 62350 is also available for the trialing procedure when the catheter is tunneled. This code is defined for implantation of a tunneled IT catheter with an external pump. However, the code definition also includes "for long-term medication administration," and the trial, by its nature, is temporary. Code 62350 also has a global period of 10 days, which can impact on billing for postprocedure visits and permanent pump implantation. An alternative is to use the spinal catheter code 62319 with modifier −22 for increased service to reflect the tunneling. Codes submitted with modifier −22 are usually reviewed by the payer; this is why documentation on the need for tunneling and the difficulty it added to the procedure may be necessary in the procedure report.

In general, physicians who perform an injection should not assign a separate E&M code on the same day unless a separately identifiable E&M service is provided. With a global period of 0 days, injections are considered minor procedures, and under global period rules, visits by the same physician on the same day that are related to the procedure are included in the payment for the procedure. However, the global fee applies only to visits that are related to the usual pre- and postoperative care for the procedure. Visits can be coded separately when a significant, separately identifiable E&M service is also performed.[17] On both of these points, the intensity of trial evaluation and monitoring may qualify for separate E&M codes, as supported by the documentation. When an E&M service is coded and billed separately on the same day as the injection, modifier −25 must be appended to the E&M code to bypass global edits. CMS has stated that a different diagnosis is not required to bill a significant and separately identifiable E&M

service provided on the same day as an injection or other procedure.[18]

Billing Compliance

CMS and other payers routinely monitor for physicians and groups with high use of modifier −25 to separately bill E&M services. This may prompt a review of records to verify that the documentation supports a significant and separately identifiable E&M service. When it does not, the payer may impose prepayment screening. Proper billing for E&M services within the global period is also a current focus of OIG review.

Surgical Implantation

Medical Necessity

The initial evaluation and results of the trial should have established whether the patient meets the specific criteria needed to proceed to permanent system implantation. Although trialing is typically a percutaneous procedure that may be appropriately performed in any number of settings, including a medical office, ASC, hospital outpatient department, or hospital operating room, permanent implantation of an IT catheter and infusion pump is true surgery and requires a formal operating room setting with laminar airflow, formal sterility protocols, and adequate space for a surgical operation. The patient may reasonably be admitted overnight or discharged the same day after the surgical implantation depending on the specific circumstances of the patient and the postoperative IT infusion. Many payers default to the outpatient setting for permanent implantation of the catheter and pump. However, inpatient admission may be justifiable because of the risk of IT opioid overdose as well as the need to adjust opioid doses immediately after pump implantation. The nature of the patient's underlying condition and the comorbidities that accompany it may also meet inpatient acuity.

If the procedure is staged and the catheter and pump are implanted in separate episodes of care, there must be a definitive clinical reason for doing so, such as the patient's inability to withstand a lengthy procedure because of co-morbidities or the decision by the implanter to trial the patient with an implanted intraspinal segment of catheter attached to an exteriorized catheter, which is in turn connected to an external pump. With this method of trialing, the implanted segment can be retained after a successful trial, sparing the patient additional catheter surgery.

Documentation

As before, key elements of initial evaluation and trialing reports should be integrated into the implantation record because the documentation for this phase must be able to stand on its own. Notations to "see prior record" should be avoided unless copies of the prior reports are incorporated into the implantation medical record and are immediately available to outside reviewers. This means that the diagnostic indications in the operative report for catheter and pump implantation should again indicate chronic intractable pain as a distinct diagnosis with a separate and specific underlying cause. The introductory section of the operative report should also include a point-by-point summary of all prior measures undertaken without adequate pain relief and a point-by-point summary of the trial results. If the procedure is being staged, both operative reports should include a statement explaining the clinical reason.

For the procedure itself, the body of the operative report should clearly identify the device components implanted, their locations, and the implantation technique. In the header of the report, it is useful to refer to the procedures in terms related to their CPT code descriptions, again bearing in mind that not all users and reviewers of the report will be physicians.

Coding

Diagnosis coding is similar to trialing, with the chronic pain code as the principal diagnosis and a code for the underlying cause of the pain as a secondary diagnosis. CPT provides codes 62350 and 62351 for permanent catheter insertion, depending on whether a laminectomy was necessary. Because the SynchroMed pump is programmable, code 62362 is used for pump implantation. If a nonprogrammable pump where to be implanted, code 62361 is available. The main coding issues arise with fluoroscopy and the initial pump filling and programming. Although some specialty societies suggest that fluoroscopy may be included in the global service for intraspinal catheter placement, there is no consensus among all relevant societies on this point. As previously stated, NCCI edits bundle the general fluoroscopy code 76000 and 76001 into code 62350 but do not bundle the more specific fluoroscopy code 77003. Many payers allow separate coding and reimbursement for 77003 with code 62350 for catheter implantation.

The initial pump filling and programming are not coded separately because the definition of code 62362 includes pump preparation and programming. This is enforced by NCCI edits, which bundle the filling and programming codes into pump code 62362.

Billing Compliance

The distinct ICD-9-CM codes for chronic pain were created in 2007, and the guideline requiring that they be sequenced as the principal diagnosis for pain management encounters went into effect at the same time. Unfortunately, some payers have not yet caught up with this policy change, and their medical policies may not include the pain codes or may require that the underlying disorder be used as the principal diagnosis. This may cause a correctly coded claim to be rejected or denied.

Because the *ICD-9-CM Official Guidelines* are mandated by HIPAA, physicians must comply with their coding and sequencing requirements. As a long-term solution for this type of denial, payer medical directors must be approached by individual physicians and by specialty societies to add the pain codes and proper sequencing instructions to their medical polices. Payers are subject to HIPAA, and the *ICD-9-CM Official Guidelines* apply to them as well.

Code 62350 for percutaneous catheter insertion and code 62362 for pump implantation both have global periods of 10 days. Code 62351 for catheter insertion via laminectomy has a global period of 90 days. In general, then, patient visits during the global time period are not separately billable because they relate to recovery from the procedure. Also note that visits for medical treatment of any complications, such as infection, are included in the global package and are not separately billable during the global period unless they require a return to the operating room.[19]

There are exceptions to billing separate E&M codes for visits during the global period.[20] These may involve visits for unrelated diagnoses or for management of the patients' underlying condition independent of the surgery. Modifier −24 is appended to the E&M code to show that the visit is unrelated to the surgery even though it occurred during the postoperative period. This bypasses global edits and allows the visit to be paid separately. Use of a different diagnosis code is usually sufficient to establish that the visit is truly unrelated to the surgery.[21] However, frequent use of modifier −24 may increase the level of scrutiny paid to the physician's billing.

For staged procedures, physicians must append modifier −58 to the code for the second-stage procedure. This indicates to payers that the procedure was staged by intention. Staged procedures are also subject to payer review because they generate two payments at 100% for both the physician and the outpatient facility rather than a discounted 50% payment for the second procedure had both procedures taken place during the same operative encounter. For this reason, documentation on the clinical need for staging is necessary in both operative reports.

Pump Refilling and Maintenance

Medical Necessity
Most payers do not allocate a fixed number of visits for pump refilling and maintenance. Instead, their medical polices indicate more generally that the frequency must be supported by the patient's clinical picture and must take into account the size of the pump.[22]

Documentation
Some payers have specific documentation requirements for refill and maintenance visits, which can serve as a template for appropriate documentation (**Box 8-6**).

The need to distinctly reassess the patient's condition must be documented, for example, if there has been a significant change in symptoms or the appearance of a new side effect. The reassessment must then be supported by documentation of an interval history, targeted examination, and elements of medical decision making.

If all or a portion of the refill and programming is rendered by the office nurse, the documentation must also indicate the physician's active participation and ongoing management of the patient's care, for example, by review of the history or programming notes. This is needed to substantiate physician billing for any services rendered by office staff. Because the CPT codes for refilling and maintenance differentiate between physicians and other professionals, there must be explicit documentation of who personally performed the service.

Coding
Although some physicians have a persistent bias against V codes, *Coding Clinic* has published that ICD-9-CM diagnosis code V53.09 is correctly used as the principal diagnosis for routine refilling and pump interrogation visits.[23] Despite the wording of its description, code V53.09 is a diagnosis code, and its use indicates that the primary reason for the encounter is attention to the device itself rather than a new issue with the patient's pain. Pain and its underlying cause are then coded as a secondary diagnosis.

For nonroutine visits, however, the condition prompting the visit is used as the principal diagnosis. This may be a pain code, a symptom code, or the underlying diagnosis depending on the nature of the condition. CPT codes 95990 and 95991 are used for pump refilling. Code 95991 is assigned only when the refilling is personally performed by the physician. In all other circumstances, code 95990 is used instead even though the physician may be present while a staff member refills the pump. For pump analysis, code 62367 is used for interrogation only, and code 62368 is used when the pump is reprogrammed. Notably, the AMA has published that pumps require programming at the time of refill, indicating that code 62368 is assigned in addition to 95990 or 95991 whenever a pump refill is performed.[24] The use of two separate codes, one for programming and one for refilling, follows instructional notes in the CPT manual and is permitted under NCCI edits.

A major issue in refilling and maintenance is whether an E&M visit code can be assigned separately. When a visit involves only routine refilling and reprogramming, even if the dosage is revised, no E&M service should be reported. However, a separate E&M code may be assigned when a significant and separately identifiable service takes place above and beyond that typically associated with a refill and maintenance visit. This may include scenarios in which, for example, the physician expends additional time and effort assessing newly developed side effects or symptoms, adjusting the patient's oral medications, distinctly reassessing the underlying condition, or evaluating an unrelated condition.[23,25] The fact that IT granuloma formation is now documented to occur over time in a significant percentage of chronic IT infusion patients may provide medical necessity for more intensive evaluation and monitoring of patients with implanted IT delivery systems.[26]

The physician must append modifier –25 to the E&M code to indicate that, as supported by the documentation, a significant and separately identifiable evaluation took place in addition to the refilling and maintenance.

In the office setting, physicians should also be certain to assign separate HCPCS II codes for the drug itself, usually either code J2275 or J2278, and the pump refill kit A4220 (**Box 8-1**). Based on Medicare precedent, many payers bundle payment for the refill kit into the payment for the refilling service. However, many make a separate payment for the drug. The drug must represent a cost to the physician to be coded and billed separately. Some payers may request an invoice.[27]

To use the J codes, the drugs must be packaged as stated in the code description. Compounded drugs cannot be coded to J2275 or J2278 but must instead be coded to J3490, unclassified drug, even if the compound is similar to or includes an off-the-shelf drug.[26,28]

Billing Compliance
Some payers have a bias against V codes as a principal diagnosis and do not include V53.09 in their medical policies, causing correctly coded claims to deny. As with the pain codes, resolution requires asking the payer to add code V53.09 to the policy.

A key compliance issue involves "incident to" services in which the physician bills for services actually rendered by a staff member, such as an office nurse, nurse practitioner, or physician's assistant. Because harsh penalties can be imposed for improper billing of "incident to" services, this can be a complex topic and often requires legal guidance. That noted, there are two general rules of thumb.[28]

The first is that there is no "incident to" billing in the facility setting. For a physician to bill pump refilling and maintenance in, for example, a hospital outpatient pain clinic, the physician must personally perform the services. If a nurse performs the services, the physician cannot bill. That is the case regardless of whether the nurse is a hospital or physician employee and regardless of whether the physician was physically present while the nurse rendered the service. The second rule of thumb is that the physician can in fact bill for refilling and maintenance performed by a staff nurse, nurse

Box 8-6: Refill, Interrogation, and Reprogramming Documentation Requirements
Pump status before and after refill
Patient's response to current dosage and rate
Reasons for any alteration in dosage and rate
New response to current dosage and rate
Reassessment of patient's overall condition and treatment goals, as needed

practitioner, or physician's assistant in the physician office if the service falls within the scope of practice of the nonphysician provider and certain requirements are met. A key requirement is "direct physician supervision."

Direct supervision means that "the physician must be present in the office suite and immediately available to provide assistance and direction throughout the time the aide is performing services." Notably, direct supervision "does not mean that the physician must be present in the same room with his or her aide" or that "each occasion of service by auxiliary personnel . . . need also always be the occasion of the actual rendition of a personal professional service by the physician." Rather, a service may be considered "incident to" when it is rendered "during a course of treatment where the physician performs an initial service and subsequent services of a frequency which reflects his/her active participation in and management of the course of treatment."

The nature of pump refilling and maintenance seems to dovetail neatly with this requirement. The initial service of implanting the pump is always performed by physicians. Patients are then seen periodically for refilling and maintenance as needed for continued relief of symptoms. As long as the physician remains actively engaged in patient care and is immediately available in the office suite during each encounter, refilling and maintenance can be performed by the office staff and billed under the physician's name. Note that code 95990 must be assigned for the pump refill when it is performed by the nonphysician provider rather than the physician.

Compounded drugs present another compliance issue. Because compounded drugs require review for individual pricing, many payers require that an invoice accompany the claim or be made available on request. Others require that the compound formula be entered onto the CMS-1500 claim form. If this information is omitted, claims may be automatically denied.

Similarly, most payers require that all components of the refilling and maintenance service, including the pump refill code, reprogramming code, drug J code, and any E&M code, be submitted together on the same claim. Claims with these codes that are billed separately for the same date may be automatically denied. As always, physicians can expect high scrutiny to be given when refill claims are routinely billed with a separate E&M visit code.

Routine Pump Replacement and Troubleshooting Device Complications

Medical Necessity

As long as the original pump implantation was adjudicated as medically necessary, scheduled replacement is routinely approved. Medical necessity is also generally not an issue for revision and removal as needed for device complications. In fact, some payers have medical policies explicitly stating that replacement, revision, and removal of infusion pumps and catheters for end of life and malfunction is de facto medically necessary.[29,30]

Documentation

For routine pump replacement, physicians should be certain to clearly document that the reason for the replacement procedure is end of battery life as opposed to a true device malfunction. Otherwise, the documentation should include the specific reasons that a device complication is suspected, such as fever or a sudden increase in the patient's pain, along with an itemization of steps taken to rule out non–device-related causes. To ensure proper coding, the documentation should specify the exact type of complication, such as a flipped pump, detached or broken catheter, catheter migration, infected pocket, or pocket erosion.

For the procedure documentation, the same template for initial implantation is appropriate for a replacement, adding a description for removing the old device.

Coding

As with routine pump refilling and maintenance, the principal diagnosis for a routine pump replacement is V53.09. ICD-9-CM also has codes specifically for device complications. Because IDDS are considered nervous system devices, complication codes 996.2 for mechanical issues, 996.63 for device-related infections, and 996.75 for all other device complications are used. The same codes are assigned regardless of whether the complication involves the pump, the catheter, or the pocket.

The AMA has published that a catheter dye study uses code 61070 and 75809 even though code 61070 is located in the CPT manual under the heading "Skull, Meninges, and Brain."[31] For a noninvasive rotor study, the common practice is to assign code 62368 for pump analysis with reprogramming plus code 76000 for simple fluoroscopy.

For replacement of the pump, the same code is used as for the initial implantation of the pump. This is because code 62362 is defined as "implantation or replacement." Similarly, codes 62350 and 62351 are defined as "implantation, revision or repositioning" of the catheter, so the same code is used for all three procedures. As with initial implantation, NCCI edits do not allow pump filling and programming to be coded separately with pump replacement.

NCCI edits generally do not allow removal of the old device to be coded separately in a pump or catheter replacement. If removal of the old pump is coded separately, NCCI edits are set up in such a way that the implantation code 62362 is actually rebundled into the removal code 62365, and only the lower RVU removal code is paid. Likewise, if removal of the old catheter is coded separately, NCCI edits rebundle the implantation codes 62350 and 62351 into the removal code 62355 so that only the lower RVU removal code is paid. The NCCI edits barring coding removal of the old device with implantation of the new device do allow an override. To override the edit and allow both codes to pay, modifier –59 is appended to the implantation code, 62362 for the pump, or 62350 or 62351 for the catheter to indicate a distinct procedural service. CMS frequently raises concerns about overuse of modifier –59 to improperly bypass NCCI edits. As a general rule, NCCI edit policy holds that modifier –59 is appropriate only when the procedures involve "different anatomical sites or different patient encounters."[32] In a pump replacement, then, use of the modifier –59 override could be justified when the pump is relocated to a newly developed pocket at a different site. For a catheter replacement, an override could be justified when the new catheter is inserted through a different access or at a different spinal level.

Billing Compliance

Medical treatment of surgical complications is included in the global package, so visits for complications that arise during the global period for the implantation procedure are not coded separately. However, the procedure is coded separately when treatment requires a return to the operating room, defined in this context as a place of service "specifically equipped and staffed for the sole purpose of performing procedures."[33] This includes a regular operating room as well as a distinct interventional radiology suite and, depending on the specific configuration, a pain clinic procedure room.

Return trips to the operating room during the global period are identified by appending modifier –78 to the procedure code for treating the complication. Use of the modifier allows the procedure to be paid separately outside of the global period, although payment is not made at 100% of the rate. Instead, payment is made for the value of the intraoperative portion only.[34] CMS divides the RVUs for all procedures into three operative portions. For example, the 2010 RVUs for catheter removal code 62355 are apportioned into 10% preoperative, 80% intraoperative, and 10% postoperative. Therefore, when 62355-78 is submitted, Medicare pays 80% of the rate. The rationale for this is that the physician is providing the intraoperative portion separately, but the preoperative and postoperative portions remain part of the global period.

Conclusion

IDDS is an extremely helpful, indeed sometimes life-saving, therapy for many patients. Although initial cost outlays are high secondary to hardware and operating room costs, IDDS has been shown to be cost-effective in well-selected patients over the long term.[35] Hopefully, government and private payers will realize the unique utility of this therapy and maintain reimbursement levels that will allow physicians to continue implanting appropriate patients and technology vendors to continue with technological improvements to drug delivery systems. By recognizing and responding to issues involving medical necessity, documentation, coding, and compliance, physicians can help bring this about.

Acknowledgement

The author would like to acknowledge Linda Holtzman, MHA, RHIA, CCS, CCS-P, CPC, CPC-H, and Medtronic, Inc.

References

1. Wang JK, Nauss LA, Thomas JE: Pain relief by intrathecally applied morphine in man. *Anesthesiology* 5:149-151, 1979.
2. Medtronic: *Neuromodulation*. Unpublished data from Medtronic Device Registration System, Minneapolis, MN, Medtronic.
3. Deer TR, Krames E, Levy RM, et al: Practice choices and challenges in the current intrathecal therapy environment: an online survey. *Pain Med* 10(2):304-309, 2009.
4. Centers for Medicare & Medicaid Services: *Final changes to the hospital outpatient prospective payment system and CY 2010 payment rates.* Regulation #CMS-1414-FC, accessed January 1, 2010, from http://www.cms.gov/ASCPayment/ASCRN/list.asp.
5. *Exclusions from coverage and Medicare as secondary payer, compilation of the Social Security Laws, Social Security Act, Title XVIII, section 1862(a)(1)(A),* accessed May 15, 2010, from http://www.ssa.gov/OP_Home/ssact/title18/1862.htm.
6. Centers for Medicare & Medicaid Services Manual System: *Infusion pumps,* Publication 100-03 Medicare National Coverage Determinations, Chapter 1, Section 280.14, Baltimore, MD, 2005, Centers for Medicare & Medicaid Services.
7. Health Insurance Reform: Standards for electronic transactions, rules and regulations. *Federal Register* 65(160):50312, 2000, accessed July 14, 2010, from http://www.access.gpo.gov/su_docs/fedreg/a000817c.html.
8. Centers for Medicare & Medicaid Services: *Proper usage regarding distinct procedural service.* Modifier 59 Article, accessed March 14, 2003, from https://www.cms.gov/NationalCorrectCodInitEd.
9. Surgeons and global surgery. *Medicare Claims Processing Manual,* Chapter 12, Section 40, Baltimore, MD, 2003, Centers for Medicare & Medicaid Services.
10. Cornell University Law School: *Civil monetary penalties* (Section 1320a-7a), *criminal penalties for acts involving federal health care programs* (Section 1320a-7b), Title 42 of the US Code, Chapter 7, accessed June 2, 2010, from http://www.law.cornell.edu/uscode/42/usc_sec_42_00001320—a007a.html and http://www.law.cornell.edu/uscode/uscode42/usc_sec_42_00001320—a007b.html.
11. United Healthcare Oxford Health Plans: *Outpatient pain management interventions.* Policy #PAIN 007.12 T1, accessed December 20, 2009, from https://www.oxhp.com/secure/policy/outpatient_pain_management_1209.html.
12. Anthem: *Implantable infusion pumps.* Policy #SURG.00068, accessed August 19, 2010, from http://www.anthem.com/medicalpolicies/policies/mp_pw_a053366.htm.
13. BlueCross BlueShield of North Carolina: *Implantable infusion pumps.* Guideline #EBG.DME0150, accessed March 10, 2010, from http://www.bcbsnc.com.
14. Coffey R, Owens M: Mortality associated with implantation and management of intrathecal opioid drug infusion systems to treat noncancer pain. *Anesthesiology* 111:881-891, 2009.
15. Anthem: *Implantable infusion pumps.* Medical Policy #SURG.00068, accessed October 21, 2009, from http://www.anthem.com/medicalpolicies/policies/mp_pw_a053366.htm.
16. Diseases of nervous system and sense organs: pain codes as principal or first-listed diagnosis. *Official Coding Guidelines for Coding and Reporting,* ICD-9-CM, Section I.C.6.a, p 32, accessed August 25, 2010, from http://www.ucdmc.ucdavis.edu/compliance/pdf/icdguide09.pdf.
17. *NCCI Policy Manual,* Version 15.3, Chapter 8, Section C.15, accessed September 19, 2010, from http://www.ncci.com.
18. Surgery and global surgery. *Medicare Claims Processing Manual,* Chapter 12, Section 40, Baltimore, MD, 2010, Centers for Medicare & Medicaid Services.
19. Payment for codes for chemotherapy administration and nonchemotherapy injections and infusions: therapeutic, prophylactic, and diagnostic injections and infusions (excluding chemotherapy), Chapter 12, section 30.5(C), and payment for evaluation and management services provided during global period of surgery: CPT modifier "–25"—significant evaluation and management service by same physician on date of global procedure, Chapter 12, Section 30.6.6(B). *Medicare Claims Processing Manual,* Baltimore, MD, 2010, Centers for Medicare & Medicaid Services.
20. Definition of a global surgical package: components of a global surgical package. *Medicare Claims Processing Manual* Chapter 12, Section 40.1(A), Baltimore, MD, 2010, Centers for Medicare & Medicaid Services.
21. Definition of a global surgical package: services not included in the global surgical package, Chapter 12, Section 40.1(B), and payment for evaluation and management services provided during global period of surgery: CPT modifier "–25"—unrelated evaluation and management service by same physician during postoperative period, Chapter 12, Section 30.6.6(A). *Medicare Claims Processing Manual,* Baltimore, MD, 2010, Centers for Medicare & Medicaid Services.
22. Billing requirements for global surgeries: unrelated procedures or visits during the postoperative period, Chapter 12, Section 40.2.A.7. *Medicare Claims Processing Manual,* Baltimore, MD, 2010, Centers for Medicare & Medicaid Services.
23. Palmetto GBA: *Implantable infusion pump for treatment of chronic intractable pain,* LCD Number L28268, accessed August 16, 2010, from http://www.palmettogba.com/palmetto/palmetto.nsf/DocsCat/Home.
24. Implantable pumps. *AHA Coding Clinic,* 2nd Quarter 1999, pp 3-4, accessed September 11, 2010, from http://thecodingclinic.com.
25. Refilling and maintenance of implantable delivery systems. *CPT Assistant* 16(7):1-3, 2006.
26. Noridian Administrative Services: *Article number A43220,* accessed September 11, 2010, from https://www.noridianmedicare.com.
27. Medtronic *neuromodulation SynchroMed EL, SynchroMed II and IsoMed implantable Infusion pumps: Food and Drug Administration, class 1 recall.* Accessed June 20, 2010, from http://www.fda.gov/MedicalDevices/Safety/RecallsCorrectionsRemovals/ListofRecalls/ucm062343.htm.
28. Palmetto GBA: *Article number A49293,* accessed August 16, 2010, from http://www.palmettogba.com/palmetto/palmetto.nsf/DocsCat/Home.

29. Covered medical and other health service: services and supplies, *Medicare Benefit Policy Manual* Chapter 15, Section 60, 2010.

30. Aetna: *Clinical policy bulletin: infusion pumps*, Number 0161. Accessed April 16, 2010, from http://www.aetna.com/cpb/medical/data/100_199/0161.html.

31. Independence Blue Cross: *Insertion of implantable infusion pumps*, Medical Policy Number 11.15.03d, accessed July 20, 2010, from http://www.ibx.com/index.jsp.

32. Medicine/Physician and Facility Reporting with Hydration and Drug Administration Procedures in the Facility 90772 (Q&A). *CPT Assistant* 18(7):13, 2008.

33. Version 15.3, Chapter 1, section E.1(d), *NCCI Policy Manual*, accessed September 19, 2010, from http://www.ncci.com.

34. Definition of a global surgical package. *Medicare Claims Processing Manual* Chapter 12, Section 40.1, 2010.

35. Adjudication of claims for global surgeries. Chapter 12, Section 40.4, *Medicare Claims Processing Manual* 2010.

II Implant Devices

Chapter 9 Methods of Trials for Consideration of Intrathecal Drug Delivery Sytems

Chapter 10 Techniques of Implant Placement for Intrathecal Pumps

Chapter 11 Programmable versus Fixed-Rate Pumps for Intrathecal Drug Delivery

Chapter 12 SynchroMed EL versus SynchroMed II

Chapter 13 Minimizing the Risks of Intrathecal Therapy

Chapter 14 Complications Associated with Intrathecal Drug Delivery Systems

9 Methods of Trials for Consideration of Intrathecal Drug Delivery Systems

Joshua Wellington

CHAPTER OVERVIEW

Chapter Synopsis: Intrathecal drug delivery systems (IDDS) may be used to treat patients with chronic pain or spasticity. A trialing period can help to predict whether treatment might ultimately be successful. The trial period may also help to determine the best drug or drug combination and delivery method. Pain is treated primarily with opioid drugs, but these agents differ in their water and fat solubility, which should be considered when determining whether to deliver to the fluid-filled epidural space or the more fatty intrathecal space. Ziconotide, a conotoxin, may also be used to treat pain. The location of delivery also affects the circulation and spread of the drug and may influence the extent of side effects. For spasticity, the γ-aminobutyric acid antagonist baclofen is the drug of choice. Patients who are candidates for IDDS typically have pain that is refractory to more conventional delivery of drugs—often the same drugs that might be delivered to the spinal cord. Therefore, a trial can also show whether the procedure will be efficacious before permanent implantation of the drug delivery pump. The method of drug delivery during the trial—whether in a bolus or a continuous application—should also be considered for the individual patient. Together, the patient and clinician should determine whether the trial should be considered a success and whether to move ahead with implantation for IDDS.

Important Points:
- The decision to trial a patient for an intrathecal drug delivery system should be taken very seriously.
- The trial can be done by epidural or intrathecal route.
- Trialing may be done with an opioid drug, nonopioid drug, or combination.
- Pain relief, function improvement, and tolerance of side effects are all components of determining the success or failure of the trial.
- The psychological aspect of the patient's well being should be considered carefully before proceeding with a permanent implant.

Clinical Pearls:
- The decision to trial a patient for an IDDS for pain control is evolving over time.
- The classic reason for trialing was for patients who failed to achieve efficacy with opioids or failed to tolerate the side effects.
- New drugs such as ziconotide allow patients who have never had opioids or who are not appropriate candidates for opioids to be considered for an IDDS.
- The patient should have stable clotting parameters and all medications impacting bleeding should be stopped or modified prior to surgery if appropriate.
- The patient should have no active systemic infections and no local infection at the trialing site.
- The need for a trial has never been proven in a prospective randomized fashion and some clinicians believe an IDDS may be placed without doing a trial. This is a controversial point.

Clinical Pitfalls:
- The patient may have excellent pain relief but may not tolerate the side effects of the chosen drug used for trialing. Failure to consider pain relief and side effects may lead to long-term failure of the therapy.
- Complications of trialing such as postdural puncture or nerve irritation may confuse the patient and the physician. In these cases, the team should consider canceling the trial and repeating it at a later date.
- The failure to use fluoroscopic guidance to place the needle or catheter may lead to a failed trial because of inability of the body to respond to drugs placed in the unintended anatomical location of the neuroaxis.
- A successful trial does not guarantee a successful permanent implant, and the patient should be counseled on the possibility of failure even if they experienced appropriate pain relief.

Establishing a Diagnosis

When considering an intrathecal drug delivery system (IDDS) as an option for patients, the clinician is faced with a number of options for trialing medications to assess for potential efficacy and side effects. A trial is the essential first step to determine whether administering medication(s) via the spinal axis will yield the hoped for results before proceeding with pump implantation. Intrathecal (IT) drug delivery is considered in patients who have been refractory to conservative treatment for spasticity or pain.

The history of trialing for IDDS has not been well documented. The techniques described in this chapter using a single bolus, multiple boluses, or catheter either via the epidural or IT route had been available long before the introduction of implanted IDDS. The first clinical implant of a programmable pump (which became the Medtronic SynchroMed pump) for IT morphine occurred in 1982. In 1988, the implantable programmable SynchroMed Pump was released for use in cancer chemotherapy. The indication for treatment of cancer pain and nonmalignant pain with IT morphine using the SynchroMed Pump was approved by the U.S. Food and Drug Administration (FDA) in 1991. The SynchroMed EL (extended-life) pump was approved by the FDA in March 1999 and voluntarily discontinued in August 2007 based on broad acceptance of the SynchroMed II pump, which was released in July 2004. With the introduction and evolution of implanted IDDS, trialing methods have similarly paralleled to assess a patient's potential response for efficacy and adverse events.

Many pain syndromes of either malignant or nonmalignant nature may be appropriate for IT drug delivery. At the point when more conservative options such as medication management or injection therapies have failed, an IDDS may provide a distinctly different and better option.

Spasticity is a pathological phenomenon of velocity-dependent increased muscle tone resulting from upper motor neuron injury or dysfunction. Although research related to spasticity has occurred for decades, it was James W. Lance who in 1970 rendered the definition most accepted today that spasticity is "a motor disorder characterized by a velocity-dependent increase in tonic stretch reflexes with exaggerated tendon jerks, resulting from hyper-excitability of the stretch reflex, as one component of the upper motor neuron syndrome."[1] Spasticity may arise as related to pathology of either spinal or cerebral origin. Spinal cord damage by trauma, ischemia, inflammation, demyelination, tumor, and so on may give rise to spasticity. The effects of spasticity are seen below the level of the spinal cord lesion. Spasticity may also result if the brain has been injured by trauma, stroke, disease (e.g., multiple sclerosis), a congenital condition (e.g., cerebral palsy), anoxia, or tumor. However, spasticity from cerebral origin can be variable such that all muscle groups may not be affected equally. There may be differences from one side to the other or from the upper to the lower extremities. Failure of descending central neural inhibition to the stretch reflex is thought to ultimately result in spasticity.

In the treatment of patients with spasticity, oral antispasmodics such as benzodiazepines, tizanidine, Dantrium, and baclofen are commonly used. However, baclofen is most commonly selected for IT delivery if a patient has failed oral therapy because of a lack of efficacy, intolerable side effects, or both.

Anatomy

Spinal anatomy as it relates to methods of trials for considering IDDS is especially relevant. As discussed in the Technique section below, a trial medication may be administered into either the epidural or IT space. Review of the anatomy as it relates to the administration of intraspinal medications is important to understand appropriate dosing as well as effects that may be expected (**Fig. 9-1**).

The spinal canal surrounding the spinal cord is composed of three layers: dura mater, arachnoid, and pia mater. The pia mater directly contacts and overlies the spinal cord. The dura mater and arachnoid are adhered together and separated from the pia mater

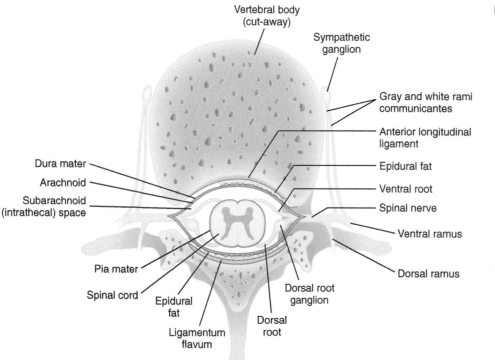

Fig. 9-1 Spinal anatomy.

Vertebral body (cut-away)
Sympathetic ganglion
Gray and white rami communicantes
Anterior longitudinal ligament
Epidural fat
Ventral root
Spinal nerve
Ventral ramus
Dorsal ramus
Dura mater
Arachnoid
Subarachnoid (intrathecal) space
Pia mater
Spinal cord
Epidural fat
Ligamentum flavum
Dorsal root
Dorsal root ganglion

by a large subarachnoid, or IT, space filled with cerebrospinal fluid (CSF). Within the bony spinal canal posterior to the dura mater and anterior to the lamina is located the ligamentum flavum. Between the dura mater and the ligamentum flavum is the epidural space, which contains fat and the posterior internal venous plexus. The IT and epidural spaces are of particular relevance for the purpose of trials.

Administration of a medication directly into the IT space allows the medication to freely mix with CSF and circulate via bulk flow throughout the spinal canal. This is especially true for hydrophilic medications such as morphine, hydromorphone, baclofen, and ziconotide. Because of low lipid solubility and high hydrophilicity, these medications enter the lipid substance of the spinal cord more slowly, thus remaining free in the CSF, allowing for circulation throughout the spinal column. This also accounts for the greater potential of hydrophilic medications to cause adverse events (e.g., sedation, nausea, vomiting, respiratory depression) because bulk flow of CSF may distribute the medication to supraspinal centers. For highly lipophilic medications such as fentanyl and sufentanil, the lipid-containing spinal cord is entered more rapidly, and medication is eliminated from the CSF quicker. Therefore, although lipophilic medications may be an option for an IDDS, a clinician must carefully consider the method of administration for a trial. For example, a single bolus would likely not yield a successful trial because safety would prohibit IT administration at any location cephalad to the L1 spinal level as discussed below. An epidural single bolus trial would potentially be feasible with a lipophilic opioid; however, the best trial method most closely resembling that of an IDDS with a lipophilic opioid would be placement of an IT catheter with the tip positioned at the spinal level of greatest nociception. For a lipophilic medication trial, anatomy can therefore have everything to do with potential success or failure.

The epidural space is a potential space located between the ligamentum flavum and the dura mater. Administration of a medication directly into the epidural space allows the medication to diffuse across the dura mater and arachnoid into the IT space. The medication may then directly act upon receptors on the spinal cord. There is also greater potential for systemic side effects as medication is also taken up by the epidural internal venous plexus.

Spinal cord anatomy is of particular importance when considering lumbar puncture for administration of an IT trial. Understanding the basics of spinal anatomy will allow the clinician to hopefully avoid causing a potentially devastating neurological injury. The spinal cord extends about 45 cm (or 18 inches) from the medulla oblongata at the base of the brain caudad through the bony spine to a level between the first and second lumbar vertebrae, where it ends as the conus medullaris. Examining the variation of position of the conus medullaris in an adult population by magnetic resonance imaging (MRI), Saifuddin et al[2] found the mean conus position at the lower third of L1 with a distribution ranging from the middle third of T12 to the upper third of L3.[2] The exception to this could be in tethered cord syndromes when a tethered filum terminale pulls the spinal cord lower in the spinal canal with the growth of the individual.[3] Recognizing that the majority of a patient population will have a conus terminating at approximately the vertebral level of L1-L2, the clinician must plan for lumbar puncture at L2-L3 or below to avoid potential complications of spinal cord injury with needle placement.

Basic Science

There are currently only three medications approved by the FDA for use with IDDS (**Box 9-1**). For discussion about the

> ### Box 9-1: Medications Approved by the U.S. Food and Drug Administration for Intrathecal Drug Delivery Systems
>
> Preservative-free morphine sulfate sterile solution
> Intrathecal baclofen injection (Lioresal)
> Preservative-free ziconotide sterile solution (Prialt)

pharmacology of these medications, please review Chapters 2, 3, and 27. Clinicians may use these medications in addition to numerous other off-label medications in IDDS. For the purpose of trials, however, single medications are usually administered. The pharmacology of morphine is based on its predominant interaction with the opioid μ-receptor. The pharmacology of baclofen is such that it is thought to bind to presynaptic γ-aminobutyric acid type B receptors (GABA-B) within the brainstem and dorsal horn of the spinal cord. The pharmacology of ziconotide is unique as a pain medication in that it is not an opioid agonist. Ziconotide was approved by the FDA in December 2004 for the management of severe chronic pain. It is a neuroactive peptide that is the synthetic equivalent of the ω conopeptide MVIIA found in the toxin secreted by the magician's cone snail *Conus magus*. The antinociceptive mechanism of action in animals by ziconotide is through inhibition of primary nociceptive afferent neurons via blockade of N-type calcium channels. Although ziconotide has been demonstrated to block human N-type calcium channels in vitro,[4] the exact mechanism of action contributing to analgesia in humans has not been elucidated.

Imaging

When considering IDDS, imaging may be quite helpful and necessary for the clinician to safely and effectively perform the trial. There are two primary imaging considerations. First, is imaging of the spine appropriate before performing a trial? Second, is imaging (fluoroscopic guidance) required during a trial?

In a patient with a known history of spinal surgery or deformity, plain radiographs, computed tomography, or even MRI may be appropriate to visualize the anatomy before needle placement. This may be especially helpful for a clinician who may be performing a blind (non–fluoroscopic guided) trial by single bolus (either epidural or IT) in the ambulatory setting. By having spinal imaging available, needle placement may be thoughtfully planned to try to avoid complications, enhance patient comfort, and ultimately ensure a technically successful trial, although this method is not recommended.

The use of fluoroscopic guidance for the placement of an epidural or IT catheter must be used when performing a trial. Not only will fluoroscopic guidance aid the clinician in the technical placement of the needle, but imaging will also allow direct visualization of the location of the catheter to verify that it is positioned at the anatomical level desired. Without imaging, it is impossible to precisely ascertain where a catheter may have gone after it has been threaded through a needle.

Guidelines

There are no current guidelines related to methods of trials for consideration of IDDS. IT medication guidelines do exist[5] but are not discussed here. Knight et al[6] described recommended doses for continuous IT catheter trials. It was suggested that morphine sulfate be initiated at 0.2 mg/day with titration to approximately 2 mg/day. Hydromorphone could be started at 0.3 mg/day and titrated to effect. A ceiling dose was not described, but clinically, either sufficient pain improvement or adverse events would bring an end to the trial. Trials were recommended over 2 to 3 days. Certainly, the starting dose of trial medication as well as the optimal dose will very likely be impacted by the dose of systemic (oral or transdermal) medication that the patient was taking before the trial. It has not been described within the literature at what dose an opioid or baclofen trial should be considered a failure. Inherently, a failed opioid trial would not obtain acceptable pain relief before intolerable side effects were present.

Fortunately, when performing a baclofen trial, objective measures do exist for assessing a patient's response. Although this has not been specified within literature guidelines, in general, IT baclofen trials via single bolus are given initially as 25 to 50 µg and do not exceed 100 µg. Pediatric dosing may be even lower with doses down to 12.5 µg.[7] Specific dosing guidelines for continuous catheter trials with baclofen have not been described.

Indications and Contraindications

The indications for considering a trial of IT drug delivery for the treatment of either spasticity or pain share similarities (Box 9-2). If a patient is not experiencing a therapeutic effect from systemic (oral, transdermal, or intravenous) medications or is experiencing dose-limiting side effects, then a trial to consider an IDDS is appropriate. For example, in a patient with spasticity caused by a spinal cord injury who is becoming sedated because of a high dose of oral baclofen (i.e., >100 mg/day) without obtaining a desired reduction in spasticity, then IT administration of baclofen via a trial would be very appropriate to assess for an IDDS. Similarly, in a patient with chronic pain who is experiencing sedation, short-term memory loss, constipation, and/or nausea without adequate analgesia because of high-dose systemic opioids, then consideration of a trial for an IDDS is certainly appropriate.

Although a patient may meet the indication criteria noted above, clinicians must be sure that a contraindication would not rule out a potential trial. Contraindications that must be weighed when selecting patients to trial for IDDS are listed in Box 9-3.[8]

In patients with either systemic or occult infections, there is risk during even a single-bolus trial of spreading infection into the spinal axis, potentially causing meningitis. This risk would be even greater with an indwelling catheter during a trial. Patients with malignant pain caused by cancer with encroachment of tumor within the spinal canal risk an unsuccessful trial because CSF may not be able to circulate and adequately distribute the medication

throughout the spinal canal. This is particularly true for hydrophilic medications and perhaps less pertinent for lipophilic medication; nonetheless, advancing tumor within the spinal canal remains a contraindication.

Particularly thin or emaciated patients are contraindicated because of concern for skin breakdown if they undergo permanent IDDS implant. An eroded pump through the skin would require urgent explant out of concern for infection at the site and potentially meningitis if left unchecked. Surgical techniques have been described, specifically subfascial pump placement, to prevent skin erosion in emaciated patients.[9] This may be particularly helpful in children undergoing implant for administration of IT baclofen for spasticity because they are generally of small stature and body habitus.

An allergy to the device materials in an IDDS or sensitivity to medications that may be used would also prohibit a potential trial. Because implantable pumps are made from inert materials such as titanium and plastic, allergy to the materials is exceedingly rare. In patients with documented sensitivities or allergies to metals, a test strip of the pump components may be obtained from the manufacturer for allergy testing before a trial. Although sensitivity or allergy to a medication (i.e., morphine) would prevent its consideration for use in a trial, another medication could certainly be used (i.e., hydromorphone or ziconotide).

Equipment

The equipment necessary for conducting a trial depends on the type of trial being conducted. Appropriate antiseptic for skin preparation, local anesthetic, needles, trial medication, and potentially an epidural or IT catheter are all materials that may be required. Fluoroscopic imaging requires the use of a fluoroscope. If trial medication is to be dispensed through either an epidural or IT catheter, an external infusion pump is also required.

Technique

The possible techniques for trialing medications when considering IDDS is varied. During the trial, the planned medication is administered to assess for efficacy and potential adverse events. A trial may be IT or epidural with advantages and disadvantages of delivering the medication into each of these spaces (Table 9-1). From this basic division, trials may be further separated into those that are single bolus, multiple single boluses over time, or administered continuously via a catheter (Fig. 9-2). The choice for how a trial is carried out may depend on the patient, the clinician, and resources within the health care system.

IT trials administering continuous medication via an indwelling catheter offer the best opportunity to assess a patient for drug efficacy versus side effects because this exactly replicates the administration route of an implanted pump. During an IT catheter trial, the catheter tip should be placed fluoroscopically at the level where the permanent catheter is planned. Similarly, for an epidural trial, the catheter tip should be placed fluoroscopically at the level of greatest nociception where placement of the permanent IT catheter is ultimately planned. Catheter tip placement is also of vital importance for IT baclofen trials; however, this is discussed in detail in Chapter 20. Of note, epidural baclofen trials have not been described in the literature.

Administering a trial in the form of a bolus, either single or multiple over time, also allows for assessment of efficacy and adverse events. There are pros and cons to bolus trials. Positive attributes include decreased cost, ability to perform in an

---

Box 9-2: Indications for Considering a Trial for Intrathecal Drug Delivery Systems

Inadequate therapeutic effect of systemic medications
Dose-limiting side effects

Box 9-3: Contraindications When Considering a Trial for Intrathecal Drug Delivery Systems[14]

Systemic infection
Occult infection
Tumor encroachment of the spinal canal
Emaciation
Allergy to the device materials
Sensitivity to medications that may be used in an IDDS

IDDS, intrathecal drug delivery system.

Table 9-1: Trialing Methods: Potential Advantages and Disadvantages

Trialing Method	Single Bolus	Multiple Boluses	Catheter
Epidural Advantages	• Quick • Inexpensive • Avoids dural puncture	• Quick • Inexpensive • Avoids dural puncture • Able to better estimate effective starting dose for IDDS	• Avoids dural puncture • Improved assessment of response over time • Able to better estimate effective starting dose for IDDS during trial titration
Disadvantages	• Not the same space (epidural vs. IT) • Not the same delivery as IDDS (bolus vs. infusion)	• Not the same space (epidural vs. IT) • Not the same delivery as IDDS (bolus vs. infusion)	• Not the same space (epidural vs. IT) • Time consuming • Expensive • Potential increased risk of complications
Intrathecal Advantages	• Quick • Inexpensive • Same space as IDDS	• Quick • Inexpensive • Same space as IDDS	• Best assessment of response over time • Best estimate of effective starting dose for IDDS during trial titration
Disadvantages	• Not the same delivery as IDDS (bolus vs. infusion)	• Not the same delivery as IDDS (bolus vs. infusion)	• Time consuming • Expensive • Potential increased risk of complications

IDDS, intrathecal drug delivery systems; IT, intrathecal.

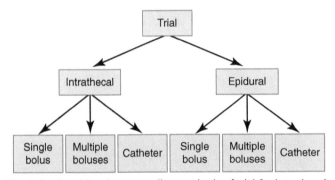

Fig. 9-2 Considerations regarding methods of trial for intrathecal drug delivery systems.

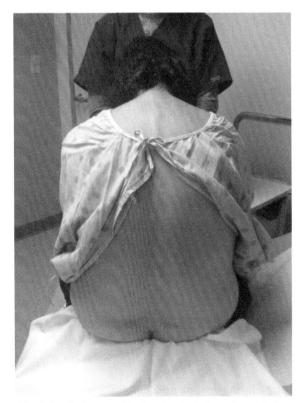

Fig. 9-3 Patient positioning for single intrathecal bolus.

outpatient setting, and ease for the patient and clinician. A negative attribute is that these methods less closely resemble the continuous infusion offered by IDDS. A bolus administered allows the patient and clinician to observe the effects of the medication, but especially when using an opioid to trial for chronic pain, the risks of adverse events are potentially greater. Because clinicians are reliant on patients' self-reports of pain, there may also be a greater potential for a placebo effect during a single bolus trial.

The technical aspects of performing a trial for IDDS depend on the type of trial. Single- or multiple-bolus trials for IT administration of the planned medication use the technique of lumbar puncture that has been well described elsewhere. **Figs. 9-3 to 9-10** demonstrate pictorially the administration of a single IT bolus. Similarly, epidural administration via a single or multiple bolus would require epidural access using techniques described previously, such as "loss of resistance."

The placement of a catheter for a trial of IDDS requires more resources, equipment, and planning than the bolus technique. **Fig. 9-11** shows basic placement of an epidural catheter. A catheter may additionally be tunneled to decrease infection risk as shown in **Fig. 9-12**. In addition to placing an epidural or IT catheter, an external infusion pump is required to administer the planned medication and allow for dose titration. If the catheter is to be placed IT, it is recommended to use the smallest gauge catheter feasible to try to avoid a postdural puncture headache (PDPH). A double-catheter technique has also been described for an IT medication trial.[10] This method involves placement of simultaneous IT and epidural catheters. The reasoning for this technique is to have the ability to treat a PDPH promptly during the trial if one develops.

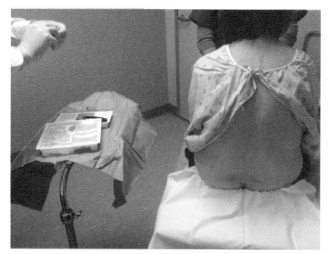

Fig. 9-4 Preparing the equipment.

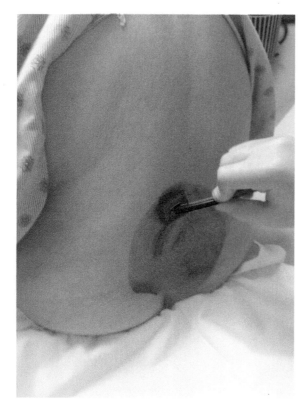

Fig. 9-5 Prepping the patient's lumbar region.

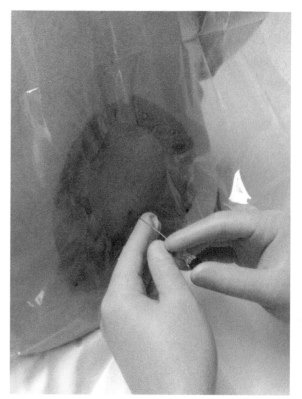

Fig. 9-6 Inserting the spinal needle.

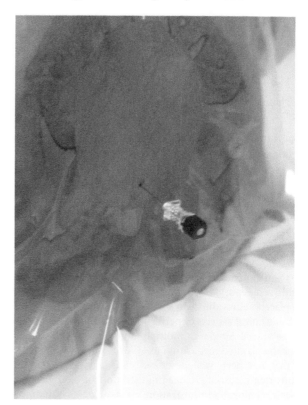

Fig. 9-7 The spinal needle is advanced until cerebrospinal fluid is obtained.

Patient Management and Evaluation

Depending on the type of trial being performed, the management as well as the evaluation of the patient may vary. The administration of baclofen versus an opioid will result in different desired effects and adverse events. The methods by which a clinician evaluates a person with spasticity versus pain during a trial also differs.

When trialing an adult patient with baclofen for spasticity using the single-bolus technique, a range of 50 to 100 µg baclofen is commonly administered. The primary endpoint for evaluation of spasticity reduction is improvement by at least 1 point on the Modified Ashworth Scale. Secondary endpoints during IT baclofen trial include functional improvement (i.e., increased gait speed,

improved gait efficiency), reduced pain, and facilitated ease of care. After the injection of baclofen, these endpoints may be evaluated over the time period of the medication's effects. The effects of a single injection of baclofen may be seen as soon as 30 minutes, usually peak around 4 hours postinjection, and resolve within

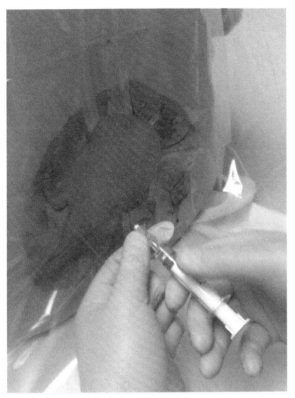

Fig. 9-8   Attaching the syringe with trial medication.

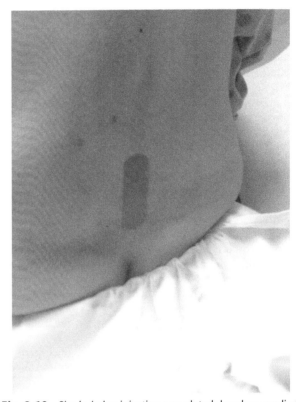

Fig. 9-10   Single-bolus injection completed; bandage applied.

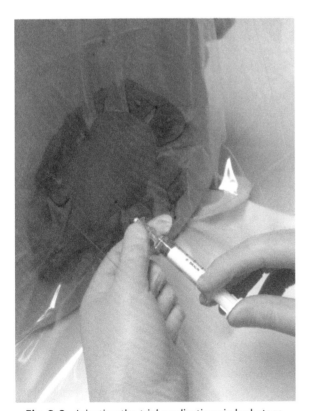

Fig. 9-9   Injecting the trial medication via barbotage.

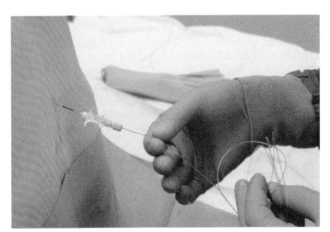

Fig. 9-11   Epidural catheter placement through a Tuohy needle.

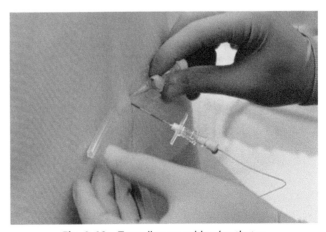

Fig. 9-12   Tunneling an epidural catheter.

about 8 hours. Therefore, the examination of a patient may occur at any point along this timeframe.

In the author's experience, examination of a patient 3 to 4 hours after a single injection allows sufficient documentation of the desired spasticity reduction. Additionally, little monitoring is required during this assessment period. It is certainly appropriate to obtain basic vital signs before any procedure, including an IT trial. It is also appropriate to have the necessary resuscitative equipment and medications available in case they are (rarely) required. In more than 100 IT baclofen single-bolus trials, no adverse events were seen with the exception of PDPHs in fewer than 5% of patients, which resolved with conservative treatment (unpublished data).

When trialing IT baclofen in children, bolus administration has been found to be adequate with doses ranging from 12.5 to 50 μg.[7] These doses are sufficient to reduce muscle tone, diminish pain, and assist ease of care. Although slight lethargy and lowered CSF pressure have been reported, respiratory depression has not. A review of the literature was unsuccessful in finding respiratory depression associated with baclofen trials in the dosing ranges noted above. There has been report of respiratory depression associated with IT baclofen bolus injections of 500 to 1000 μg for the treatment of tetanus[11]; however, this is 10 times the usual dosing range of trials for spasticity.

Although single-bolus IT baclofen trials are often performed because of their ease and cost, a continuous catheter trial offers the potential to most closely mimic how a patient will respond with an IDDS. This is a distinct advantage over bolus trials even though catheter trials are more time consuming and expensive. Catheter trials entail placement of a catheter (either epidural or IT, as discussed previously in the Technique section) with dose titration usually over 1 to 3 days. This may occur in the inpatient or outpatient setting, depending on the resources of the health system. Currently, guidelines recommending the duration of a continuous catheter trial for baclofen or opioids do not exist, so this remains at the discretion of the clinician. Ultimately, the duration of a continuous catheter trial would likely depend on the response of the patient to the trial medication or the presence of adverse events that would halt the trial. Of note, baclofen trials are covered in detail in Chapter 22.

Managing and evaluating a patient during an opioid trial carries different considerations than for an IT baclofen trial. The appropriate dose for either an epidural or IT opioid trial must be individualized for each patient based on his or her systemic medication dose, age, and medical comorbidities. Conversion for systemic morphine doses to intraspinal doses has been described by Krames[12] and is generally accepted for clinical use (**Fig. 9-13**). Further equianalgesic

conversion of morphine to hydromorphone is on a five to one basis.

The greatest concern in patient management during an opioid trial is avoidance of respiratory depression. Although these concerns are well documented in acute and perioperative pain literature, there is little or no literature studying respiratory depression associated with bolus or catheter trials in opioid-tolerant patients with chronic pain, malignant or nonmalignant. One prospective, randomized, double-blind, dose-response study examining the opioid related side effects after IT morphine single bolus was found upon literature search.[13] However, this study used opioid-naïve patients with chronic nonmalignant back pain who received a range of 0.015 to 0.25 mg IT via a single bolus. Clinically significant respiratory depression (respiratory rate <6 breaths/min) was not reported. Although respiratory depression certainly remains a concern, in the opioid-tolerant population that undergo an epidural or IT trial, there is likely less risk involved than in the opioid-naïve population. Of the two potential trial methods, bolus or continuous catheter, a bolus trial carries a greater potential risk of adverse events, including respiratory depression due to a higher C_{max} (maximum concentration) from administration of the dose all at once.

Another significant issue related to evaluation of opioid trials is that results depend on the patient's and physician's interpretation of response and as well as expectations. When assessing pain, there is an unfortunate lack of objective measures to lead the patient and clinician to determine what is a "successful" trial versus a "failure."

In general, the expectations for a successful trial should be the reduction of at least 50% of the patient's typical pain compared with before the trial. Clinicians often additionally assess for functional improvement during a trial. This may include discussing with the patient whether during the trial it was noted that ambulation, activities of daily living, and instrumental activities of daily living were performed with greater ease. By using additional functional markers as criteria for a successful trial, a degree of objectivity is introduced into an otherwise subjective interpretation.

Another method for assessing a patient's response during a trial is to evaluate for a decrease in the need for breakthrough pain medication. For example, if a patient typically uses five or six tablets of a given immediate-release medication throughout the day for breakthrough pain and this is reduced to one or two tablets per day during the trial period, this reduction in dose is objective evidence that may indicate a positive trial. It has not been described by how much breakthrough pain medication should be reduced during a trial to assist with interpreting a trial as successful. This ultimately would be at the discretion of the clinician and likely not used as sole criteria for deciding whether a trial is successful. Rather, this information could be used in conjunction with subjective reductions in the report of pain along with functional improvement.

The subjectivity with which how opioid trials may be interpreted may lead to improper patient selection and the implantation of IDDS that will yield poor outcomes. This would be very unfortunate because data exist demonstrating the efficacy of IDDS over comprehensive medical management.[14] However, a clinician who strives to gather the best data available by assessing a patient's pain reduction, functional improvement, and reduction in breakthrough pain medication will likely have the greatest opportunity for appropriately evaluating a patient and interpreting a trial as a success or failure.

A variety of methods have been described to trial ziconotide. A recent review of ziconotide trialing methods identified three techniques: bolus injection, limited-duration infusion, and continuous

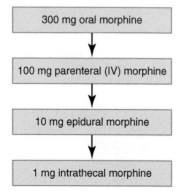

Fig. 9-13 Intraspinal morphine conversion ratios. IV, intravenous.[5]

300 mg oral morphine

↓

100 mg parenteral (IV) morphine

↓

10 mg epidural morphine

↓

1 mg intrathecal morphine

infusion via an IT catheter.[15] Results found that patients often obtained successful analgesia during trialing regardless of the trial method. Although all three options described are viable for ziconotide trials, further controlled studies comparing each method are needed.

Outcomes Evidence

Attempt has been made by the author to cite evidence throughout this chapter as relevant to the section topics. As directly related to this chapter's topic, there are no systematic reviews, retrospective or prospective studies, or case reports discussing outcomes as related to the various methods of trials for consideration of IDDS.

Risk and Complication Avoidance

A number of potential risks and complications may be associated with trials for an IDDS, depending on the type of trial method performed. Some of these risks have already been outlined. Whether proceeding with a bolus trial or a continuous catheter trial, potential complications may be classified as mechanical (related to the technique or equipment), pharmacological (the medication used), and medical (e.g., infection, edema, anticoagulation).

Mechanical complications may occur during needle placement for either an epidural or IT bolus trial. There are additional risks if a catheter is placed. With either trial method (bolus versus catheter), neurological injury, bleeding, infection, or PDPH could occur. Even if a clinician is performing an epidural trial, an accidental dural puncture could result in headache. Certainly, if a dural puncture is planned, then the likelihood of a PDPH may be greater. Although this is written about extensively within the obstetrical literature, there is a paucity of data regarding planned (nonaccidental) dural puncture for the purpose of a trial for IDDS and whether this may result in a PDPH. It has been demonstrated that use of a blunt-tip needle (i.e., Sprotte) versus a beveled cutting needle (i.e., Quincke) reduces the incidence of PDPHs.[16]

Pharmacological complications associated with a trial could also occur. A patient may have an allergic reaction to the trial medication. A patient could be accidentally overdosed by either receiving a planned single-bolus dose that was too high or if a concentration error was made in preparing the medication, thereby giving the patient a much higher dose than ordered. If a patient is undergoing a catheter trial, erroneous programming of the external pump could also result in an overdose.

Medical complications could occur on many levels. Contamination of the trial medication could inadvertently cause a devastating infection. The patient may have the adverse event of edema caused by the trial medication (seen most commonly with opioids). Bleeding is usually self-limited, but in patients who are anticoagulated, further challenge is placed on the clinician to conduct a safe trial. Evidence-based guidelines exist for guidance regarding patients receiving antithrombotic or thrombolytic therapy.[17]

Although it is probably less likely a concern during a trial, patients receiving IT opioids have been found to have changes in their neuroendocrine function.[18] The majority of patients developed hypogonadotropic hypogonadism with fewer developing central hypocortisolism. These changes were seen in patients receiving long-term IT therapy; hormone replacement improved these effects. However, because a trial is potentially the beginning of the road of lifelong therapy, this should at least be discussed with patients.

In summary, methods of trials for consideration of IDDS are varied, and the chosen method for any given person will likely depend on the patient, clinician, and health care system. The manner in which a trial is conducted is of utmost importance to ensure the greatest chance of success for the therapy and ultimately the patient. Putting all of the elements in place for a trial allows the patient to potentially experience what will become a life-changing therapy.

References

1. Lance JW: Spasticity: disordered motor control. In Feldman RG, Young RR, Koella WP, editors: *Symposium synopsis*, Chicago, 1980, Year Book, p 485.
2. Saifuddin A, Burnett SJ, White J: The variation of position of the conus medullaris in an adult population. A magnetic resonance imaging study. *Spine* 23(13):1452-1456, 1998.
3. Fitz CR, Harwood Nash DC: The tethered conus. *Am J Roentgenol Radium Ther Nucl Med* 125(3):515-523, 1975.
4. Bleakman D, Bowman D, Bath CP, et al: Characteristics of a human N-type calcium channel expressed in HEK293 cells. *Neuropharmacology* 34(7):753-765, 1995.
5. Deer T, Krames ES, Hassenbusch SJ, et al: Polyanalgesic Consensus Conference 2007: recommendations for the management of pain by intrathecal (intraspinal) drug delivery: report of an interdisciplinary expert panel. *Neuromodulation* 10:300-328, 2007.
6. Knight K, Brand F, Mchaourab A, et al: Implantable pumps for chronic pain: highlights and updates. *Croat Med J* 48(1):22-34, 2007.
7. Hoving MA, van Raak EP, Spincemaille GH, et al: Intrathecal baclofen in children with spastic cerebral palsy: a double-blind, randomized, placebo-controlled dose-finding study. *Dev Med Child Neurol* 49(9):654-659, 2007.
8. Krames ES, Olsen K: Clinical realities and economic considerations: patient selection in intrathecal therapy. *J Pain Symptom Manage* 14(3 suppl):S3-S13, 1997.
9. Albright AL, Turner M, Pattisapu JV: Best-practice surgical techniques for intrathecal baclofen therapy. *J Neurosurg* 104(4 suppl):S233-S239, 2006.
10. Burton AW, Hassenbusch SJ: The double-catheter technique for intrathecal medication trial: a brief technical note and report of five cases. *Pain Med* 2(4):352-354, 2001.
11. Saissy JM, Demazière J, Vitris M, et al: Treatment of severe tetanus by intrathecal injections of baclofen without artificial ventilation. *Intensive Care Med* 18(4):241-244, 1992.
12. Krames ES: Intraspinal opioid therapy for chronic nonmalignant pain: current practice and clinical guidelines. *J Pain Symptom Manage* 11(6):333-352, 1996.
13. Raffaeli W, Marconi G, Favelli G, et al: Opioid-related side-effects after intrathecal morphine: a prospective, randomized, double-blind dose-response study. *Eur J Anaesthesiol* 23(7):605-610, 2006.
14. Smith TJ, Staats PS, Deer T, et al: Randomized clinical trial of an implantable drug delivery system compared with comprehensive medical management for refractory cancer pain: impact on pain, drug-related toxicity, and survival. *J Clin Oncol* 20(19):4040-4049, 2002.
15. Burton AW, Deer TR, Wallace MS, et al: Considerations and methodology for trialing ziconotide. *Pain Physician* 13(1):23-33, 2010.
16. Strupp M, Schueler O, Straube A, et al: "Atraumatic" Sprotte needle reduces the incidence of post-lumbar puncture headaches. *Neurology* 57(12):2310-2312, 2001.
17. Horlocker TT, Wedel DJ, Rowlingson JC, et al: Regional anesthesia in the patient receiving antithrombotic or thrombolytic therapy: American Society of Regional Anesthesia and Pain Medicine Evidence-Based Guidelines (third edition). *Reg Anesth Pain Med* 35(1):64-101, 2010.
18. Abs R, Verhelst J, Maeyaert J, et al: Endocrine consequences of long-term intrathecal administration of opioids. *J Clin Endocrinol Metab* 85(6):2215-2222, 2000.

10 Techniques of Implant Placement for Intrathecal Pumps

Asokumar Buvanendran, Matthew Jaycox, and Timothy R. Deer

CHAPTER OVERVIEW

Chapter Synopsis: Surgical placement of an intrathecal (IT) catheter and pump in a patient who has had a successful trial needs meticulous attention. This chapter details patient position and various approaches to IT catheter placement and discusses the options for pump location and placement. The risks and benefits for the location of the pump placement and measures that can be undertaken to avoid common complications are also discussed.

Important Points:
- The patient should be carefully selected for IT drug infusion before the technical aspects of the procedure are considered.
- The location of the pump should be considered before implant based on patient comfort, anatomy, and surgical challenges.
- The catheter and needle should be placed using a paramedian approach with a needle placement below the conus when possible.
- The catheter should be secured with both a purse-string suture and an anchor to the surrounding tissue.
- Pocketing should be carefully planned to ensure it places the pump in the appropriate tissue plane with an appropriately sized pocket to accommodate the pump volume without tension or laxity.
- Surgical sterility needs to be maintained at all times.

Clinical Pearl: The pain physician should check for the presence of CSF frequently during the surgical procedure.

Clinical Pitfall: Lack of CSF from the side port before closing the pump site necessitates re-exploring the entire catheter and connections of the catheter to the pump to ensure free flow of CSF.

Introduction

Chief among the considerations regarding intrathecal (IT) drug pump implantation technique are patient positioning (e.g., lateral decubitus vs prone); type of anesthetic; IT needle entry point; eventual catheter tip location; site of pump placement; and a knowledge of the patient's lumbar spine anatomy, including history of any prior spine surgery or pathology.[1,2] The technique to place a permanent pump and catheter should be performed in an operating room under sterile conditions. Intravenous antibiotics should be administered and should cover skin flora based on susceptibilities in the local environment.

Site of Pump Implantation

In the majority of patients, the only anatomical location that can reasonably accommodate the size of the pump is the lower quadrant of the left or right abdomen. Thus, most patients are positioned in the lateral decubitus fashion to allow for exposure of this field. In select patients, one may choose to implant the reservoir pump in the posterior flank (**Fig. 10-1**). There are some considerations that may drive one toward favoring this latter site. For instance, if a patient is morbidly obese with a large panniculus, anchoring the pump to adequately prevent flipping or rotation may be very difficult, if not impossible. If the anchoring fascial layer cannot be reached reliably without proceeding beyond a depth of 2.5 cm, communication with the device and accessing the refill port postoperatively may be

compromised.[1,3] This complication may be mitigated therefore by posterior flank implantation above the buttock, where there is often less excess tissue. Another consideration occurs in the case of re-implantation because of a pump pocket wound infection or painful pump site. In the case of a prior wound infection, re-implantation into the prior wound site is ill advised, so one is left with the contralateral abdomen or the posterior flank.[4] The relative proximity of the lower abdomen to the groin must be considered given the prior history of infection; therefore one may choose to place the pump at a pocket site away from this area. A painful pump site that is not caused by mechanical disruption of the pump by bony prominences such as the costal margin or iliac bone may be addressed by relocation of the pump to the posterior flank. This is a technically simpler procedure than relocation to the contralateral abdomen, which would require replacement of part if not the whole catheter. The posterior flank is easier from a purely technical surgical standpoint, given that the patient will be positioned prone. However, patient interaction with the device postoperatively may be more difficult. In patients who have had extensive surgery in the abdomen such as those with visceral tumors, the abdomen may not be an option, but this is a rare clinical situation. Thus, most patients will have the IT pump implanted in the lower quadrant of the left or right abdomen and as a consequence will be positioned in the lateral decubitus position.

Before choosing the site, one should have a discussion with the patient regarding pump site location. The anatomic constraints are

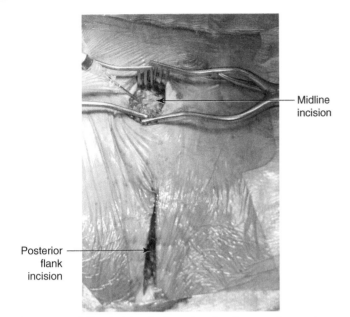

Fig. 10-1   Midline incision for intrathecal catheter and posterior flank.

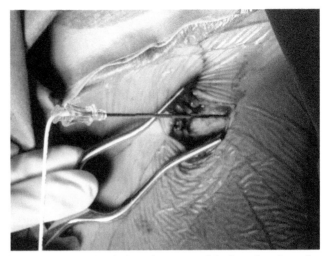

Fig. 10-2   Dissection before placement of the intrathecal needle and catheter.

the bony borders of the iliac crest, the symphysis pubis, and the costal margin. None of these should come in contact with the pump when the patient is seated because of discomfort and risk of damage to the pump or catheter.[1,3,5] Therefore marking the patient in the seated or standing position should be done preoperatively. Non-anatomic constraints include the patient's waistline and belt line and should be taken into account during marking. With the rise in popularity of patient-activated medication bolusing remotes, patients may have a preference for abdominal placement on their own left- or right-handedness. Having a sample of such a bolusing device available to the patient preoperatively may aid their decision. In patients with advanced scoliosis, the physician should consider the rib to pelvic angle and the potential for progression of the scoliosis over time.

When the pump is implanted in the lower abdominal quadrant below the belt line, it is also important to not place the pump too deep because it may lead to problems in interrogation and refilling of the pump. The pump pocket incision should be made to approximate the size of the pump. The incision can be carried down to the rectus fascia in thin patients. This is followed by tunneling through the subcutaneous tissues from the pump pocket to the posterior incision. This must be done carefully to prevent accidental puncture of the peritoneum and possibly pleura.

Type of Anesthesia

With regards to anesthesia, most favor local anesthesia with sedation because it allows rapid recovery after the procedure, as well as quick assessment of neurological status intraoperatively if any concern arises.[1,3] Permanent placement can be performed under local, spinal, or general anesthesia, but general anesthesia is usually chosen to ensure a more pleasant experience for the patient. Pressure points must be adequately padded and cared for to allow the patient to lie comfortably. If general anesthesia is chosen, ideally muscle relaxation would be held until after needle and catheter instrumentation of the spine is complete to allow for assessment of neurological status.[3,6] The absence of muscle relaxants will not always predict nerve irritation, and vigilance should be given to the

needle placement and catheter course by careful fluoroscopic guidance.

Surgical Technique

If the lateral decubitus position is selected for implantation, the side desired for abdominal pocketing should be upright. The surgical field should be widely prepped and draped well outside of the planned incision. The C-arm fluoroscope should be draped in a sterile fashion and positioned to provide a true anteroposterior view of the spine. Fluoroscopy can be used to identify the L2-L3, L3-L4, or L4-L5 levels. A level below the terminal portion of the spinal cord is recommended when possible. The entry level chosen will be guided partly by ease of access as determined from fluoroscopy and ideally would be below the level of the spinal cord (L1). Most advocate entry at L2-L3 or L3-L4 because entry above these levels may risk spinal cord trauma, and entry below at L4-L5 or L5-S1 may lead to catheter malfunction as a result of the greater mobility of the spine at this level.[1,2,6] However, spine pathology and prior lumbar surgery may make this impractical and necessitate a more cephalad entry point such as the thoracic spine. If a high catheter is planned, one may not be able to adequately thread the catheter all the way from the lumbar region. Such approaches may carry increased risk to the spinal cord but may be necessary for a successful outcome.

After the entry level is chosen, the approach of the needle will be in a paramedian fashion, starting 2 cm laterally, at a shallow angle of approximately 30 to 45 degrees and 1 to 1.5 vertebral bodies below the intended interlaminar space selected for dural puncture. Having the catheter enter in a paramedian approach avoids the midline structures of the spinous processes and may reduce wear and tear on the catheter.[1,2,6] In addition, the catheter will have to pass through several layers of paravertebral muscle with this approach, which may mitigate the risk of persistent dural leak around the catheter.[3]

When considering entry into the spinal fluid, two approaches exist. The implanter could either make a 5-cm longitudinal incision in the skin just lateral to midline (**Fig. 10-2**) down to the dorsolumbar fascia and then when completed access the IT space using a Tuohy needle within the wound. Alternatively, one may percutaneously access the IT space using a Tuohy needle, document good cerebrospinal fluid (CSF) flow, and then following catheter

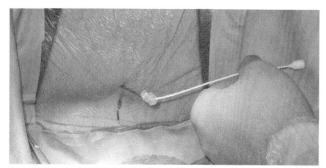

Fig. 10-3 Placement of the intrathecal needle and catheter before skin incision.

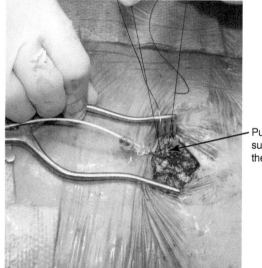

Purse-string suture around the needle

Fig. 10-5 Purse-string suture placed around the intrathecal needle.

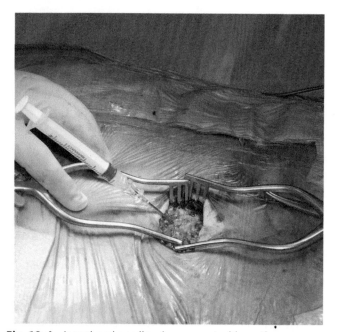

Fig. 10-4 Intrathecal needle advancement with continuous aspiration for cerebrospinal fluid.

placement through the needle (**Fig. 10-3**), incise down to the dorsolumbar fascia using a needle-within-incision technique. The first approach confers the advantage of being able to achieve hemostasis relatively easily using electrocautery before needle placement without the obvious risk of a nearby metal needle implanted in the spinal space.[1] In addition, with this technique, if accessing the IT space proves unexpectedly difficult, one may need to lengthen the incision, which could be undesirable.

When percutaneously approaching the dura in a paramedian fashion, the stylet of the needle should be kept in place and oriented with the bevel parallel to the longitudinal dural fibers to minimize the risk of persistent dural leak. After the dura is punctured, the stylet should be removed, and appropriate CSF backflow (**Fig. 10-4**) should be observed. A radiopaque guidewired catheter should be advanced carefully through the needle. Lateral fluoroscopy should demonstrate the catheter passing within the IT space. If the catheter must be withdrawn, it should not be done so through the introducer needle because this may shear or fracture the catheter.[1] When the tip of the catheter is at the desired location, the free end of the catheter should be secured to the drape with a rubbershod. If appropriate based on the approach taken, a 5-cm vertical incision should be made, incorporating the needle, and it should

be advanced to the dorsolumbar fascia, exposing the adjacent supraspinous ligament. The edges of the incision should be gently undermined using blunt dissection to allow for a smooth fascial plane for the anchoring hardware to rest in and to permit gentle bending of the catheter.

Before removing the needle, a purse-string suture should be placed with a non-absorbable suture (**Fig. 10-5**). The strategy for securing the catheter varies with some tying the suture after catheter removal and some before removal, with both techniques being acceptable. The CSF flow should be confirmed after the needle and stylet are removed and the suture is secured. Care should be taken to remove the needle and radiopaque guidewire together in one motion.[1-3,6] At this point, provided the intraspinal tip of the catheter is in an appropriate location, one may provide neuraxial anesthesia to the patient. This is a controversial method of providing anesthesia and should only be used in those with experience and comfort with spinal anesthesia. The majority of clinicians prefer to continue with monitored anesthesia care with supplemental sedation. If the clinician chooses to use a spinal approach, the local anesthetic may be administered through the in situ catheter using a 24-gauge angiocatheter inserted into the end of the IT catheter lumen.[1] This may provide superior patient comfort. A total of 7.5 to 10 mg of bupivacaine is usually sufficient for the remainder of the case, but the risks of this method should be considered.[1]

Attention is now turned to anchoring the catheter. Using a heavy nonabsorbable suture, such as 2-0 Silk or Ethibond, an anchoring suture is placed into the fascia as near as possible to the catheter entry point. The manufacturer-supplied anchor is slid over the catheter and secured to the fascia using the previous anchoring suture (**Figs. 10-6** and **10-7**). There are multiple different anchoring systems available, and securing of the anchor needs to be tailored to the specific model used. In general, though, the stitch should be secured to the fascia first and then to the anchor itself (**Fig. 10-7**). After it has been secured, good CSF flow from the catheter is redocumented and the catheter's end is clamped to prevent further CSF loss. The wound is irrigated and then packed with antibiotic-soaked gauze.

One should then direct attention to the lower quadrant of the abdomen and the desired pump pocket site (**Fig. 10-8**). If operating alone, it is advisable to place the IT catheter first and then fashion

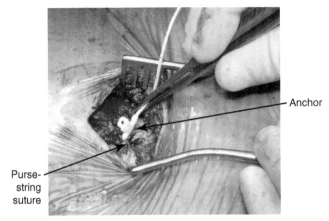

Fig. 10-6 Purse-string suture knot after intrathecal needle is removed.

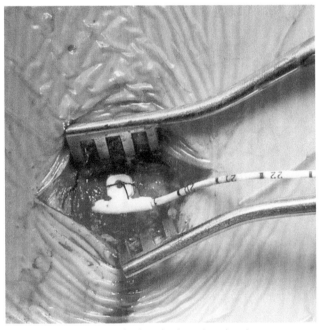

Fig. 10-7 Anchoring the intrathecal catheter.

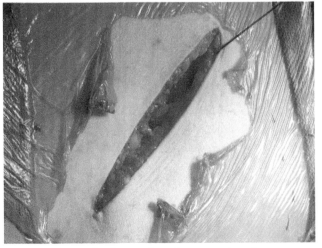

Fig. 10-8 Preparation of pump pocket site.

the pump pocket second. Then if the IT space is unable to be accessed or the catheter unable to be threaded, one is not left with an empty subcutaneous pump pocket.[1] The skin to be incised should be localized. A 10- to 12-cm transverse incision is made down to the subcutaneous layer beneath the superficial fatty plane of Camper's fascia and the membranous plane of Scarpa's fascia. The base of the pocket will usually be the fascia of the external oblique or the rectus abdominis, although some favor a subfascial placement in very thin patients.[1,2,7] Using blunt dissection, a subcutaneous pocket is fashioned in this plane big enough to accommodate the size of the chosen pump. Wrapping unwound gauze around a gloved hand can provide traction to aid in this task. Meticulous hemostasis will reduce the risk of postoperative hematoma and can be achieved using electrocautery.[4] The pocket should be created in a caudad direction and should be eccentric with regards to the incision. Therefore, the incision should not overlie the refill port on the device. If the refill port is clear of the incision, it will be easier to locate and feel. The superior edge of the incision is gently undermined for about 2 to 3 cm to reduce tension for eventual closure. The pocket can be size tested using the pump device, but in general, if one can fit four fingers up to the palm, the pocket is large enough. The pocket should be sufficiently large to permit placement of the pump device without difficulty but tight enough to prevent excess mobility of the pump. After it has been created, the pocket is irrigated and packed with antibiotic gauzes. Some authors are now favoring the placement of iodine-soaked gauzes at the wound edges to reduce the risk of infection.[6,8]

Next, attention should be turned to tunneling and passing the catheter. If the exposed catheter is long enough to reach the subcutaneous pump pocket and still allow for two tension-relief loops to be placed under the pump, then there is no need for extension tubing. If not, the distal tip of the catheter will need to be cut and spliced to connector tubing using a connector mechanism. In the former case, the malleable tunneler is used to tunnel from the midline back incision to the pump pocket site, and the spinal catheter is passed to the pump pocket (**Fig. 10-9**). With the catheter tunneled and passed, adequate CSF flow from the distal end is document. The catheter is then pulled through the tunnel to the pump pocket. It is very important to save any excised portions of catheter for volumetric calculations. Failure to do so could lead to a dosing error during the initial priming bolus of the catheter.

Next, the IT drug pump is prefilled with the desired medication, and the catheter extension or connector is secured to the pump. Unless it is a sutureless system, the connection should be reinforced to the pump using 2-0 silk ligatures. The sideport of the pump is accessed and CSF is withdrawn to ensure integrity of the system (**Figs. 10-10** and **10-11**).

Before placing the pump within the pocket, anchoring sutures must be placed within the base of the pocket (**Fig. 10-12**). The programmable pump will have metal anchoring loops around its circumference through which these anchoring sutures may be passed. These anchoring sutures should be made of heavy nonabsorbable suture and should be placed into the fascia. Two anchoring sutures are required to prevent rotation, and a minimum of three are required to prevent flipping.[1,3] Ideally, four anchoring sutures are placed into the base of the pocket. Alternatively, one may use a Dacron pouch placed around the pump. The Dacron pouch will ultimately endothelialize, assisting in forming a fibrous capsule around the pump. This will secure the pump but may make it difficult to remove in the future and may result in extensive scarring, making catheter revision or removal difficult in future surgeries.

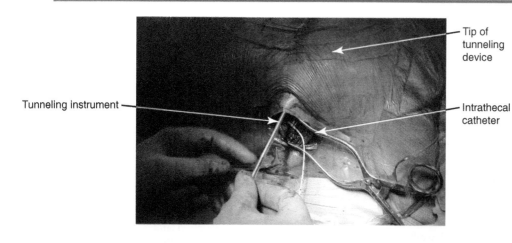

Tip of
tunneling
device

Tunneling instrument

Intrathecal
catheter

Fig. 10-9 Tunneling from the
spinal incision to the abdominal
pocket site for the pump.

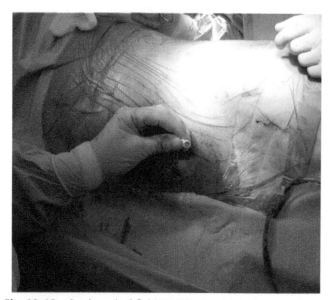

Fig. 10-10 Cerebrospinal fluid (CSF) is visualized after tunneling
the CSF from midline to the pocket site.

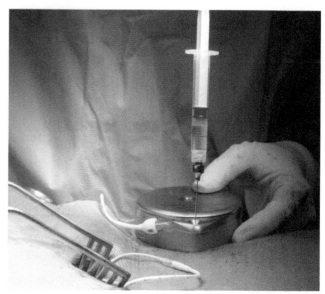

Fig. 10-11 Cerebrospinal fluid is aspirated from the side port of
the pump before anchoring.

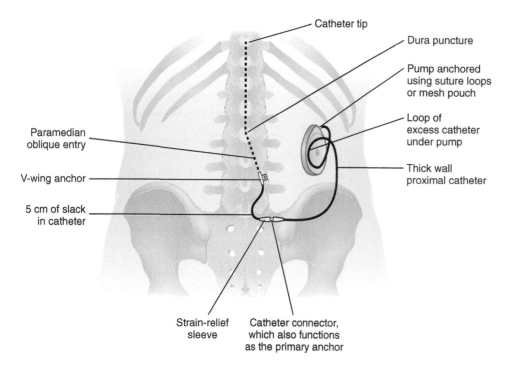

Catheter tip

Dura puncture

Pump anchored
using suture loops
or mesh pouch

Loop of
excess catheter
under pump

Thick wall
proximal catheter

Paramedian
oblique entry

V-wing anchor

5 cm of slack
in catheter

Strain-relief
sleeve

Catheter connector,
which also functions
as the primary anchor

Fig. 10-12 Suggested placement of
intrathecal catheter and pump
position.

One should adopt a uniform orientation system when implanting pump devices to allow for ease of troubleshooting in the future. The pump sideport may be oriented toward the 3, 9, or 12 o'clock positions. However, orienting the sideport toward 12 o'clock may have it underlie the scar, which could make sideport access difficult in the future. With the sideport of the pump oriented toward the umbilicus, the position of the metal anchoring rings roughly corresponds to the 2, 4, 8, and 10 o'clock positions within the pocket. With the anchoring sutures in place, the free ends of the sutures are passed through the metal rings on the side of the pump and the pump is suspended down into the pocket. The excess catheter is carefully coiled beneath the pump; the practitioner must avoid capturing the catheter within the anchoring sutures.[1,2,9] The anchor sutures are carefully tied off one by one, making sure after each that the catheter or connector has not been ligatured in the process. Failure to tuck the coils of catheter beneath the pump risks puncture of the catheter during pump refills later.[9]

After the pump has been securely anchored in place, a clinician may aspirate CSF from the sideport to demonstrate integrity of the system. At this point, one may even elect to perform a sideport myelogram using iodinated contrast under fluoroscopy, checking for any extravasation of contrast medium along the catheter's length. The risk of placing contrast should be considered before performing a myelogram. When the practitioner is satisfied with the pump and catheter, the wounds should be copiously irrigated with antibiotic irrigation.

The incisions are then carefully closed. An inverted interrupted layer of 2-0 absorbable suture is used for the primary fascial layer of both incisions. If the patient is particularly thin, this layer may include the deep dermal layer, or one may close this latter layer in a running continuous fashion using 3-0 absorbable suture. The skin edges can then be closed using a 4-0 monofilament in a running subcuticular fashion. Steri-Strips can be used to reinforce the apposition. If skin tension is a problem, surgical staples may be used for reinforcement. Or, alternatively, one may close the dermal and skin layers using interrupted horizontal mattress sutures for added strength. This is done with nonabsorbable 3-0 monofilament such as nylon. The wounds are dressed with gauze and transparent sterile dressing. Application of an abdominal binder in the recovery room will reduce the likelihood of seroma accumulation.[2,7]

The pump is programmed to the desired continuous setting. It is also then instructed to deliver a priming bolus. The purpose of this priming bolus is to the clear the catheter and internal pump tubing of CSF and infuse the drug to the tip of the catheter. This usually corresponds to approximately 0.4 mL of the infusion but should be calculated based on catheter length and drug concentration. Errors in volumetric calculation of the catheter may lead to unintended overpriming of the catheter with subsequent delivery of a depot of medication to the CSF. Therefore, this must always be done in a monitored setting.

Conclusion

The implantation of an IT pump has many integral parts. These include patient selection, preoperative assessment, implantation of the pump, and postoperative management. This chapter has given an overview of the technical aspects of pump implantation, but the other parts of the process should be carefully considered and carried out with vigilance. Methods described in this chapter should be used when possible, but the need to adapt techniques should be individualized based on patient needs.

References

1. Follet KA, Burchiel K, Deer T, et al: Prevention of intrathecal drug delivery catheter-related complications. *Neuromodulation* 6:32-41, 2003.
2. Knight KH, Brand FM, Mchaourab AS, et al: Implantable intrathecal pumps for chronic pain: highlights and updates. *Croat Med J* 48:22-34, 2007.
3. Staats P: Intrathecal drug delivery systems. In Raj P, editor: *Interventional pain management: image guided procedures*, ed 2, Philadelphia, 2008, Saunders Elsevier, pp 519-528.
4. Follet KA, Boortz-Marx RL, Drake JM, et al: Prevention and management of intrathecal drug delivery and spinal cord stimulation infections. *Anesthesiology* 100:1582-1594, 2004.
5. Dickerman RD: The role of surgical placement and pump orientation in intrathecal pump system failure: a technical report. *Pediatr Neurosurg* 38:107-109, 2003.
6. Albright AL: Best practice surgical techniques for intrathecal baclofen therapy. *J Neurosurg* 104:233-239, 2006.
7. Vender JR, Hester S, Waller JL, et al: Identification and management of intrathecal baclofen pump complications: a comparison of pediatric and adult patients. *J Neurosurg* 104:9-15, 2006.
8. Choi S, McComb JG, Levy ML, et al: Use of elemental iodine for shunt infection prophylaxis. *Neurosurgery* 52:908-913, 2003.
9. Fluckiger B, Knecht H, Grossman S, et al: Device-related complications of long-term intrathecal drug therapy via implanted pumps. *Spinal Cord* 46:639-643, 2008.

11 Programmable versus Fixed-Rate Pumps for Intrathecal Drug Delivery

Devin Peck and Sudhir Diwan

CHAPTER OVERVIEW

Chapter Synopsis: Intrathecal drug delivery systems (IDDS) for chronic pain have been shown to be safe and effective for properly selected patients who have pain intractable to opioid medication or who experience severe side effects. IDDS can be maintained by an implantable pump device with either a programmable or fixed-rate delivery schedule. Programmable pumps allow for more complex delivery schedules and for patient-controlled bolus delivery. Fixed-rate machines, in contrast, cannot be controlled by the practitioner; even the drug dose must be altered by changing the medication's concentration in the pump chamber. Ultimately, the patient and clinician should work together to determine the most appropriate delivery system.

Important Points:
- Intrathecal drug pumps may be appropriate in patients with inadequate pain control with oral opioids or those in whom an adequate dose is limited by side effects.
- Available pumps can be divided into programmable and fixed-rate models.
- Programmable pumps can be set by the practitioner to deliver medication at a desired rate.
- Programmable pumps offer the option of complex dosing schedules and patient-administered boluses.
- Fixed-rate pumps are set by the manufacturer to infuse at a constant rate that cannot be altered by the practitioner.
- The dose of fixed-rate pumps is controlled by changing the concentration of the medication within the pump chamber.
- There exist advantages and disadvantages to both programmable and fixed-rate pumps.
- The ultimate decision of which type of pump to implant is based on the individual needs of the patient and the preferences and comfort level of the physician.

Clinical Pearls:
- IDDS can be an essential tool in the treatment of chronic pain and spasticity.
- These systems may be appropriate for patients in whom opioid side effects preclude the attainment of a therapeutic dose.
- The two main classes of intrathecal pump systems are fixed-rate systems and programmable systems.
- Fixed-rate systems are potentially lower profile and may be powered without a battery, thereby obviating additional surgical procedures for battery changes.
- Programmable systems offer a great deal of flexibility in dosing and may allow complex dosing regimens, frequent noninvasive dose changes without reservoir refills, and patient-controlled bolus dosing.

Clinical Pitfalls:
- Careful patient selection is essential for successful implantation of an IDDS as patients require close long-term or lifelong follow-up.
- Careful calculation of proper intrathecal dosing is essential to maintain safety.
- Fixed-rate intrathecal pumps are most appropriate for use in patients with a stable level of pain and drug requirement over time; however, this may be difficult to predict with any certainty.
- Programming errors are possible with programmable pumps, which can lead to under- or overdosing patients.
- Patients with programmable systems may theoretically require closer follow-up and the availability of a clinician programmer in any geographic area to which they travel.

Introduction

The treatment of chronic pain can present many challenges. In some patients, escalating dose requirements make oral opioid therapy ineffective or impractical. In some cases, side effects from these medications may limit the patient from reaching a therapeutic dose. In these cases and others, the implantation of intrathecal drug delivery systems (IDDS) may be appropriate.

Such systems are used to deliver medications directly into the intrathecal space. In most cases, opioids are selected as the sole infusate or as part of a combination of medications for intrathecal infusion. When delivered in this manner, opioid medications act at receptors located in the substantia gelatinosa in the dorsal horn of the spinal cord. Because they are delivered directly into the intrathecal space and do not pass through the circulatory system to arrive there, side effects are reduced compared with other delivery routes. In addition, the effective dose can be profoundly reduced.

Table 11-1: Fixed-Rate Pumps versus Programmable Pumps

	Fixed-Rate Pumps	Programmable Pumps
Battery	No	Yes
Programmability	No	Yes
Presence of propellant	Yes	No
Availability of models with side port	Yes	Yes
Advantages	No battery replacement surgery required (may be more cost-effective), smaller profile device, larger capacity reservoir possible	Applicable to wider range of pain syndromes, easy to change medication dosage, availability of patient-controlled bolus administration
Applications	Stable chronic pain syndromes, hepatic artery infusion of chemotherapy, subcutaneous insulin therapy, antibiotic infusion for osteomyelitis	Chronic malignant or nonmalignant pain, refractory spasticity

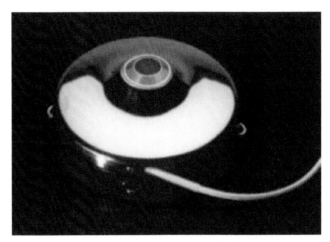

Fig. 11-1 Codman 3000 implantable drug pump.

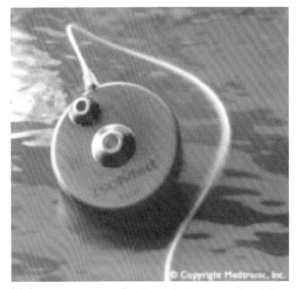

Fig. 11-2 IsoMed constant flow drug infusion system. Copyright Medtronic, Inc.

For example, the estimated equianalgesic dose of oral to intrathecal morphine is 300 to 1.[1]

There exist two main classes of IDDS: programmable pumps and fixed-rate pumps (**Table 11-1**). Programmable pumps can be set by the practitioner to deliver medication at a desired rate or programmed so a patient can deliver an intermittent bolus by self-administration. Fixed-rate pumps are set by the manufacturer to infuse at a constant rate that cannot be altered by the practitioner. When dose changes are desired, the concentration of the medication contained within the pump chamber can be changed.

Current and Future Options

The first pump approved for intrathecal drug delivery was the Infusaid Model #400 pump, which was a fixed-rate system and is no longer available. Subsequent to this, the Codman 3000 pump (**Fig. 11-1**) and the Medtronic IsoMed pump (**Fig. 11-2**) were approved for use. Both of these represent fixed-rate systems. The only programmable pumps available as of this writing are the Medtronic SynchroMed pumps. These include the SynchroMed EL (**Fig. 11-3**) and newer SynchroMed II pumps (**Fig. 11-4**).[2]

In the near future, more options are anticipated to come on the market. For example, a clinical trial is currently underway to evaluate the safety and efficacy of a new device known as the Prometra intrathecal pump system. This pump has been designed by Medasys Technologies and would represent the second novel programmable IDDS. In addition, new fixed-rate systems are currently undergoing clinical trials for U.S. Food and Drug Administration approval in the United States. These include the AccuRx Constant Flow pump (**Fig. 11-5**) designed by Advanced Neuromodulation Systems and the Archimedes pump (**Fig. 11-6**) designed by Codman. Both of these pumps are already available in Europe.[2]

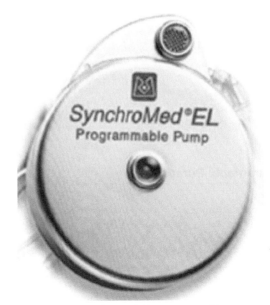

Fig. 11-3 SynchroMed EL programmable pump.

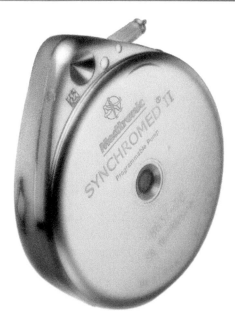

© Medtronic, Inc. 2008

Fig. 11-4 Medtronic SynchroMed II programmable pump. Copyright Medtronic, Inc.

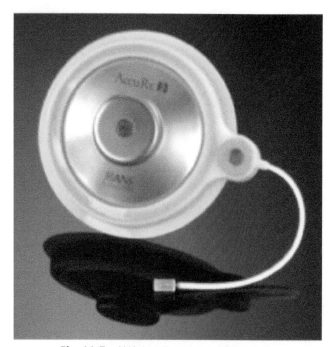

Fig. 11-5 ANS AccuRx constant flow pump.

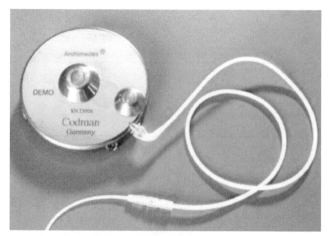

Fig. 11-6 Codman Archimedes Constant Flow pump.

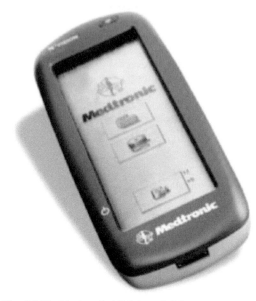

Fig. 11-7 Medtronic N'Vision clinician programmer.

Programmable Pumps

Overview

Programmable pumps can be used to treat malignant and nonmalignant chronic pain, spasticity, and hepatic or intravenous (IV) infusion. The infusion of sterile preservative-free morphine into the intrathecal space may be used to treat chronic, intractable pain that has failed other therapeutic methods.[3] Intrathecal infusion of baclofen can be used for the treatment of severe spasticity.[4] Programmable pumps may be used for the intravascular infusion of chemotherapeutic agents for the treatment of cancer.[5] Finally, the treatment of chronic infectious processes such as osteomyelitis can be facilitated by the IV infusion of antibiotics.[6]

Equipment

Programmable IDDS consist of an implantable, programmable pump, an intrathecal catheter, and an external device used to program the pump[3] (**Fig. 11-7**). Pumps vary in terms of the dimensions of the pump, the volume of the drug reservoir, the presence of a port allowing access to the catheter, and a reservoir valve.

The external programmer is a handheld device that communicates with the implanted pump through a programming head via coded radiofrequency signals. It provides a noninvasive method to interrogate and program the pump. Information is therefore both sent to and received from the pump in this way.[5]

Programming

Several factors can be programmed into the pump and allow the clinician to tailor therapy to each specific patient. These factors include:

- Identifying information for the patient
- Date and time that current settings were initiated

- Type and concentrations of the medication(s) contained within the pump reservoir
- Infusion mode
- Dose of medication delivered per unit time (usually per day)
- Volume of medication contained within the reservoir
- Volume at which the low reservoir alarm will sound
- Clinician-delivered bolus doses
- Patient-delivered bolus doses

Immediately after implantation of the pump, it must be programmed with the initial settings. In addition, a priming bolus must be programmed to account for the dead space contained within the intrathecal catheter. Reprogramming can then be carried out on an as-needed basis. Reprogramming must take place after a refill of the medication reservoir; with any pump flow studies; or if the clinician wishes to change the dose, concentration, or type of medication delivered.[5]

Different infusion modes can be programmed that specify dosing schedules for the infusion pump. These modes indicate the dose of medication to be delivered at a specified rate (per hour or per day) and over a specified duration of time. The modes are:

1. Stopped pump mode: Pump is turned off, but saved data are retained.
2. Single-bolus mode: Delivers a specified dose over a specified time period and then returns to the stopped pump mode.

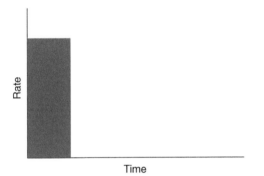

3. Simple continuous mode: A continuous infusion of medication is delivered at a daily dose specified by the programmer.

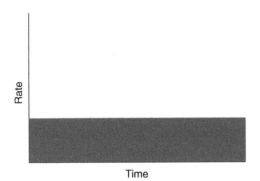

4. Single bolus + simple continuous mode: A single bolus is delivered. When completed, the pump reverts to simple continuous mode.

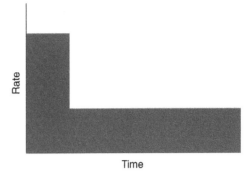

5. Periodic bolus mode: A bolus dose is specified and is delivered at the maximum rate. The programmer automatically calculates the duration of the bolus based on the dose specified. Boluses are intermitted with "delay periods" during which the pump runs at the minimum rate for a specified time period.

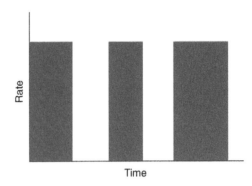

6. Complex continuous mode: A sequence of two to 10 subprograms with a specific dose, rate, and duration is delivered and repeated, typically in a 24-hour pattern.[5]

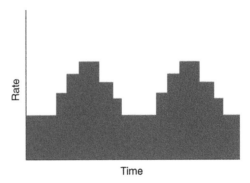

Fixed-Rate Pumps

Overview

Fixed-rate intrathecal pumps can be used to infuse pain medication into the intrathecal space in the same fashion as programmable pumps. These pumps are set during the manufacturing process to deliver a constant volume of solution per unit time.[5] The Medtronic IsoMed pump, for example, is available in flow rates over the range of 0.3 to 1.3 mL/day.[7] These devices can be used to infuse pain medication into the intrathecal space to treat patients with chronic pain refractory to other therapies. In addition, they are often used for the IV infusion of chemotherapeutic agents for patients with malignancies. One of the applications of these pumps is the infusion of floxuridine into the hepatic artery of patients with colorectal cancer metastatic to the liver.[8] When used for the treatment of chronic pain, these pumps are most appropriate for patients who experience stable pain that is not expected to change over time.[9] As one might expect, this greatly limits the application of these pumps in patients with chronic pain.

Equipment

The equipment involved in the implantation and operation of a fixed-rate intrathecal pump system is much the same as that required for a programmable system. The obvious difference is the absence of an external device to program the pump flow rate. The system consists of the pump itself, which contains a reservoir to store the medication, and a specialized catheter designed for intrathecal implantation.[9] Although programmable pumps are mechanical in nature and powered by a battery, fixed-rate systems are driven instead by either an injected pressurized gas or by an elastomeric diaphragm.[10] The flow rate of the infusate is determined by the diameter of the orifice through which it flows. The flow rate is therefore an intrinsic part of the pump design and cannot be changed.

Advantages and Disadvantages of Programmable and Fixed-Rate Intrathecal Pumps

Advantages of Programmable Pumps

The advantages afforded by programmable intrathecal pumps lie in their adaptability. In a vast majority of cases, chronic pain is a dynamic phenomenon. Even in the case of long-standing chronic pain syndromes, the character, quality, location, and intensity of pain can change. This change may be caused by progression or regression of existing pathology, the development of new pathology, or a change in the central processing and integration of the painful experience by the patient.

A programmable system allows the clinician to easily alter the dose of medication delivered to the patient without making any changes to the medication contained within the pump reservoir. Therefore, in the case that a patient experiences an increase in pain or reports inadequate pain control, the external programming device can be used to increase the flow rate and thus the delivered dose.[5] A programmable system may be most appropriate for implantation in patients who require frequent dose adjustments during their pump trial.[11]

One characteristic of chronic pain that complicates management is the phenomenon of acute exacerbations that may be superimposed on a continuous baseline experience of pain. When traditional oral opioid therapy is used to treat patients with such a pattern of pain, a long-acting compound is often used along with a short-acting medication for intermittent breakthrough pain. In the case of intrathecal opioid therapy, the option exists for the use of bolus dosing administered by the patient with the use of a handheld device. This can be useful in the treatment of such superimposed breakthrough pain.[12]

When a patient experiences pain in a variable yet predictable pattern, a complex-continuous dosing program can be used.[5] For example, if the patient reliably experiences his or her worst pain in the morning, this can be accounted for by programming the pump such that it will automatically run at a higher flow rate in the early morning and then change to a lower flow rate for the afternoon hours.

Disadvantages of Programmable Pumps

The flexibility afforded by a programmable system can also present dangers. The ability of the clinician to alter the dosing schedule opens the door to programming errors. These errors can result in underdosing the patient, which can lead to inadequate pain control and even withdrawal. A more serious error may result in overdosing, which can lead to an increase in side effects or even life-threatening complications.[3,5]

A greater number of variables that can be customized leads to a greater potential for human error. For example, the date and time in the programmer's internal clock must be accurate so the low reservoir alarm date is accurate. The volume of medication in the reservoir must also be programmed accurately by the clinician; otherwise, the refill date will be incorrect. If the volume is overestimated, there is a risk that the pump will run out of medication before the low reservoir alarm sounds, raising the possibility of abrupt cessation of dosing.[5]

Telemetry—that is, communication between the external programmer and the implanted pump—must be functioning properly for any programming changes to be made. For example, if the pump is placed too deeply in the patient (a maximum depth of 1.5 in or 3.8 cm), there will be difficulty establishing a connection.[5] This can lead to situations of under- or overdosing, particularly in the immediate post-implant period when adjustments may be needed to find the appropriate dose. In addition, if telemetry is not functioning properly, it becomes impossible to stop the pump in the case of an emergency.

Close follow-up of a patient with a programmable IDDS is paramount to safe and effective use of the system. Meticulous documentation, both digital and hard copy, must be maintained for every pump interrogation, pump refill, or change in dosing. Aspects of the patient's life once taken for granted, such as travel or relocation, take on new dimensions of complexity. The availability of qualified clinicians in any new geographic area is a concern. Patients must therefore be provided with updated documentation of the status of their pump, including current settings, reservoir volume, and medication and concentration.

Advantages of Fixed-Rate Pumps

The advantages of fixed-rate intrathecal pumps stem for the most part from their simplicity. Because no programming is required on the part of the clinician, many of the complexities that make management difficult are not a factor. For example, there is no danger of programming errors that might have the potential to lead to under- or overdosing. Because management of the pump is simplified, concerns about the availability of a qualified clinician to manage the pump are lessened. In this sense, patient relocation or travel become less concerning.

Fixed-rate pumps do not contain batteries. Instead, pressurized gas in a chamber located behind the reservoir pushes the medication through the catheter.[7,13] This allows for a smaller profile device, which is an attractive feature from a cosmetic perspective and may simplify implantation. In addition, fixed-rate pumps do not require periodic battery changes as do programmable pumps. This reduces the patient's exposure to repeated surgical procedures and may reduce cost in the long term.[13]

Disadvantages of Fixed-Rate Pumps

The indications for implantation of a fixed-rate intrathecal pump system are more limited compared with programmable systems, and patient selection may be more challenging. These systems are appropriate for patients with stable pain syndromes. That is, their level of pain should not be anticipated to change significantly over a period of time.[9] In most cases, this requires that a clear pathophysiology and etiology of their pain syndrome be well elucidated before implantation. In many cases, however, this may be difficult or impossible. In addition, it may be impossible to predict with any certainty a stable course for any pain syndrome. In most cases, chronic pain is a dynamic phenomenon, both over the long and short terms.

In the event that a patient with a fixed-rate pump experiences a change in his or her level of pain, a change can be made to the delivered dose of pain medication. However, this requires an adjustment of the concentration or type of medication in the pump.[7,9,12] This process is, of course, more involved than a simple reprogramming, a process that requires little prior preparation and does not require that the clinician obtain new medications that may need to be custom compounded by a pharmacist. Finally, in the event of an emergency, it may be difficult to stop the infusion of medication by a fixed-rate pump because there is no external programming device available to do so via telemetry.

It is important to note, however, that a review of patients with programmable pumps revealed that 94.1% of these patients were in fact receiving infusions in simple continuous mode at their most recent visits, essentially mirroring the capabilities of a fixed-rate device.[14] However, over the course of the period of time examined by the study, 41.7% of patients had at least at one time been managed by more complex, programmable infusion schedules.[14] An analysis of more than 1600 pump implantations by multiple practitioners examined dose adjustment practices for patients with fixed-rate pumps. The effective dose for patients with fixed-rate pumps was found with an average of 2 to 6 dose adjustments over a period of 1 to 6 months. Those with programmable systems were reported to require 5.3 ± 3.5 adjustments over 3 to 6 months.[11] The process can be further simplified if dose adjustments are made to coincide as often as possible with scheduled reservoir refills.

Conclusions

IDDS can be an indispensable tool in the management of patients with chronic pain. They may be appropriate in patients with inadequate pain control with oral opioids or those in whom an adequate dose is limited by side effects. Practitioners may opt to implant a device with programming capabilities or one with a fixed flow rate. Several advantages and disadvantages of each type of system can be listed. Ultimately, this decision is often based on the results of a pump trial, the individual needs of the patient, and the preferences and comfort level of the physician.

References

1. Lamer TJ: Treatment of cancer-related pain: when orally administered medications fail. *Mayo Clinical Proc* 69(5):473-480, 1994.
2. Krames E: *Implantable technologies.* Englewood, CO, 2011, National Pain Foundation.
3. Turner JA, Sears JM, Loeser JD: Programmable intrathecal opioid delivery systems for chronic noncancer pain: a systematic review of effectiveness and complications. *Clin J Pain* 23(2):180-195, 2007.
4. Burchiel KJ, Hsu FP: Pain and spasticity after spinal cord injury: mechanisms and treatment. *Spine* 26(24 suppl):S161, 2001.
5. Medtronic, Inc: *SynchroMed® infusion system clinical reference guide for pain therapy.* Minneapolis, MN, 2001, Medtronic, Inc.
6. Meani E, Romanò C: Treatment of osteomyelitis by local antibiotics using a portable electronic micropump. *Rev Chir Orthop Reparatrice Appar Mot* 80(4):285-290, 1994.
7. Medtronic, Inc: *IsoMed® implantable constant-flow infusion pump technical manual.* Minneapolis, MN, 2008, Medtronic, Inc.
8. Homsi J, Garrett CR: Hepatic arterial infusion of chemotherapy for hepatic metastases from colorectal cancer. *Cancer Control* 13(1):42-47, 2006.
9. Medtronic, Inc: *IsoMed® constant-flow infusion system clinical reference guide for pain therapy.* Minneapolis, MN, 2006, Medtronic, Inc.
10. Bedder MD: Intrathecal analgesics, choice of system. In Krames ES, editor: *Neuromodulation*, ed 1, St. Louis, 2009, Elsevier, pp 457-465.
11. Faaberg J, Koulousakis A, Staats PS: Clinical protocols for titrating constant flow implantable pumps in patients with pain or spasticity. *Neuromodulation* 8(2):121-130, 2005.
12. Ilias W, le Polain B, Buchser E, et al: Patient-controlled analgesia in chronic pain patients: experience with a new device designed to be used with implanted programmable pumps. *Pain Pract* 8(3):164-170, 2008.
13. Codman and Shurtleff, Inc: *Codman® 3000 Implantable Constant-Flow Infusion Pump.* Raynham, MA, 2008, Codman and Shurtleff, Inc.
14. Staats P, Whitworth M, Barakat M, et al: The use of implanted programmable infusion pumps in the management of nonmalignant, chronic low-back pain. *Neuromodulation* 10(4):376-380, 2007.

12 SynchroMed EL versus SynchroMed II

Rajpreet Bal, Sudhir Diwan, and Jeffrey Loh

CHAPTER OVERVIEW

Chapter Synopsis: With the rise of intrathecal drug delivery systems for chronic pain has come the development of several models of pump delivery systems. This chapter compares the technical details of these models, namely the SynchroMed EL and SynchroMed II pumps produced by Medtronic. The updated SynchroMed II pump now in production is the superior pump. Considerations include the material makeup and overall design of the device. During implantation, attention must be given to certain requirements for the machine to function properly and safely. For example, the device must be warmed to body temperature before implantation. Some of the technical details must be understood by the patient because certain activities or manipulations could harm or displace the device. Each pump is outfitted with several chambers that control how the drug is delivered to the spinal cord. Several strengths and weaknesses of the pump devices are discussed.

Important Points:
- SynchroMed EL pumps are not manufactured anymore.
- The telemetry of the SynchroMed EL pump requires a magnet to be place over the reservoir to communicate.
- The magnet is not required for telemetry of SynchroMed II reservoirs.
- Telemetry of SynchroMed EL does not show more than one drug of the mixture, while SynchroMed II will show individual drug descriptions of all medications in the mixture.

Clinical Pearls:
- SynchroMed EL Pump
  - Two different pump volumes: 10 and 18 mL
  - Consists of three sealed chambers; one for the reservoir propellant, the second for an electronic module and battery, and the third for a peristaltic pump and drug reservoir
  - Can be used for both intrathecal and intravascular use
  - Compatible for neuraxial use with preservative-free morphine sulfate, ziconotide, and baclofen, or intravenous infusion with chemotherapeutic medications
  - Drug stability, specifically with narcotics and baclofen, has been shown to be 90 days in duration
  - Capable of administering four different medication modes: single bolus, continuous infusion, complex continuous infusion, and periodic boluses
- SynchroMed II Pump
  - Two different pump volumes—20 mL and 40 mL—but with comparable thickness to the SynchroMed EL pump
  - Improved accuracy of flow rates until the pump reservoir reaches 1 mL
  - Drug stability shown to be 180 days duration with morphine and baclofen
  - Uses a three-roller pump system with radiopaque ball markers, allowing the clinician to track roller rotation when performing a roller study
  - Drug reservoir uses a pressure diaphragm, which allows for immediate aspiration of medication from the reservoir
  - Multiple modes of administering medications; simple continuous infusion, a single bolus, a flex infusion, or a minimum rate infusion mode.
  - Improved memory capacity capable of storing patient demographics, catheter and pump information, multiple drug information, and physician notes

Clinical Pitfalls:
- SynchroMed EL Pump
  - Pump life span based on consumption of battery life, which can vary between 3 and 7 years
  - Lack of a bacterial filter on the side access catheter port
  - Pump flow becomes less accurate below a pump reservoir volume of 2 mL
  - The recommended alarm volume is not sufficient to prevent severe withdrawal symptoms
  - Pump must be warmed to body temperature before implantation for proper function
  - Minimal memory with which to store patient and drug information
- SynchroMed II Pump
  - Admixtures of drugs shown to potentially generate drug impurities that can result in pump damage and pump stalls
  - Life span is dictated by both battery life as well as motor revolutions, with high infusion rates associated with a shorter pump life
  - Pump function can become impaired if exposed to radiation, lithotripsy, or any drastic changes in pressure or temperature
  - Lack of a bacterial filter on the side access catheter port
  - Slower transmission time between the pump and programmer because of greater amount of data transmission

Introduction

Many different clinical pain states exist; as such, various modalities of pain management have been developed to effectively target chronic pain. One of the specific modalities devised as a method for the treatment of chronic pain is the administration of intrathecal (IT) pain medications. Although the clinician has many different routes of administration of medications, the use of IT drug delivery systems (IDDS) has become one of the more common techniques used by pain physicians today.[1] This chapter addresses the development of the Medtronic SynchroMed EL and SynchroMed II programmable infusion pumps, specifically seeking to highlight the differences between these two IT infusion pumps.

SynchroMed EL Pump

The Medtronic SynchroMed EL (**Fig. 12-1**) and SynchroMed II programmable infusion pumps both administer IT medications in the same route of delivery. However, many of the specifics between these two pumps differ upon close comparison (**Fig. 12-2**). At this time,

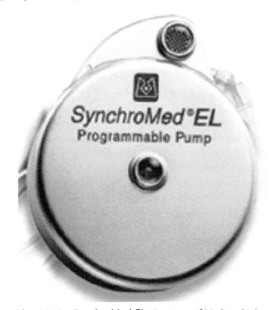

Fig. 12-1 SynchroMed EL. Courtesy of Medtronic, Inc.

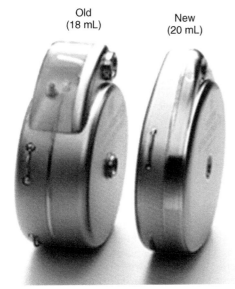

Old (18 mL)   New (20 mL)

Fig. 12-2 Pump sizes comparison. Courtesy of Medtronic, Inc.

the SynchroMed EL pump is no longer manufactured by Medtronic and has been replaced by the newer SynchroMed II model.

The SynchroMed EL system is a titanium-based pump designed in two different reservoir volumes, 10 and 18 mL, with the 10-mL pump indicated for use in a smaller patient with an insufficient body mass or in a patient who desires a smaller, lower profile pump. Although the SynchroMed EL pump lists the reservoir volumes as 10 and 18 mL, the actual usable reservoirs for this pump are 8 and 16 mL, respectively. As expected, SynchroMed EL pumps have different weights; 185 and 223 g for the 10- and 18-mL pumps, respectively. Based on Medtronic guidelines,[2,3] the SynchroMed EL pump has a life span of 6.5 years; however, the true life span depends on consumption of the battery, which can vary between 3 and 7 years in duration.

Both versions of the SynchroMed EL pump demonstrate precisely controlled infusion flow rates, with accuracy until the pump reservoir reaches 2 mL. When the reservoir volume decreases below 2 mL, pumps may exhibit a decrease in actual flow rate compared with the programmed flow rate, resulting in potential loss of clinical effect or drug withdrawal symptoms.[4] The SynchroMed EL pump is compatible for neuraxial use with preservative-free morphine sulfate, ziconotide, and baclofen as medications for the treatment of patients with chronic pain. The SynchroMed EL pump is also compatible with the intravenous (IV) infusion of chemotherapeutic medications such as floxuridine, doxorubicin, cisplatin, or methotrexate for the treatment of patients with primary or metastatic cancer as well as the IV infusion of clindamycin for the treatment of those with osteomyelitis. Based on manufacturer guidelines, overall drug stability, specifically with narcotics and baclofen, has been shown to be 90 days in duration with the SynchroMed EL infusion pump.[3,5] However, drug stability and life span within the SynchroMed EL pump truly depend on the medication being infused.[6]

SynchroMed EL Pump Design

The design of the SynchroMed EL infusion pump consists of three sealed chambers. One chamber contains the reservoir propellant, the second chamber contains a hybrid electronic module and battery, and the third chamber contains a peristaltic pump and drug reservoir (**Fig. 12-3**). The peristaltic pump, which forces medications from the reservoir to the administration site, consists of a two-roller model, with pumping action mediated through electronic circuitry. This pump is designed so that a reservoir valve prevents further introduction of fluid into the reservoir when capacity is reached. The actual construct of the reservoir valve is a volume-activated design, such that an expanding drug reservoir bellows pulls the valve stem onto a metal seat to form a seal.

The SynchroMed EL pump contains a side catheter access port for drug administration or diagnostic purposes accessible with the use of a 25-gauge needle. The design of the catheter access port consists of a mesh screen over the catheter access port. This side catheter access port does not contain a bacterial filter, so the clinician must maintain strict, sterile conditions when accessing this port.

SynchroMed EL Pump Implantation

Before implantation, certain precautions must be conveyed to the patient to prevent damage to the pump. Direct exposure of radiation must be avoided because therapeutic radiation may damage the electronic circuitry of the pump, ultimately causing cessation of pump function. Lithotripsy should be avoided because the effects on the pump are unknown. Patients are also cautioned to avoid certain physical activities that may directly damage the

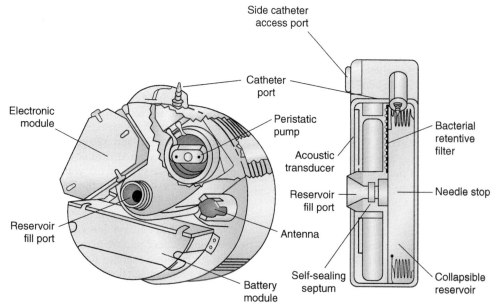

Fig. 12-3 Pump mechanics. Courtesy of Medtronic, Inc.

implant site or device. Manipulation of the pump through the skin must be avoided because this action can result in catheter disconnection, angulation, and kinking. Any activities that involve pressure or temperature changes can affect the infusion rate and disrupt function of the SynchroMed EL pump. Thus, scuba diving, saunas, hot tubs, hyperbaric chambers, and long-duration flights are scenarios during which patients should exercise caution.[7]

To ensure proper use of this infusion pump, the SynchroMed EL pump should be first warmed to body temperature before implantation. Failure to warm the pump to body temperature before emptying and initial filling procedures can result in incomplete emptying and subsequent overfilling of the reservoir, which can lead to activation of the reservoir valve. The SynchroMed EL pump has also been shown to improperly infuse at a temperature below 35° C. Thus, if not adequately warmed, the programmed purge bolus may not remove air in the pump tubing and fluid pathway. In addition, before implantation of the SynchroMed EL pump, the practitioner must first perform a pump purge of the system to prevent overpressurization of the pump. Failure to comply with any of these steps can result in an overinfusion of medication, which can potentially result in serious injury or death to the patient.

When implanting the SynchroMed EL pump, the pump must lie 1 inch (2.5 cm) or less in depth from the surface of the skin. A pump implantation depth greater than 1 inch results in inhibited access to the pump's septum and potential interference with the programming telemetry. Before suturing the pump into place, one should verify that the implanted pump's center reservoir fill port and side catheter access port are easy to palpate and that the catheter will not become twisted or contorted. To reduce any post-implant issues, the catheter should also be secured away from the center reservoir fill port and side catheter access port. To ensure proper placement, most SynchroMed EL pumps provide suture loops with which to secure the pump. In certain situations in which suture loops are not provided on the SynchroMed EL pump, a mesh pouch is instead provided to anchor the pump into a fixed location.

SynchroMed EL Pump Programming

After implantation, the SynchroMed EL pump can be programmed to administer medications through various methods. The pump can be programmed to administer a single bolus, a continuous infusion, a complex continuous infusion, or a periodic bolus. Single-bolus administration will administer a specific medication dose for a specified period of time. With a continuous infusion, medication is administered continuously at a specified rate. Similarly, the complex continuous infusion administers medication continuously between two and 10 variations, with each variation programmed for a specified duration of time. Finally, with periodic boluses, the infusion pump administers a prescribed dose of medication for a determined period at regular intervals. In between periodic boluses, the SynchroMed EL pump must infuse a minimal flow of 1.8 μL/hr to prevent catheter occlusion. Because of the increased risk of catheter occlusion in the vascular environment, single-bolus and periodic bolus administration are not recommended for intravascular infusion.

The SynchroMed EL pump is designed to store the pump model, patient identification, and a single drug identification with the concentration, the infusion mode, and the calibration constant (i.e., the number of electrical pulses required by the peristaltic mechanism to dispense 1 μL of fluid). Out of the storable information, each pump is capable of being programmed to store the date and time a prescription was entered. The clinician is also capable of programming the reservoir volume and the low reservoir alarm settings. After it is activated, each alarm occurs at specific intervals (between 4 and 16 sec) until deactivated by the programmer via telemetry. The low battery and low reservoir alarms are single-tone alarms that occur at intervals depending on the pump flow rate; a higher flow rate results in an alarm with shorter intervals than a lower flow rate.

Some of the disadvantages of the SynchroMed EL pump are that programming of patient identification is capable of storing only three characters and that the drug name storage can hold only five characters. In addition, when stopping the SynchroMed EL pump using the programmer therapy stop key, the clinician must be

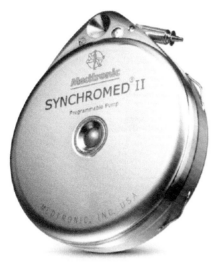

© Medtronic, Inc. 2008

Fig. 12-4 SynchroMed II infusion pump. Courtesy of Medtronic, Inc.

aware that the pump does not obtain or provide pump status information and that the pump will decrease its infusion rate to 0 μL/day.[3]

SynchroMed II Pump

The SynchroMed II infusion pump (Fig. 12-4) is also a titanium-based pump designed to hold two different drug reservoir volumes. Unlike the SynchroMed EL pump, the SynchroMed II has reservoir volumes of 20 and 40 mL. Although the SynchroMed II pump comes in reservoir volume sizes twice the size of the SynchroMed EL, the thickness of the SynchroMed II 20-mL pump (19.5 mm) is actually smaller than the SynchroMed EL pump thickness of 21.6 mm. Even the 40-mL SynchroMed II pump thickness of 26.0 mm is marginally larger than the SynchroMed EL pump. Thus, for a pump of roughly the same size, the SynchroMed II pump contains nearly double the amount of deliverable drug. Although the reservoir volumes of the SynchroMed II pump are listed as 20 and 40 mL, this pump has a usable reservoir volume of 19 and 39 mL for the two pumps, respectively. This difference of 1 mL between usable and listed reservoir volume in the SynchroMed II pump is an improvement on the 2-mL difference between usable and listed volumes for the SynchroMed EL pump. As expected with two different size pumps, the 20- and 40-mL SynchroMed II pumps have different weights of 165 and 215 g for the 20- and 40-mL pumps, respectively. Based on Medtronic guidelines,[8] the SynchroMed II pump is indicated to have a life span of 7 years, which is similar to the 6.5 year life span of the SynchroMed EL pump. However, the true life span is again dictated by the life of the battery as well as motor revolutions, with high infusion rates associated with a shorter pump life.

The SynchroMed II pump demonstrates precisely controlled infusion flow rates, with accuracy until the pump reservoir reaches 1 mL, which is the reason for this pump's usable reservoir volumes of 19 and 39 mL. At volumes below 1 mL, the pump flow rate rapidly decreases before finally stopping. Thus, clinicians must be aware of loss of medication effects or withdrawal symptoms. Based on Medtronic guidelines,[8] the SynchroMed II pump is similar to the SynchroMed EL pump in terms of medications compatible for administration. IT infusions of sterile, preservative-free morphine

sulfate, ziconotide, and baclofen as well as intravascular infusion of chemotherapy, floxuridine, and methotrexate for the treatment of cancer have all been shown to be compatible in the SynchroMed II infusion pump. Overall drug stability, specifically with morphine and baclofen, has been shown to be 180 days with the SynchroMed II infusion pump, which is twice the duration seen with the SynchroMed EL pump.

Of note, admixtures of drugs should be avoided for use in the SynchroMed II pump. Admixing drugs has been shown to potentially generate drug impurities that can alter a drug product's stability and result in pump damage and pump stalls caused by pH changes.

SynchroMed II Pump Design

The SynchroMed II pump delivers medications using the same basic mechanics found within the SynchroMed EL pump. Drug enters the pump through the reservoir fill port and passes through the reservoir valve into the pump reservoir. Battery-powered electronics and motors precisely infuse medication using peristaltic action. However, unlike the SynchroMed EL, the SynchroMed II uses a three-roller system with radiopaque ball markers, which allows the clinician to track roller rotation when performing a roller study. Another change used in the SynchroMed II pump is the use of a pressure-activated reservoir, unlike the volume-activated valve found in the SynchroMed EL pump. As the drug reservoir fills, a pressure diaphragm in the SynchroMed II flattens, causing a spring to push the pump's valve stem onto a metal seat to form a seal. The benefit of this design allows for immediate release of the seal upon aspiration by a clinician, unlike the SynchroMed EL, which requires continuous aspiration and time for release of the reservoir valve.

The SynchroMed II pump is also designed with a catheter access port for drug administration and diagnostic purposes. The size of the catheter access port on the SynchroMed II is slightly larger than the port found on the SynchroMed EL pump, allowing for use of a 24-gauge or smaller needle. The design of the port is a single-hole, funnel design that provides easier access of the port compared with the mesh screen found on the SynchroMed EL pumps. As with the SynchroMed EL pump, the SynchroMed II pump side catheter access port does not contain a bacterial filter, so the clinician must use a bacterial-retentive filter and strict, sterile precautions when injecting or aspirating through this port (**Tables 12-1** and **12-2**).[2,8]

SynchroMed II Pump Implantation

Although the SynchroMed EL pump requires certain precautions before implantation into a patient, the SynchroMed II pump has improved upon some of these issues. Unlike the SynchroMed EL pump, the SynchroMed II pump does not require warming of the pump or a pump purge before implantation of the pump for proper device function. The SynchroMed II pump, however, does require certain precautions that should be followed to prevent pump damage after implantation. Patients should avoid exposing the SynchroMed II pump to high temperatures, commonly found in hot showers, steam rooms, saunas, tanning beds, and so on, which can result in an overinfusion of medication and potentially serious side effects. Activities that require excessive twisting or stretching should be avoided because sudden, excessive, or repetitive bending, twisting, bouncing, or stretching can damage the components and require surgical revision or replacement of the device. These activities can also dislodge or occlude the catheter, resulting in a change in infusion rate, resulting in clinically significant side effects. Patients should avoid manipulating or rubbing the

Table 12-1: Pump Comparisons[2]

	SynchroMed EL Pump	SynchroMed II Pump
Reservoir volume	10-mL pump: 1.2 mL 18-mL pump: 2.4 mL	20-mL pump: 1.4 mL 40-mL pump: 1.4 mL
pump	10-mL pump: 105 mL 18-mL pump: 125 mL	20-mL pump: 91 mL 40-mL pump: 121 mL
Reservoir port	4.75 mm	6.8 mm
Pump rollers	Two rollers	Three rollers
Reservoir valve	Volume-activated valve Releases upon continuous aspiration	Pressure-activated valve Releases upon aspiration immediately
Alarms	One tone indicates low reservoir volume and low battery Two tones indicate pump memory error	Critical alarm indicates empty reservoir, end of service, motor stall, >48 hours of stopped pump duration, memory error Noncritical alarm indicates low reservoir volume, noncritical memory error, elective replacement error
Warming	Warm to body temperature before implantation	Not indicated
Pump purge	Required to confirm operation before implantation	None and purge infusion mode not available
Information management	Stores mode, patient identification (three letters), concentration (five letters), infusion, calibration constant	Stores patient demographics, catheter and pump information, drug (five names up to 25 letters), concentration and infusion, physician notes, time-stamped log, calibration constant
Radiopaque identifier	None	Used to identify pump model under fluoroscopy
Longevity at 0.5 mL/day	≈6.5 years	≈7 years

Table 12-2: Programming Comparisons[2]

	SynchroMed EL Pump	SynchroMed II Pump
Programmer models	8840, 8821, 8820, 8810	8840 N'Vision
Magnet accessory	Required on 8840 N'Vision	Do not use
Infusion	Complex continuous infusion	Flex infusion mode available that allows two different drug delivery patterns in a 7-day week
Bridge bolus	Only programmed with simple continuous infusion and for a limited duration	Programmed in simple and flexible infusion modes Minimum rate infusion mode available
Programmer stop key	No pump status obtained before stopping Programs to 0 μL/day	Pump status obtained before stopping Programs to minimum rate of 6 μL/day

the pump into place, the clinician must ensure that the reservoir fill port is anteriorly oriented and that the reservoir fill port and catheter access port will be easily accessible after implant.[9] The SynchroMed II only comes with suture loops for implantation, so the clinician should ensure that no sutures lie directly over the reservoir fill port or the catheter access port because misplaced sutures could impede entrance to the catheter access port or reservoir.[10]

SynchroMed II Pump Programming

After implantation, the SynchroMed II pump has multiple programmable delivery modes by which to administer medications. The most common modes include a simple continuous infusion, a single bolus, a flex infusion, or a minimum rate infusion mode. The delivery mode for a simple continuous infusion or a single bolus is the same as that of the SynchroMed EL pump. The flex infusion found on the SynchroMed II pump is similar to the complex continuous infusion mode found on the SynchroMed EL pump. However, this infusion mode is capable of delivering a sequence of up to 13 independent steps of varying doses, rates, and durations over a fixed basal rate for each 24-hour period in a range of 1 to 7 days. Thus, the flex infusion improves upon the complex continuous infusion by allowing the clinician to increase the number of independent steps from 10 to 13 as well as allowing different dosing patterns each day, unlike the same daily dosing pattern found on the SynchroMed EL pump. Although both pumps use a minimum infusion rate (SynchroMed EL 0.048 mL/day), the SynchroMed II pump can infuse a minimum rate of 0.006 mL/day which is one-seventh the minimum volume infused by the SynchroMed EL pump. The SynchroMed II pump also uses a stopped pump mode not found on the SynchroMed EL where the pump stops its pump motor and discontinues its infusion. However, after 48 hours, a critical alarm sounds to alert the patient and clinician of potential damage to the pump. Thus, it is recommended to use a minimum infusion rate to maintain tubing patency.

Similar to the SynchroMed EL pump, the SynchroMed II pump is designed to store background information about the pump. With the SynchroMed II pump, the clinician is capable of storing patient

pump or catheter through the skin. Manipulation can cause skin erosion, component damage, catheter disconnection, kinking, or dislodgement and result in drug or cerebrospinal fluid leakage into the surrounding tissue. Manipulation may also cause pump inversion, making refill of the pump impossible. Patients should also avoid radiation exposure to prevent system damage or operational changes.[2,8]

When implanting the SynchroMed II pump, the pump must lie 1 inch (2.5 cm) or less in depth from the surface of the skin, the same requirement as the SynchroMed EL pump, to allow for access to the pump's reservoir and catheter access port. When suturing demographics, pump information, catheter information, drug identification, drug concentration, physician notes, time-stamped event logs, the infusion prescription, and the calibration constant. Although the SynchroMed EL pump is capable of storing only three letters for patient identification, the SynchroMed II pump is capable of storing a patient's full name, as well as his or her address and telephone number. Another improvement in the SynchroMed II pump is the ability to store five drug names, with each drug name able to consist of up to 25 characters. The SynchroMed II's pump programming also allows for recording of individual drugs with their concentrations and can store physician notes, providing a means of communication to other clinicians. However, with the improvements made in the SynchroMed II pump's programming system comes an increased time required for transmission of data between the pump and programmer. A typical programming interrogation takes roughly 30 seconds, and a pump update may last between 30 and 90 seconds.[2,8]

The alarm system of the SynchroMed II pump has also been modified compared with the SynchroMed EL pump. The SynchroMed II pump consists of two different alarm tones with a 3-second, two-tone alarm representing a critical alarm and a second, single-tone alarm representing a noncritical alarm. Examples of critical alarms include an empty reservoir, end of service, motor stall, stopped pump duration greater than 48 hours, and a critical pump memory error. Noncritical alarms include low reservoir volumes, elective replacement indicator, and a noncritical pump memory error. Finally, unlike the SynchroMed EL pump, when stopping the SynchroMed II pump through the use of the stop key, the SynchroMed II pump will provide the clinician with the pump status before shutdown and will also program the pump to the minimum infusion rate of 0.006 mL/day, effectively preventing pump occlusion.[8]

Conclusion

Although both the SynchroMed EL and SynchroMed II pumps provide an effective means by which to administer an IT or intravascular infusion of medications, the SynchroMed II pump acts to improve upon many of the shortcomings found with the SynchroMed EL pump (see **Tables 12-1** and **12-2**). With recent developments in interventional pain techniques, IDDS are an important part of the chronic pain treatment algorithm. The overall improvements made upon the SynchroMed II ultimately enhance the ease of use for clinicians as well as ease of maintenance required by patients. The similarities in both the pumps are in route of delivery, battery life span, medications, and physical restrictions recommended to patients to prevent pump damage after implantation. The differences in the two pumps enhance the safety profile of the SynchroMed II pump. The SynchroMed II pump has a more efficient design resulting in larger drug reservoir volume, drug stability, larger refill port, flexible infusion, and improved programming and alarm system. Through this chapter, one hopefully gains a

better understanding of these two pumps, specifically with respect to both pumps' structural and programming designs.

Future

Despite the improvements in the IDDS that has helped us to deliver medications where the receptors are, thereby minimizing the side effects and improving pain control, the risks involved with programming error can be life threatening. Also, the inability to interrogate the IT pump by a transtelephone system for monitoring and programming such as those used for implantable cardiac pacemakers and defibrillators via a remote station makes it difficult to help patients in times of emergency. Currently, the pump cannot be interrogated until either a health care provider goes to the patient or the patient goes to the hospital. The constantly evolving microprocessor-based, all-digital technology using interactive telemonitoring may help solve this problem in the future. These devices are inherently very expensive and put a huge final burden on the health care system. Because of the high costs of these devices, many developing countries are still far from benefitting from the state-of-the-art IDDS. Hopefully, governing societies and manufacturing industries will make collaborative efforts toward making these devices affordable to large parts of the world, including developing countries.

References

1. Belverud S, Mogilner A, Schulder M: Intrathecal pumps. *Neurotherapeutics* 5(1):114-122, 2008.
2. Medtronic, Inc: *SynchroMed EL/SynchroMed II programmable pump comparison*, Minneapolis, MN, 2006, Medtronic, Inc.
3. Medtronic, Inc: *Medtronic SynchroMed EL implant guide*, Minneapolis, MN, 2006, Medtronic, Inc.
4. Rigoli G, Terrini G, Cordioli Z: Intrathecal baclofen withdrawal syndrome caused by low residual volume in the pump reservoir: a report of 2 cases. *Arch Phys Med Rehabil* 85(12):2064-2066, 2004.
5. Classen AM, Wimbish GH, Kupiec TC: Stability of admixture containing morphine sulfate, bupivacaine hydrochloride, and clonidine hydrochloride in an implantable infusion system. *J Pain Symptom Manage* 28(6):603-611, 2004.
6. Bennett G, Serafini M, Burchiel K et al: Evidence based review of the literature on intrathecal delivery of pain medication. *J Pain Symptom Manage* 20(2 suppl):S12-S36, 2000.
7. Cheng JF, Diamond M: SCUBA diving for individuals with disabilities. *Am J Phys Med Rehabil* 84:369-375, 2005.
8. Medtronic, Inc: *Medtronic SynchroMed II Implant Guide*, Minneapolis, MN, 2006, Medtronic, Inc.
9. Ethans K: Intrathecal baclofen therapy: indications, pharmacology, surgical implant, and efficacy. *Acta Neurochir Suppl* 97(Pt 1):155-162, 2007.
10. Follett KA, Naumann CP: A prospective study of catheter-related complications of intrathecal drug delivery systems. *J Pain Symptom Manage* 19(3):209-215, 2000.

13 Minimizing the Risks of Intrathecal Therapy

Joshua P. Prager

CHAPTER OVERVIEW

Chapter Synopsis: Although intrathecal drug delivery systems (IDDS) for chronic pain or spasticity have undergone significant technical and clinical improvements in their 30 years, they still carry serious inherent risks. These risks can be minimized with careful attention to the implantation procedure itself, the choice of delivery device, and the medications to be administered. Some perioperative risks include infection, spinal damage during implantation, and development of granulomas at the catheter tip. But analysis of the literature and comparison with spinal stimulation procedure revealed that the serious or even lethal side effects of opioid drugs present the most significant risk for perioperative mortality. IDDS has shifted from a short-term therapy for pain relief in terminal patients to a long-term option for pain management. Another side effect of IDDS that may be overlooked is long-term modification of the neuroendocrine and immune systems, including reproductive hormones. Considering these risks, IDDS requires careful attention to patient selection and acute awareness of risk management techniques by the clinician.

Important Points: Intrathecal therapy has been practiced for almost 3 decades. Despite its demonstrated advantages, IT therapy also carries risks. Since the first reservoir for IT drugs was implanted in 1981, experts have continuously worked to maximize the advantages and minimize the risks. Ongoing management of patients with complex pain problems is often time consuming and difficult, hence vigilance remains the watchword. The diagnosis, treatment, and prevention of complications should include an algorithm that is intended to improve efficacy and safety. The opioid morphine and the nonopioid antiinflammatory drug ziconotide are the only Food and Drug Administration (FDA)-approved analgesics for IT therapy. Most commonly used, morphine has shown higher morbidity and mortality when compared with the spinal cord stimulator for similar chronic pain conditions. The Polyanalgesic Consensus Conference 2007 recommended starting with lower doses and escalating slowly when beginning IT therapy. IT catheter tip inflammatory mass granuloma remains the most serious risk of the therapy due to the potential for neurological deficits. Regular surveillance and immediate investigation of new complaints of increased pain, weakness, or both may prevent serious sequelae like permanent paralysis. Literature also indicates that long-term IT opioid therapy more profoundly influences neuroendocrine functions than oral opioid therapy. The dedicated effort of experts has produced numerous consensus statements and guidelines to facilitate IT therapy.

Clinical Pearls: IT therapy has been used successfully in long-term pain management for patients with various chronic malignant and nonmalignant pain syndromes. The common side effects of morphine therapy usually occur soon after starting the IT therapy and resolve within a few months. The clinician must be skilled to implant the device, and recognize and manage perioperative complication to maximize the advantage of IT therapy. Device-related perioperative complications can be minimized by meticulous surgical techniques and thorough training in pump surgery. When starting IT therapy, high-risk patients should be monitored for 24 hours in a hospital setting. Whenever possible, start with lower dosage and escalate slowly to minimize drug-related complications. Consider ziconotide for neuropathic pain syndrome when appropriate. Follow the Polyanalgesic Algorithm for Intrathecal Therapies to decide the line and choose medication(s), concentrations, and combinations. Be vigilant and establish protocol to investigate new pain with or without neurological symptoms to diagnose and manage granuloma early. If granuloma is detected, withdraw the catheter tip approximately 2 cm from the mass to prevent its growth. If neurological deficits do not improve, surgical removal of the mass is required. Consider neuroendocrinal investigation if the patient shows decreased libido and/or any other evidence of hypogonadotropic hypogonadism or hypocorticism.

Clinical Pitfalls: For IT therapy, drug compounding is the common practice. Compounding is a complicated practice with high risk of infection if attention is not paid to sterile techniques. Drug compounding should be carried out as per United States Pharmacopoeia (USP) and American Society of Health-System Pharmacists (ASH) guidelines. Catheter failure, migration, or disconnection may cause acute withdrawal symptoms. Hormonal changes have been reported with long-term IT therapy that may necessitate hormone replacement therapy. Granuloma, an inflammatory but noninfectious mass that is prevalent in patients requiring high concentrations of opioids, can cause severe neurological deficits if not recognized and managed early. So far granuloma has not been reported with the use of intrathecal ziconotide, while morphine and hydromorphone are the two most commonly reported drugs to cause granuloma. Reducing the drug concentration may reduce the incidence of granuloma formation.

Introduction

Experience with tens of thousands of cases[1] over almost three decades, improved drug delivery systems,[2] and new pharmacological regimens[3] have made intrathecal (IT) therapy an effective treatment for intractable pain in appropriately selected patients.

Indeed, IT therapy has been used successfully in long-term pain management for patients with failed back surgery syndrome, complex regional pain syndrome, spinal stenosis, osteoporosis with compression fractures, pancreatitis, phantom limb pain syndrome, and peripheral neuropathies.[4] Despite its demonstrated advantages, however, IT therapy also carries risks. These can be broadly categorized as relating to the implantation procedure, the delivery device, or the medications administered intrathecally.[2]

Since the first reservoir for IT drugs was implanted in 1981,[5] expert panels have convened periodically to assess outcomes, address therapeutic limitations, review the medical literature, survey current practices, discuss standards of care, and write clinical practice guidelines.[3,4,6-8] Their work highlights several concepts that deserve attention. First, to maximize advantages and minimize risk to patients, clinicians must be aware of the potential complications of IT therapy and recognize those who are most at risk during its long-term application. Second, IT therapy requires the experience of a skilled physician for placement and perioperative management.[4] IT therapy is technically challenging, requiring knowledge of IT opioids (ITOs) and pharmacology as well as proper use of infusion devices.[9] In addition, ongoing management in patients with complex pain problems is time consuming and difficult.[10] Third, most of the known risks of IT therapy can be managed effectively, but *vigilance* remains the watchword.[4]

This chapter reviews the major complications associated with IT therapy. The first is perioperative morbidity and mortality, usually attributable to opioid administration or equipment implantation. As with any opioid therapy, medication-related side effects can be serious, even lethal. The common side effects of morphine therapy usually occur soon after starting therapy and generally resolve within a few months with medical management.[6] Referring physicians and patients should know, however, that there is a risk of fatality with ITO therapy, especially soon after implantation.[9] Catheter tip inflammatory masses (granulomas) also pose a potentially serious risk to patients receiving IT therapy. The 2007 Panel Consensus Recommendations for IT Granuloma Diagnosis, Treatment, and Prevention include an algorithm intended to reduce the risk of this complication.[8] Attention is now being given to effectively managing the profound effects of long-term ITO therapy on neuroendocrine function.[11] Strategies for implementing and managing IT therapy, developed through clinical experience and research, can minimize the risk to patients while offering the very real benefit of pain relief.[4,9]

Perioperative Morbidity and Mortality

In February 2006, a cluster of three deaths within 1 day of pump implantation drew attention to the potential risk of ITO therapy for patients who did not have cancer.[12] Whereas a randomized controlled clinical trial supported the safety of IT therapy compared with comprehensive medical management to treat cancer pain,[13] no such trial has been conducted for noncancer pain. Yet the majority of patients now being treated with IT therapy do not have cancer. The deaths prompted a comparison of mortality rates for IT therapy, spinal cord stimulation (SCS), lumbar discectomy in a community hospital, and Medicare lumbosacral spine surgery.[12] Mortality was higher for patients receiving IT therapy—0.088% at 3 days after implantation, 0.39% at 1 month, and 3.89% at 1 year—than for the SCS (0.011% at 3 days) and the lumbar discectomy (0.059% in hospital) groups. However, Medicare patients undergoing lumbosacral spine surgery had a higher early mortality rate (0.52% in hospital) than patients treated with IT therapy.

Further examination of the three sentinel fatalities and six others identified in a systematic literature and database search revealed some similarities.[12] In every case, opioid or central nervous system depression was a primary or contributing cause of death. Eight of nine patients died within 24 hours of pump implantation, pump replacement, or catheter revision. One patient died within 48 hours of hospital discharge. In seven of the nine cases, patients were receiving higher starting doses of morphine or morphine-equivalent hydromorphone than are recommended for opioid-naïve patients on the Infumorph label (0.2 to 1.0 mg/day). (Preservative-free morphine sulfate, commercially available as Infumorph from Baxter and Astramorph from AstraZeneca, is the only opioid approved by the FDA for IT therapy.) Thorough comparison of these patients with the group treated with SCS indicated that excess mortality resulted from opioid therapy rather than from age or gender differences. This conclusion is consistent with analysis of a postmarket safety database (ePCR) maintained by Medtronic.[12] Physicians reported a confirmed or suspected drug overdose in 25 of 88 (28.4%) deaths within 3 days of pump implant, refill, replacement, programmed dose change, or catheter revision in noncancer patients. Overdosing was thus the most frequent reported cause of death. The nuances of drug choice and administration are discussed later in the section on medication-related side effects.

The ePCR database also contained information regarding 41 pumps that were returned for analysis after early fatalities.[12] Abnormalities were detected in eight pumps (19.5%), including battery depletion ($n = 2$), reservoir septum damage ($n = 2$), pump memory errors ($n = 2$), broken motor screws ($n = 1$), and residue on gears ($n = 1$). None of these conditions lead directly to drug overdose; in fact, most caused the infusion to cease.

Device-related perioperative morbidity and mechanical failure can be minimized by meticulous surgical technique and thorough training in pump operation. Consensus guidelines for limiting risk appear in **Box 13-1**.[4] The most common catheter-related complications are associated with suboptimal implantation technique, although the impact of these complications may be delayed beyond the perioperative period.[2] Catheter-pump misconnection or leakage and kinking, displacement, or obstruction of the catheter can all have serious consequences.[4] Because there are no programming safeguards to prevent potentially fatal overdose, clinicians should be skilled in pump programming and troubleshooting.[9]

To reduce the incidence of perioperative complications, the Polyanalgesic Conference 2007 recommended that vulnerable patients be monitored for 24 hours in a hospital setting when starting IT therapy or changing doses or drugs.[3] Their list of vulnerable patients included elderly and very young patients, opiate-naïve patients, and patients with poor cardiac function or respiratory reserve. In-hospital monitoring was not considered necessary for simple dosing changes or low-dose introduction of new medication.

Box 13-1: Guidelines for Minimizing the Risk of Perioperative Morbidity[4]

- Begin intrathecal therapy with a safe starting dose even if that dose does not provide effective pain relief.
- Avoid the use of concomitant central nervous system depressants during the immediate postimplantation period.
- Become an expert in pump construction and programming.
- Personally supervise initial pump programming.
- Avoid excessively concentrated solutions at the start of therapy to minimize the delay of drug effects associated with slow infusion rates.
- Calculate the time at which new drug will first enter the intrathecal space and ask patients and caregivers to be especially vigilant for side effects during that time.
- Avoid using conversion tables to determine starting doses because these tables have no scientific basis and could lead to lethal drug overdose.

Medication-Related Side Effects

The opioid morphine sulfate and the nonopioid antiinflammatory drug ziconotide (Prialt, Azur Pharma) are the only FDA-approved analgesics for IT therapy. Although this review concentrates on these approved first-line medications, numerous other medications have been used clinically.[4] The Polyanalgesic Algorithm for Intrathecal Therapies[14] lists hydromorphone as a first-line choice; fentanyl, bupivacaine/clonidine as second-line choices in combination with opioids; sufentanil as a fourth-line choice; and ropivacaine, bupivacaine, midazolam, meperidine, and ketorolac as fifth-line choices. A number of experimental agents are considered sixth-line choices, including gabapentin, adenosine, octreotide, Xen2174, CGX-1160, and Am336.[7]

Almost all IT drug side effects are mediated by opioid receptors.[6] A drug's hydrophilicity or lipophilicity controls the speed and extent of absorption, which in turn determines whether side effects are localized or occur as cerebrospinal fluid (CSF) ascends cephalad. Morphine, which is highly hydrophilic, migrates slowly, and its effects linger. This pattern of IT morphine metabolism and distribution produces slower onset and longer lasting antinociception but also tends to amplify side effects. Hydromorphone, also a first-line choice based on preclinical and clinical evidence, acts more quickly and is more potent than morphine because of greater lipophilicity.[3] Although hydromorphone activates more than one type of opioid receptor, it produces fewer metabolites than morphine and distributes less widely, traits that may explain its having fewer side effects. Common side effects of IT morphine therapy are listed in **Table 13-1**. Note that the most frequently occurring side effects appear near initiation, are eminently treatable, and generally resolve during the first 3 months of IT therapy.

Before the nine fatalities described earlier,[12] the most serious side effects of IT therapy were believed to be associated with prolonged, high-dose opioid administration.[10] The investigation prompted by those cases demonstrated that early mortality occurs at a rate of approximately one per 1000 implants or component replacement procedures and that great care should be taken in selecting drugs and dosing regimens to prevent overdosing.[12] In theory, the mandate has always been to fine tune the opioid dose until achieving maximal analgesia with minimal side effects.[10] In practice, finding the appropriate balance between pain relief and side effects proves more complicated. Individual variation exists in patients' responses to opioids and no ceiling dose has ever been established.[15] In addition, conversion of large oral opioid doses to equivalent IT doses can be problematic.[9] Nor is there a true conversion factor for switching from one IT medication to another. Consequently, the Polyanalgesic Consensus Conference 2007 recommends starting with extremely low doses and escalating slowly when beginning IT therapy or changing from one medication to another.[3] Table 13-2 lists the panel's recommendations for the drug concentrations and doses used in IT therapy. During dose escalation, the panel recommended dosing increases of 20% to 30%, guided by each individual's needs and tolerance, at once-weekly intervals for frail or elderly patients and at more frequent intervals for younger, robust patients.

Ziconotide, the most recently FDA-approved drug for IT therapy, has been used effectively to treat neuropathic, nociceptive, and mixed neuropathic and nociceptive pain.[4] At the 2007 Polyanalgesic Consensus Conference, ziconotide was upgraded to a first-line medication. Its most common side effects are memory impairment (11.3%), dizziness, nystagmus and speech disorder (8.5%), nervousness and somnolence (7% each), and abnormal

Table 13-1: Incidence and Management of Side Effects Associated with Intrathecal Morphine Therapy

Side Effect	Incidence	Treatment
Pruritus	0% to 100%[25] 14% for long-term ITT[26]	Easily treatable with mu antagonist naloxone
Nausea and vomiting	30% with acute ITT[25] ~21% in long-term ITT[26]	Antiemetics Improved by lowering dose
Urinary retention	42%[27] to 80%[28] ~3% in long-term ITT[26] Dose dependent More common in men with enlarged prostates	Cholinomimetic agents (e.g., bethanechol)
Constipation	30%[26]	Stool softener, bowel stimulant, or laxatives
Edema (preexisting venous insufficiency and edema are relative contraindications to ITT[29])	3%[26] to 16%[30]	Leg raising, elastic stockings, compressive air pumps, salt and fluid restrictions, diuretics
Mental status change (sedation and lethargy, paranoid psychosis, catatonia, euphoria, anxiety, delirium, hallucination)	10% to 14% in long-term ITT[26]	Lower opiate dose first Treat sedation with psychostimulants (modafinil), neuroleptics (haloperidol), or benzodiazepines (lorazepam)
Sexual dysfunction	68.8% in women, 95.8% in men[11] Caused by opioid-induced hypogonadism	Lower opiate dose Rotate opioids Prescribe HRT
Respiratory depression	Cause of some fatalities soon after the start of IT[12]	Start ITT with low dose Monitor vulnerable patients for 24 hours after start or change of ITT[3] Readily reversed with naloxone or nalbuphine

HRT, hormone replacement therapy; ITT, intrathecal therapy.
Adapted from Ruan X: Drug-related side effects of long-term intrathecal morphine therapy, *Pain Physician* 10:357-365, 2007.

Table 13-2: Polyanalgesic Consensus Panelists Recommendations for Intrathecal Drugs Concentrations and Doses[3]

Drug	Maximum Concentration	Maximum Daily Dose
Morphine	20 mg/mL	15 mg
Hydromorphone	10 mg/mL	4 mg
Ziconotide	100 µg/mL	19.2 µg
Fentanyl	2 mg/mL	No known upper limit
Sufentanil	50 µg/mL	No known upper limit
Bupivacaine	40 mg/mL	30 mg
Clonidine	2 mg/mL	1.0 mg

gait (5.6%).[16] These side effects do not appear to be dose dependent but perhaps correlate to infusion rate.[4] A low starting dose (0.5 µg/day) and slow dose titration (not >0.5 µg/day) to a low mean dose may ameliorate the side effects seen in several placebo-controlled studies of ziconotide.[17] Ziconotide therapy can be interrupted or halted without causing serious withdrawal symptoms.[18]

Sudden loss of analgesia or lack of pain moderation during dose escalation deserve thorough investigation. Pump (battery) failure, catheter disruption, or human programming and dosing errors can all cause sudden cessation of drug delivery, which with baclofen can be life threatening.[3] Opioid tolerance may also be at fault.[10] Using a systematic troubleshooting algorithm ensures that clinicians do not overlook possible causes of ineffective treatment.[19] The clinician and patient should periodically assess treatment goals to be certain they are still being met.

Inflammatory Masses (Granulomas)

IT catheter tip inflammatory masses (granulomas) remain one of the most serious risks of IT therapy.[3] The first report of granuloma associated with IT therapy occurred in 1991,[20] 10 years after implantable pumps were introduced.[8] A survey published in 1998 found that 31 of 519 respondents (6%) had patients who developed neurological sequelae or granulomas after catheter implant.[21] By November 2000, 41 cases had been described in the medical literature or reported to regulatory authorities or manufacturers.

Neurological deficits result from the size of the inflammatory mass rather than from any neurotoxic effects of medication. Damage caused by granulomas can include sensory loss, impaired bowel and bladder function,[8] and permanent paralysis.[4] A possible cause-and-effect relationship has been posited between granuloma formation and morphine sulfate or hydromorphone. Granuloma formation in beagles was associated with lumbar CSF morphine concentrations of 40 µg/mL.[8] Animal data tied granulomas to higher total daily dosage as well as longer-term treatment, with a granuloma incidence of 0.4% after 2 years and 1.16% after 6 years. Animal data failed to define a dose that did not incite IT granuloma formation. However, adding clonidine at more than 0.25 mg/day to 1.5 mg/day morphine prevented mass formation in animals.[10]

Granuloma formation in humans is far less predictable than in animals, and its incidence is more difficult to calculate.[22] In a survey of practice choices in IT therapy, 55 of 83 respondents had treated at least one patient who developed a granuloma.[23] Sixty-six percent of the respondents had a patient experience temporary or permanent neurological injury because of a granuloma. A recent retrospective longitudinal study of 56 consecutive patients examined the factors believed to be associated with granuloma

formation.[22] Four of 56 (7%) patients developed granulomas, equivalent to 0.009 events per patient year. The study documented a significant correlation between opioid dose ($r = 0.275$; $P<0.05$), yearly increase in dose ($r = 0.433$; $P<0.05$), and granuloma formation. No correlation was found between flow rate ($r = 0.056$) or opioid concentration ($r = 0.214$) and granuloma formation, although concentration had been implicated in other studies. All patients who developed granulomas had opioid doses smaller than 10 mg/day, so this side effect occurs with relatively small morphine doses. Despite its greater solubility, diamorphine proved no better than morphine in preventing granulomas.

Patients with granulomas may present with motor or sensory dysfunction or require more medication for pain relief.[8] Breakthrough pain is as likely to signal granuloma formation as tolerance to opioids. No evidence suggests that one type of catheter or material is associated with granuloma, although some patients do seem more susceptible to granuloma formation than others. These include younger patients receiving higher morphine doses. Regular surveillance and immediate investigation of any complaint of new pain, weakness, or rapid escalation in dose facilitate early diagnosis, which may prevent serious sequelae, including permanent paralysis. Inflammatory masses can be treated with minimally invasive techniques if discovered early. Magnetic resonance imaging remains the gold standard for catheter imaging, even for patients who are also receiving clonidine. However, a computed tomography myelogram through the pump is more cost-effective.

Treatment of a granuloma consists of withdrawing the catheter tip approximately 2 cm from the mass to prevent its growth.[8] Many masses disappear after the catheter tip is withdrawn. If symptoms decrease, the catheter tip should be scanned again in 6 months. To avoid creating a new granuloma, the 2007 Consensus Panel recommends decreasing the dose of opioid or changing to fentanyl or sufentanil. If symptoms persist, the clinician should discontinue the infusion, change to saline, and empty the drug reservoir. It may be necessary to treat withdrawal signs and symptoms, especially for patients receiving clonidine or baclofen. If neurological signs and symptoms worsen, surgical removal of the mass may become necessary.

Hormonal Changes

Long-term ITO therapy profoundly influences neuroendocrine function.[11] Two major hormonal systems are primarily affected, the hypothalamic–pituitary–adrenal axis and the hypothalamic–pituitary–gonadal axis.[10] Before the advent of ITO therapy, hormonal effects were studied chiefly in heroin addicts and patients on methadone maintenance. In this population, opioids decreased libido and aggression, caused menstrual irregularities or amenorrhea, and caused galactorrhea.[24] The effects of long-term treatment of chronic pain with ITOs were less well known.

Abs et al[11] compared the endocrine consequences of long-term ITOs in 73 patients (29 men and 44 women) being treated for nonmalignant pain with 20 patients being treated for a comparable pain syndrome without opioids. In men treated with ITOs, the serum testosterone level, free androgen index, and serum luteinizing hormone (LH) level were significantly lower ($P < 0.001$ in all cases) than in the control group. In women treated with ITOs, the serum LH, estradiol, and progesterone levels were lower than in the control group. The 18 postmenopausal women had significantly decreased serum LH ($P < 0.001$) and follicle-stimulating hormone ($P < 0.012$) levels compared with the control group. Decreased libido was noted in 23 of 24 men (95.8%) and 22 of 32 women (68.8%). This effect seems to be more pronounced with IT therapy than with oral opioids. Men and women treated with ITOs had significantly lower 24-hour urinary free cortisol excretion ($P = 0.003$), peak cortisol response to insulin-induced hypoglycemia ($P = 0.002$), insulin-like growth factor ($P = 0.002$), and peak growth hormone response to hypoglycemia ($P = 0.010$) than people in the control group. Thyroid function and prolactin levels were normal in the opioid-treated group, but they had significantly decreased high-density lipoprotein (HDL) cholesterol levels ($P = 0.041$) and a significantly increased total-to-HDL ratio ($P = 0.008$) compared with the control group. Hormone replacement therapy restored libido in most patients treated with ITOs but not uniformly or completely. The calcium channel blocker ziconotide does not alter testosterone production.[3]

Opioids also exert immunomodulatory effects on both the innate and adaptive immune systems, indirectly or directly through opioid-like receptors on immune cells.[10] Prolonged opioid therapy suppresses immune function more than short-term exposure, and abrupt withdrawal of opioids can induce immunosuppression. Different opioids may act on the immune system differently; for example, methadone is reportedly less immunosuppressive than morphine. These observations are confounded by the fact that pain by itself can impair immune function. So patients whose pain is not being alleviated may be subject to immune system dysfunction apart from any opioid action.

Given that a high percentage of patients treated with ITOs also develop hypogonadotropic hypogonadism or hypocorticism, patients' endocrine levels and function should be carefully monitored during IT therapy. An unfavorable lipid profile may also need to be treated.

Minimizing Risk

Decades of experience with IT therapy for intractable pain have confirmed both its advantages and its drawbacks. Once reserved for short-term pain relief in terminal patients, IT therapy now offers the hope of diminished pain to patients who expect to live for years. The risk-to-benefit calculation changes for this new population. Clinicians can minimize risk by selecting appropriate patients for IT therapy and by following the experience-based guidelines listed in **Box 13-1**. Because IT therapy is both technically challenging and time consuming, practitioners should be prepared to invest time in their own training and in managing patients. The dedicated effort of experts has produced numerous consensus statements and guidelines that facilitate IT therapy. Their work will continue to guide the application of this valuable therapy.

Conclusions

IT therapy has provided pain relief in tens of thousands of cases. The very serious but relatively rare side effects demand vigilant oversight, prompt diagnosis, and quick resolution. The most common side effects usually occur near the start of treatment, are readily managed, and resolve within a short time. Improved drug delivery systems and new pharmacological regimens hold the promise of greater success and fewer risks to appropriately selected patients in the future.

References

1. Krames ES, Olson K: Clinical realities and economic considerations: patient selection in intrathecal therapy. *J Pain Symptom Manage* 14(3 suppl):S3-S13, 1997.

2. Follett KA, Burchiel K, Deer T, et al: Prevention of intrathecal drug delivery catheter-related complications. *Neuromodulation* 6(1):32-41, 2003.

3. Deer T, Krames ES, Hassenbusch SJ, et al: Polyanalgesic Consensus Conference 2007: recommendations for the management of pain by intrathecal (intraspinal) drug delivery: report of an interdisciplinary expert panel. *Neuromodulation* 10(4):300-328, 2007.

4. Deer TR, Smith HS, Cousins M, et al: Consensus guidelines of the selection and implantation of patients with noncancer pain for intrathecal drug delivery. *Pain Physician* 13:E175-E213, 2010.

5. Onofrio BM, Yaksh TL, Arnold PG: Continuous low-dose intrathecal morphine administration in the treatment of chronic pain of malignant origin. *Mayo Clin Proc* 56:516-520, 1981.

6. Ruan X: Drug-related side effects of long-term intrathecal morphine therapy. *Pain Physician* 10:357-365, 2007.

7. Deer TR, Krames E, Hassenbusch S, et al: Future directions for intrathecal pain management: a review and update from the Interdisciplinary Polyanalgesic Consensus Conference 2007. *Neuromodulation* 11(2):92-97, 2008.

8. Deer TR, Krames E, Hassenbusch S, et al: Management of intrathecal catheter-tip inflammatory masses: an updated 2007 consensus statement from an expert panel. *Neuromodulation* 11(2):77-91, 2008.

9. Rathmell JP, Miller MJ: Death after initiation of intrathecal drug therapy for chronic pain. *Anesthesiology* 111:706-708, 2009.

10. Ballantyne JC, Mao J: Opioid therapy for chronic pain. *N Engl J Med* 349:1943-1953, 2003.

11. Abs R, Verhelst J, Maeyaert, et al: Endocrine consequences of long-term intrathecal administration of opioids. *J Clin Endocrinol Metab* 85:2215-2222, 2000.

12. Coffey RJ, Owens ML, Broste SK, et al: Mortality associated with implantation and management of intrathecal opioid drug infusion systems to treat noncancer pain. *Anesthesiology* 5(3):881-891, 2009.

13. Smith TJ, Staats PS, Deer T, et al: Randomized clinical trial of an implantable drug delivery system compared with comprehensive medical management for refractory cancer pain: impact on pain, drug-related toxicity, and survival. *J Clin Oncol* 20:4040-4049, 2002.

14. Manichikanti L, Boswell MV, Datta S, et al: Comprehensive review of therapeutic interventions in managing chronic spinal pain. *Pain Physician* 12:E123-E198, 2009.

15. Galer BS, Coyle N, Pasternak GW, Portenoy RK: Individual variability in the response to different opioids: report of five cases. *Pain* 49:87-91, 1992.

16. Webster LR, Fisher R, Charapata S, Wallace MS. Long-term intrathecal ziconotide for chronic pain: an open-label study. *J Pain Symptom Manage* 37:363-372, 2009.

17. Fisher R, Hassenbusch S, Krames E, et al: A consensus statement regarding the present suggested titration for Prialt (ziconotide). *Neuromodulation* 8:153-154, 2005.

18. Wallace MS, Charapata SG, Fisher R, et al: Intrathecal ziconotide in the treatment of chronic nonmalignant pain: a randomized, double-blind, placebo-controlled clinical trial. *Neuromodulation* 9:75-86, 2006.

19. Krames E: Intraspinal opioid therapy for chronic nonmalignant pain: current practice and clinical guidelines. *J Pain Symptom Manage* 11(6):333-352, 1996.

20. North RB, Cutchis PN, Epstein JA, Long DM: Spinal cord compression complicating subarachnoid infusion of morphine: case report and laboratory experience. *Neurosurgery* 29:778-784, 1991.

21. Schuchard M, Lanning R, North R, et al: Neurologic sequelae of intraspinal drug delivery systems. Results of a survey of American implanters of implantable drug delivery systems. *Neuromodulation* 1:137-148, 1998.

22. Duarte RV, Raphael JH, Southall JL, et al: Intrathecal inflammatory masses: is the yearly opioid dose increase an early indicator? *Neuromodulation* 13:109-113, 2009.

23. Deer TR, Krames E, Levy RM, et al: Practice choices and challenges in the current intrathecal therapy environment: an online survey. *Pain Med* 10(2):304-309, 2009.

24. Malik SA, Khan C, Jabbar A, Iqbal A: Heroin addiction and sex hormones in males. *J Pak Med Assoc* 42:210-212, 1992.

25. Chaney MA: Side effects of intrathecal and epidural opioids. *Can J Anaesth* 42:891-903, 1995.

26. Anderson VC, Burchiel KJ: A prospective study of long-term intrathecal morphine in the management of chronic nonmalignant pain. *Neurosurgery* 44(2):289-300, 1999.

27. Winkelmuller M, Winkelmuller W: Long-term effects of continuous intrathecal opioid treatment in chronic pain of non-malignant etiology. *J Neurosurgery* 85:458-467, 1996.

28. Bailey PL, Rhondeau S, Schafer PG, et al: Dose-response pharmacology of intrathecal morphine in human volunteers. *Anesthesiology* 79:49-59, 1993.

29. Aldrete JA, Couto da Silva JM: Leg edema from intrathecal opiate infusions. *Eur J Pain* 4:361-365, 2000.

30. Anderson VC, Cooke B, Burchiel KJ: Intrathecal hydromorphone for chronic nonmalignant pain: a retrospective study. *Pain Med* 2(4):287-297, 2001.

14 Complications Associated with Intrathecal Drug Delivery Systems

Maruti Kari, Matthew Jaycox, and Timothy R. Lubenow

CHAPTER OVERVIEW

Chapter Synopsis: Intrathecal drug delivery systems (IDDS) for the treatment of chronic pain or spasticity carries significant inherent risks associated with surgical implantation of the delivery device in addition to the risks associated with opioid drugs. Many risks can be minimized with appropriate precautions. As with any surgical procedure to treat pain, proper patient selection can improve the chances of success and reduce the potential for poor outcomes or complications. Surgical risks include infection, bleeding, and neurological damage, all of which can be avoided with careful attention or immediate treatment. Mechanical risks include those associated with the catheter or the pump itself. This chapter outlines the ways that these complications may present and how they might be treated. Drug-related side effects with IDDS mirror those with systemic delivery, but spinal delivery may have more rapid or severe consequences because of its central delivery.

Important Point: Strict attention to asepsis and surgical technique is essential.

Clinical Pearl: Perform procedure initially with monitored anesthesia care and inject small doses of intrathecal bupivacaine through the catheter for surgical anesthesia once the intrathecal device is placed.

Clinical Pitfall: Performing an intraspinal trial with opiates while the patient continues to take the usual opioid dose may lead to the incorrect observation that the patient had a positive response to trial.

Introduction

The discovery of opiate receptors in the spinal cord in 1973 provided a scientific rationale for intraspinal delivery of opioid drugs.[1-3] Basbaum et al[4] described the descending pain inhibition system in the substantia gelatinosa. This observation laid the groundwork for the findings of Wang et al,[5] who reported the successful use of intrathecal (IT) morphine for treatment of intractable cancer pain in 1979. This report by Wang et al was a factor in increased utilization of spinal opioids. The use of intraspinal opioid infusions to treat chronic benign and cancer pain has continued to evolve and increase. With the increase in use of intrathecal drug delivery systems (IDDS), we are able to discern the various complications associated with this evolving technique.

Complications associated with IDDS can be categorized into surgical, mechanical, and drug-related complications.

Surgical Complications

As with any surgical procedure, bleeding, neurological injury, infection, and wound dehiscence can complicate the implantation of IDDS. Cerebrospinal fluid (CSF) leaks, seroma in the implant pocket, and malpositioning of the pump are other complications that are more specific to the implantation of these devices.

Bleeding

Intraoperative bleeding generally occurs from ineffective local hemostasis during the procedure. It is important to identify and correct systemic factors before surgery by reviewing preoperative medications for prescribed anticoagulants, herbal (e.g., garlic, ginkgo, and ginseng), and over-the-counter medications that can increase the risk of bleeding.[6] Factors that impact bleeding include medications, hepatic disease, dysfunction or lack of platelets, and clotting factor disorders. Patients who are anticoagulated are not candidates for this type of procedure until the coagulation parameters return to normal. The American Society of Regional Anesthesia and Pain Medicine guidelines (Third Edition, 2010) for anticoagulant for neuraxial analgesia should be followed to decrease the risk of spinal or epidural hematoma.[6] In rare occasions, even if all the above considerations of coagulation parameters being within therapeutic range are normal, these patients can bleed, and it is vital to recognize an epidural hematoma. Epidural hematoma, depending on the extent and neurological examination, requires prompt surgical intervention.

Neurological Injury

Neurological injury, although rare, is a very serious complication that can result from trauma to the spinal cord during the IT placement of the catheter.[7] Emphasis is on prevention. A thorough and complete neurological examination should be performed to establish a good baseline neurological status in all patients before the procedure. Imaging modalities such as radiography, magnetic resonance imaging (MRI), and computed tomography (CT) myelograms can help delineate the anatomy of the proposed insertion site. Furthermore, these can also help identify pathological structures such as metastatic lesions of the spine, potential sites for compression fractures, scoliosis, and stenosis that can potentially increase the risk of neurological injury during catheter insertion or after the procedure. If resistance is encountered while advancing the catheter, we recommend that the catheter be withdrawn completely with the needle (to prevent catheter shearing) and insertion attempted at a different level under fluoroscopic guidance. Placement of IT catheters can be difficult at times because these patients are positioned laterally, and obesity makes it more challenging. A postprocedure neurological examination should be performed and well documented. If any new signs or symptoms are noted after the procedure, they should be immediately evaluated further, if necessary, with imaging studies. Severe symptoms or signs may necessitate removal of the catheter while further evaluation is underway. There is significant controversy if the IT catheter should be placed with patients under general anesthesia or monitored anesthesia care to prevent neurological injury to patients.

Infection

Infections related to this procedure can be categorized into superficial and deep and are more common in the first 15 to 45 days after the procedure.[8-11] The rate of incidence of infection has been reported to vary anywhere between 0% and 9%.[12,13] Pediatric patients with cerebral palsy and cancer patients were found to have higher incidence rates of infections possibly because of disturbances in their immunological function.[12,14,15] The presence of feeding tubes and colostomies in this patient population also contributes to the increased risk of infections.[8] Placement of the IT pump on the side opposite to that of the ostomy site and a subfascial rather than a subcutaneous implantation may decrease the rate of infections in these patients.[15,16]

Superficial infections mainly affect the skin incision site and the subcutaneous tissue. Clinical features of superficial infections include erythema; tenderness; swelling; and increase in temperature; purulent drainage at the implant site; and elevated white blood cell (WBC) count, C-reactive protein, and erythrocyte sedimentation rate. Patients whose immune systems are compromised because of their primary disease may not present with fever or elevated WBC counts. Occasionally, it is difficult to distinguish infections at the implant site from local irritation. If in doubt, incision drainage and inspection is warranted or ultrasound-guided aspiration of fluid may be indicated. In many cases, the clinician can observe the patient very closely over several days to determine the origin of the pathology. When symptoms are persistent or severe, further investigation is warranted. The most common pathogens associated with IDDS infections include *Staphylococcus aureus*, *Escherichia coli*, and *Proteus mirabilis*.[8] Wound and blood culture should be obtained, and broad-spectrum antibiotics should be initiated while awaiting the culture results. After the pathogen is identified, antibiotics specific to that pathogen should be administered. Deep infections may involve the soft tissues surrounding the pump, the catheter tract, and the meninges. Meningitis may present with severe nausea and vomiting, headaches, nuchal rigidity, fever, and elevated WBC counts.[12] When deep infections are suspected, samples of the fluid around the pump, CSF, and blood should be sent for cultures and sensitivity testing. CSF samples can be obtained from the side port of the device in addition.[15] Such serious systemic infections warrant admission to a hospital, immediate removal of the hardware, wound debridement, and treatment with broad-spectrum antibiotics specific to the pathogen. Delayed treatment can result in severe sepsis and even shock in these patients. On rare occasions, the CSF may not be infected, but the implanted pump content may be infected, and intravenously administered antibiotics will not reach the implanted device. In these situations,

there are very few case reports of placing the antibiotic into the implanted device to be infused to the CSF of the patient with success in clearing the infection in the implanted device. However, this requires extreme coordination between the infectious disease physicians and the interventional pain physician.

Measures to Prevent Infection Several measures can be taken to prevent infections associated with IT pump implantations. Appropriate prophylactic antibiotics, in an appropriate dose, should be administered preoperatively starting within 60 minutes before the incision.[17,18] The site should be cleaned and prepped with chlorhexidine or by an a povidone–alcohol solution. With draping the field, a sterile barrier such as Ioban should be used. Surgeons may wish to double glove during the draping maneuver and then discard the outer gloves before incision.[12,15,19] The pump should be handled only by the surgeon and scrub nurse.[8] It should be filled with the desired medication before implanting the device rather than filling through the skin after implantation. The implant pocket should be thoroughly irrigated before and after implantation using antibiotic irrigation solution.[12,15] Meticulous attention to hemostasis to minimize hematoma and seroma formation is essential.[12] This includes the use of topical thrombin with or without Gelfoam pledgets and oversewing the bleeding vessels with a figure-of-eight suture technique. Strict attention to sterile technique is important for all members of the implant team. When the patient is in the lateral decubitus position, several surgical issues become more problematic. Instruments may slide off the patient, and in an attempt to catch them, members of the surgical team may contaminate themselves by dropping their hands below waistline level. It is more prudent to allow the instrument or suction device to fall and replace it rather than risk contaminating the field. Using the C-arm to visualize the anteroposterior view in the lateral decubitus position requires the C-arm to come underneath the table, and with this maneuver brings a contaminated object close to the field. It is necessary to cover the C-arm coming up from the bottom with a half sheet or other suitable drape to keep the field sterile.[12] Finally, the use of cyanoacrylate adhesive (Dermabond) to seal the wound edges before placing the dressing may improve wound healing by preventing bacteria from migrating into the newly created incision after surgery.

Patients with a high index of suspicion for postoperative infection can benefit from obtaining nasal swabs preoperatively looking for methicillin-resistant *S. aureus*. For patients who have had a history of staphylococcal infections, the preoperative use of topical mupirocin (Bactroban) may be necessary.[12,16,20,21] The first postoperative follow-up visit should be within 7 days of the procedure. It is recommended that the first pump refill procedure be scheduled at least 2 to 4 weeks after the implant date. All refills should be done using proper sterile technique. Finally, patients should be educated regarding the symptoms and signs of infection and care of the implant site.

Cerebrospinal Fluid Leaks

CSF leaks can occur at the site of the dural puncture or from the catheter itself because of fractures, punctures, migration, or dislodgement of the catheter or the connection to the pump.[22,23] Occasionally, CSF can leak from around the properly inserted catheter. During the procedure, the catheter is threaded through a Touhy needle that is larger in diameter than the catheter, and when the needle is removed after the catheter is in place, CSF tends to leak around the catheter.[22,24] In most cases, this leak is self-limiting.[23] When the leak is persistent or occurs through the incision, the surgical wound should be revised.[22] Suturing the catheter to the fascia using "tobacco sac suture" was found to decrease the

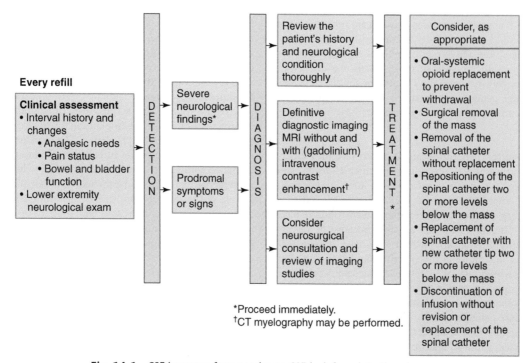

Initiation of IT analgesia
- Place catheter tip below conus medullaris (L1-L2), if possible.
- Use the lowest dose or concentration of opioid needed to treat and maintain analgesia.
- Consider nonopioid analgesic (clonidine, bupivacaine) coadministration to decrease IT opioid exposure.

Baseline information
- Complete neurological history
- Detailed neurological exam
- Radiographic documentation of catheter tip location

Every refill

Clinical assessment
- Interval history and changes
  - Analgesic needs
  - Pain status
  - Bowel and bladder function
- Lower extremity neurological exam

DETECTION

Severe neurological findings*

Prodromal symptoms or signs

DIAGNOSIS

Review the patient's history and neurological condition thoroughly

Definitive diagnostic imaging MRI without and with (gadolinium) intravenous contrast enhancement†

Consider neurosurgical consultation and review of imaging studies

TREATMENT*

Consider, as appropriate
- Oral-systemic opioid replacement to prevent withdrawal
- Surgical removal of the mass
- Removal of the spinal catheter without replacement
- Repositioning of the spinal catheter two or more levels below the mass
- Replacement of spinal catheter with new catheter tip two or more levels below the mass
- Discontinuation of infusion without revision or replacement of the spinal catheter

*Proceed immediately.
†CT myelography may be performed.

Fig. 14-1   CSF hygroma from persistent CSF leak from intrathecal space.

incidence of CSF leaks in one study.[25] Large CSF leaks can lead to persistent headaches. The incidence of such postdural headaches has been reported to vary from 1% to 30%.[22,26] The first line of management of such headaches is medical using medications such as oral or parenteral caffeine, sumatriptan, and theophylline.[26-30] If headaches persist, then an epidural blood patch can be performed. This involves injecting 15 to 20 cc of autologous blood into the epidural space to seal the puncture site. This should preferably be performed under fluoroscopy to avoid damage to the catheter and to ensure the injected blood is as close as possible to the suspected leak.[22,23] Epidural blood patches have a high success rate in treating patients with postdural headaches but have associated complications such as back pain and infection.[22,23,26]

CSF leaks along the catheter or at the pump connection site can cause CSF hygromas that are sterile collections of CSF in the subcutaneous tissues (**Fig. 14-1**). These are usually self-limiting as well as long as the source of the leak resolves.[31] CSF hygromas should not be aspirated because doing so can introduce pathogens and can potentially cause meningitis. If aspiration is necessary because of the size of the hygroma, strict adherence to sterile precautions is essential.[23]

Wound Dehiscence
Wound dehiscence can occur secondary to improper pump positioning, poor suture technique, or significant weight loss after implantation (**Fig. 14-2**) or implanting a pump that is larger than the subcutaneous pocket, infection, and excessive "twiddling" of

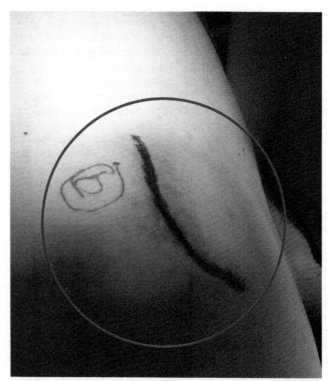

Fig. 14-2   Skin over the intrathecal pump is minimal because of post-surgical weight loss.

the pump by the patient.[23] Proper surgical technique, choosing an appropriately-sized pump, and patient education can help reduce the incidence of this complication.[7,12,14,32]

Device-Related Complications

These can be categorized as catheter-related and pump-related complications. Catheter-related complications include kinking, fractures, dislodgement from the pump or from dural entry site, migration, occlusion, and catheter-tip granuloma. Pump-related complications include pump failure, battery failure, overfilling, and torsion or pump rotation within the pocket.

Catheter-Related Complications

Problems with the catheter are more common than pump malfunctions.[13] Kinks, fractures, migration, occlusion, and dislodgement of the catheter can cause inadequate analgesia, CSF leaks, trauma to the spinal cord, or withdrawal symptoms.[13] Plain radiographic films can help detect dislodged, fractured, or disconnected catheters but are not reliable for detecting minor leaks, breaks, and kinks.[22] Visualization of the flow of a nonionic radiocontrast dye injected in the side port of the pump under direct fluoroscopy can help detect occlusion, kinks, minor leaks, and dislodgement of the catheter[31] (**Fig. 14-3**). Management of catheters that fracture, occlude, or dislodge requires surgical removal (**Figs. 14-4 and 14-5**) and replacement.[22] Kinks can be relieved by surgically freeing the catheter from scar tissue or replacing it with a new catheter. Catheter-related issues can be prevented by placement under direct fluoroscopic guidance and avoiding the mobile sections of the lumbar spine.[22]

Catheter-Tip Granuloma

Catheter-tip granuloma is an inflammatory mass that develops at the tip of the IT catheter that may produce extrinsic compression of the spinal cord, resulting in neurological sequelae of varying severity.[33] The actual incidence of this entity is difficult to establish; the reported incidence, based on various case studies, ranges from 0.1% to 0.5%.[34] The granuloma is composed of acute and

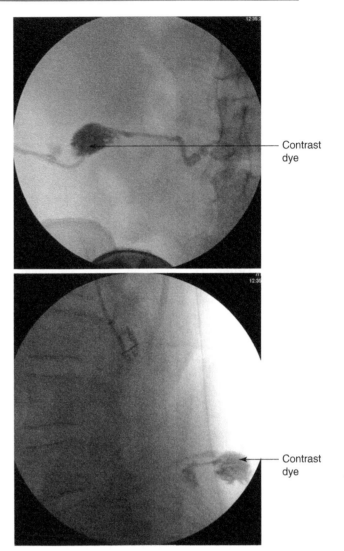
Contrast dye

Contrast dye

Fig. 14-4 Placement of intrathecal catheter and connection with previously implanted catheter.

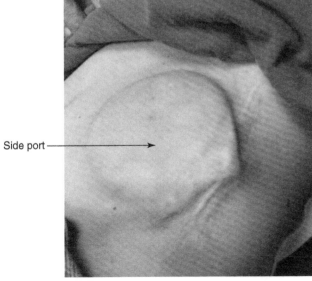
Side port

Fig. 14-3 Extravasation of contrast dye from intrathecal catheter.

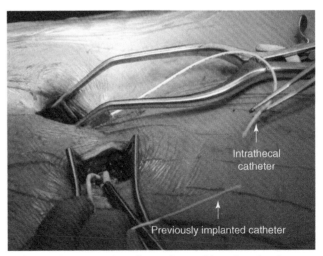
Intrathecal catheter

Previously implanted catheter

Fig. 14-5 Connection of two pieces of intrathecal catheter.

chronic inflammatory cells such as the macrophages, neutrophils, and monocytes, granulation tissue, and sometimes fibrotic tissue.[33,35] The IT catheter-tip granuloma was first reported in literature in 1991.[36] Since then, several reports have appeared describing this entity. In 2002, Hassenbusch et al[37] formed an expert panel that reviewed the available data and formulated an algorithm for the management of catheter-tip granulomas. The panel recommended prevention strategies, as well as emphasized the need for further animal and clinical research that would help better understand the formation of these granulomas[37] (**Fig. 14-6**).

Risk Factors

The risk factors associated with the development of catheter-tip granulomas can be attributable to the IT drug, dose and concentration, flow rates, catheter-tip location, type of delivery, and patient characteristics.[38]

Intrathecal Drugs IT catheter-tip masses were initially reported in patients receiving morphine infusions for chronic cancer and noncancer pain. It is now known that morphine and other opioid analgesics infused intrathecally can cause these masses over time.[33,38] Morphine, hydromorphone, and baclofen IT infusions, alone or in combination with other analgesics, were reported most commonly to be associated with catheter-tip granulomas. The incidence of IT granulomas with fentanyl is very low but has been reported. The only exceptions are IT sufentanil and ziconotide infusions.[38] The addition of IT clonidine to the existing IT analgesic was initially thought to prevent the IT catheter-tip granulomas, but more recent evidence suggests no such benefit.[37]

Dose and Concentration It is now known that the higher the concentration or the dose of the IT drug, the higher the incidence of granuloma formation.[33] It is uncertain if this problem will arise in all patients when exposed to high concentrations or if certain patients have predisposing factors.

Flow Rate Lower flow rates of IT drug infusions may be associated with increased incidence of granulomas when the concentration of the infusate is high. However, this may not be the case when the concentration of the IT drug is low or is delivered in bolus mode.[38,39] Further study is warranted.

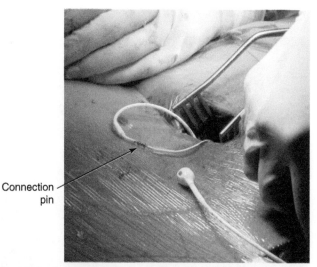

Connection
pin

Fig. 14-6 Algorithm for the management of catheter-tip granulomas. IT, intrathecal; MRI, magnetic resonance imaging.

Catheter-Tip Location Catheter tips are most commonly placed in the low thoracic or lumbar spaces. Not surprisingly, granulomas have been reported to be more commonly located in these spaces. However, granulomas have occurred with the catheter tip in cervical spaces and conus medullaris as well, suggesting that there is no one area that is better than the rest.[37,38] Nonetheless, the consensus is that the catheter tip should be located in the thoracic or lumbar spaces because these are larger spaces with greater CSF flow, allowing for greater dilution of the IT drug and thereby reducing the inflammatory response. Also, if a granuloma were to form in a space as tight as the cervical segments, the chances of spinal cord compression would be much higher with resultant potentially more severe neurological consequences. The problem with placing the catheter below the spinal cord in the conus medullaris is that the IT drug infusion is farther away from the target site, resulting in inadequate analgesia, especially when lipophilic opioids are used.[37,38]

Placement of the catheter tip dorsal to the cord as opposed to a ventral placement has been anecdotally cited as being better because it enables easier management of a granuloma if one were to form. However, there is no evidence to support or refute this practice, and at this time, it is only a matter of clinical expertise or preference.

Type of Delivery Both continuous infusion and frequent boluses of IT drugs are associated with granuloma formation.[38] There have been no comparative studies to date to examine which delivery route is superior.

Patient Characteristics Not all patients with high concentrations or dosages of IT drug infusions develop granulomas. Therefore, it postulated that some patients are more "susceptible" than others based on possible differences in CSF quantity and flow rates. However, at this time, there is no reliable way to predict who is a "susceptible patient."[38]

Clinical Presentation and Management Patients who develop catheter-tip granulomas may present with breakthrough pain or change in the character of their chronic pain and decreased analgesia requiring frequent and large dose escalations. They also present with focal sensory and motor neurological features or in extreme cases may present with paresis or bladder and bowel incontinence indicating severe spinal cord compression. No matter what the presentation, a thorough neurological examination followed by imaging studies should be performed. MRI with gadolinium contrast is the imaging study of choice.[38] A granuloma associated with IT infusion is located at the catheter tip, is extramedullary, and is isointense with the spinal cord.[39,40] A hyperintense mass with a hypointense rim indicates spinal cord compression with cord inflammation and edema.[40] CT myelogram is another valuable imaging study that can help detect these masses and associated cord compression. The nonionic radiocontrast agent can be injected through the CSF port of the device, and the spread of the agent can be visualized using CT images.[40,41]

Patients with increasing pain, sudden loss of analgesia, new pain, with or without neurological impairment should be imaged either with MRI (T1-weighted with gadolinium) or CT myelography.[40,42] If there is no mass on the imaging study, then the dose can be increased or one can add an adjuvant or adjust the catheter tip. If a mass is detected, then the catheter tip should be withdrawn out of the mass, and the dose or concentration of the IT drug should be reduced. One can also change the IT drug from morphine or hydromorphone to sufentanil or ziconotide. If no improvement in symptoms is noted, then the patient should be weaned off of the IT medication, and the pump should be filled with saline. This should cause the mass to regress in 2 to 5 months.[37] One should be aware that this can precipitate acute withdrawal if adequate replacement is not provided and could even be life threatening, especially in patients who were receiving IT baclofen or clonidine. Patients should be re-imaged within 6 months to evaluate the mass. If a small mass is still present, catheter removal or replacement should be considered. For patients with severe neurological impairments and imaging evidence of a mass with spinal cord compression, immediate surgical removal of the mass along with the IT device is recommended.[38]

Prevention, Risk Assessment, and Surveillance The average time to the development of a catheter-tip mass is anywhere between 2 months and 5 years. The shortest time to the development of an IT catheter-tip granuloma reported in literature was 27 days from the start of the infusion. As already mentioned, high concentrations, high daily doses, and low flow rates of IT morphine or hydromorphone infusions increase the risk of developing a catheter-tip granuloma.[38] Continuous infusions or frequent boluses were found to increase the risk as well. Prevention of the development of a catheter-tip granuloma entails reducing these risks as much as possible while maintaining adequate analgesia. Using lower concentrations, lower dosages, avoiding low flow rates, and switching to safer IT drug alternatives may help prevent granuloma formation. Similarly, patients receiving higher doses or concentrations at lower flow rates should be stratified as being at higher risk.[38] Providers should be vigilant for symptoms and signs that may indicate a developing IT granuloma in these patients. A focused clinical examination at every refill visit may help detect these clinical features early in the course. Patients at lower risk should be examined once a year. Imaging studies such as MRI are indicated if the clinical examination suggests neurological changes or there is a decrease in effective analgesia or significant dose escalation.[38]

Pump-Related Complications

As stated previously, pump-related complications include pump failure, battery failure, torsion, overfilling, and refilling errors.[22,31] Pump failure can result from using a drug that is incompatible with the pump. This can damage the catheter system internal to the pump.[22,23] The electronic telemetric receiver captures programming changes and resets the pump to the new settings. If this receiver fails, the pump will not accept the new settings.[22] The median battery life of a pump ranges from 48 to 60 months, and this can be affected by the settings at which the pump is programmed to deliver the drug. Mechanical failure of the pump or the battery can be managed by removing the old pump, and replacing it with a new one.[22] Torsion of the pump within the pump pocket can cause the catheter to be disconnected, kinked, or dislodged from the IT space. This can be prevented by anchoring the pump using four nonabsorbable sutures.[13] Overfilling the pump can cause pump failure because of excessive pressure and can also result in an overdose. This can be prevented by using manometric systems that are provided in the manufacturer refill kits.[22] Refilling errors such as programming the wrong concentration of the drug, using the wrong drug, or injecting the drug into the side port of the pump can all cause an excessive dose to be delivered to the patient, resulting in severe respiratory depression, cardiovascular collapse, seizures, or death. If an overdose is recognized, the pump should be aspirated of all the medication and filled with saline. The patient should be admitted to an intensive care unit for close monitoring, supportive therapy, and opioid reversal if required. Refilling errors can be minimized by allowing only staff trained in refilling techniques to perform these procedures. If locating the central refilling port is difficult in a patient, one should attempt to refill the pump under direct fluoroscopic visualization to prevent accidental injection of the side port.[22] More recently, ultrasound guidance has been suggested to facilitate identification of the central reservoir port.

Intrathecal Drugs and their Side Effects

Drug that are most commonly used for IT delivery via programmable pumps include opiates, baclofen, and ziconotide. Clonidine and bupivacaine are also used as adjuvant drugs in combination with opiates. Commonly used opiates include morphine, hydromorphone, fentanyl, and sufentanil. Side effects related to the IT drugs vary in severity based on the dose and concentration of drug or drugs being infused.

Opiates

IT opioids cause side effects that are similar to the oral opiates, but the incidence of these side effects is much lower in comparison. Within the class, morphine has a higher incidence of side effects than fentanyl, sufentanil, or hydromorphone when delivered intrathecally. This is because of the hydrophilic properties of morphine, which cause it to migrate cephalad with the CSF flow.[43] This may also be attributable to a much more extensive experience with morphine in the literature and may not represent the clinical reality. More study is needed to evaluate comparative risks. Fentanyl, sufentanil, and to some degree hydromorphone, on the other hand, are lipophilic and therefore get absorbed quickly into the spinal cord, where they attach to the opiate receptors. IT morphine has a slow onset and longer duration of action for the same reason as mentioned above, but fentanyl and hydromorphone have quick onset and shorter duration of action.[43]

Nausea and Vomiting Nausea and vomiting occur, presumably, because of the cephalad migration and interaction of IT opiates with chemoreceptor trigger zone (CTZ) (area postrema).[44,45] The incidence of nausea and vomiting has been reported to be as high as 30% with acute administration and 21% with long-term infusion.[43,46] They can also occur because of delayed gastric emptying or vestibular sensitization induced by these drugs. Positional changes tend to exacerbate these symptoms in some patients.[47-49] Ondansetron, droperidol, hydroxyzine, and prochlorperazine help counter nausea and vomiting associated with CTZ activation. In patients with vestibular sensitization, meclizine, promethazine, and scopolamine have been found to be effective. Metoclopramide enables the peristalsis of the gastrointestinal (GI) tract, thus helping with nausea and vomiting associated with delayed gastric emptying. When symptoms are exacerbated with positional changes, meclizine, scopolamine, and promethazine can help.[50,51] In patients with severe nausea or vomiting, a combination of these medications may be required in addition to lowering the dose of the IT medication.

Pruritus Cephalad migration of the IT opiate and the ensuing interaction of these drugs with the trigeminal nucleus in the superficial medulla have been presumed to cause pruritus.[52] From the trigeminal nucleus, the neural signals travel down via the cervical spinal cord to the substantia gelatinosa of the dorsal horn, which then elicits the "itch reflex."[53,54] Patients generally develop tolerance to pruritus in 1 to 2 weeks of the initiation of IT opiate infusion.[51]

Low-dose naloxone infusion provides symptomatic relief without loss of analgesia. Nalbuphine, a μ-receptor antagonist and a κ-receptor agonist, has also been used to relieve pruritus.[51] Although histamine plays no role in the mechanism for pruritus secondary to IT opiates, antihistamines have been found to provide good relief from pruritus as well.[43]

Urinary Retention The incidence of urinary retention after acute IT opiate administration has been reported to be as high as 42% to 80%. Elderly men with enlarged prostates are particularly at high risk for developing this complication.[55,56] The incidence with long-term infusions is much lower at 3%.[48] The mechanism involved in the development of urinary retention is thought to be attributable to the agonistic action of IT opiates at the μ- and the δ-opioid receptors in the lower spinal cord that decreases the sacral parasympathetic outflow to the detrusor muscles.[57] This relaxes the bladder, causing difficulty in voiding urine. Urinary retention can be readily reversed by naloxone, but this also reverses the analgesia. Cholinomimetic drugs such as bethanechol can relieve urinary retention.[58]

Constipation Opiates have been known to decrease the motility of the GI tract and prolong the intestinal transit time. Interaction with the opioid receptors in the spinal cord rather than systemic absorption has been cited as the possible mechanism for constipation.[59,60] Stool softeners along with bowel stimulants should be administered initially. One can then add a laxative such as mineral oil or glycerin suppository to the regimen.[61] Domperidone and metoclopramide are prokinetic drugs that induce peristalsis and thus may help relieve constipation. Oral naloxone has also been found to be helpful despite its low bioavailability via this route.[62]

Respiratory Depression Respiratory depression secondary to IT opioids is rare but can be life threatening. Risk factors that predispose patients receiving IT opiates via programmable pumps include advanced age, concomitant use of sedatives, coexisting respiratory or neurological disease, high doses, and use of more lipophilic opiates.[52] Another cause of respiratory depression is inadvertent injection of some of the concentrated opiate subcutaneously or inadvertently through the catheter access side port of the pump.[52] Respiratory depression can be managed by admitting the patient for close monitoring, stopping the IT infusion until the patient stabilizes, supportive therapy such as supplemental oxygen, and in severe cases parenteral naloxone. Naloxone boluses should always be titrated to effect to prevent precipitating severe withdrawal symptoms.[63] One should also be aware that a continuous low-dose naloxone infusion may be required depending on the opiate used because the half-life of naloxone may be shorter than that of the opiate and therefore a naloxone bolus may wear off, causing relapse of the respiratory depression caused by the residual opiate.[64]

Hormonal and Sexual Abnormalities IT administration of opiates has been associated with hypogonadotropic hypogonadism; growth hormone deficiency; hypocortisolism; reduced libido; and in men, difficulty maintaining an erection. These changes are not dependent on the dose or duration of IT opioid administration. It is recommended that serum lipids, 24-hour urinary cortisol, and serum androgen or estrogen levels be monitored regularly in patients receiving IT opioids. Replacement with testosterone, estrogen, and corticosteroids should be initiated if levels of these hormones are low.[65]

Weight Gain and Edema The mechanism of this adverse reaction to IT opiates is unknown but may be related to hormonal changes affected by the opiates.[51] Opiates in high doses likely adversely decrease serum aldosterone in some patients, which in turn leads to sodium and water retention. Some patients may require diuretic therapy.[61] In some cases, the symptoms are severe enough to warrant discontinuation of IT therapy and removal of the pump.

Sedation and Mental Status Changes These are common with oral, intramuscular, and intravenous opioid use, especially in elderly and opioid-naïve patients. However, these side effects are very rare with IT infusions, and patients quickly develop tolerance to them.[64]

Baclofen

IT infusions of baclofen can cause sedation and weakness and can lead to falls. The withdrawal syndrome of baclofen can be very severe and life threatening if untreated. Seizures, rigidity, myoclonus, and death can result from acute baclofen withdrawal.[66] The clinical condition of acute baclofen withdrawal mimics malignant hyperthermia with high fevers, muscle rigidity, and rhabdomyolysis. Patients and their families should be educated regarding the clinical features of baclofen withdrawal. Patients should also be provided with oral prescriptions for baclofen to be used promptly in the event of a withdrawal. Dantrolene has been found to decrease the incidence of rhabdomyolysis that may occur because of severe muscular rigidity during acute baclofen withdrawal.[66]

Clonidine

IT clonidine can cause hypotension, dizziness, and falls, and acute withdrawal can cause severe rebound hypertension.[67]

Bupivacaine

IT bupivacaine can cause excessive numbness, motor blockade, cardiotoxicity with accidental intravascular delivery, and hypotension.[68,69]

Pharmacological side effects can be minimized and patient outcomes can be improved by early recognition, close monitoring, lower starting doses, slow titration, and aggressive management of side effects when they occur.

Conclusion

Our ability to control pain with IDDS has advanced significantly over the past 20 years with the introduction of more sophisticated pumps and a wider range of medications for use. Concurrent with that is the need to minimize complications associated with this technique. Careful adherence to proper surgical technique and understanding the pharmacology of the intraspinal medications used are necessary for one to achieve this endpoint.

References

1. Pert CB, Snyder SH: Opiate receptor: demonstration in nervous tissue. *Science* 179:1011-1104, 1973.
2. Yaksh TL, Rudy TA: Analgesia mediated by a direct spinal action of narcotics. *Science* 192:1357-1358, 1976.
3. Atweh SF, Kuhar MJ: Autoradiographic localization of opiate receptors in rat brain. I. Spinal cord and lower medulla. *Brain Res* 124:53-67, 1977.
4. Basbaum AI, Clanton CH, Fields HL: Opiate and stimulus-produced analgesia: functional anatomy of a medullospinal pathway. *Proc Natl Acad Sci U S A* 73:4685-4688, 1976.

5. Wang JK, Nauss LA, Thomas JE: Pain relief by intrathecally applied morphine in man. *Anesthesiology* 50:149-151, 1979.

6. Horlocker TT, Wedel DJ, Rowlingson JC, et al: Regional anesthesia in the patient receiving antithrombotic or thrombolytic therapy: American Society of Regional Anesthesia and Pain Medicine evidence-based guidelines (third edition). *Reg Anesth Pain Med* 35(1):64-101, 2010.

7. Aprilli D, Bandschapp O, Rochlitz C, et al: Serious complications associated with external intrathecal catheters used in cancer pain patients: a systematic review and meta-analysis. *Anesthesiology* 111:1346-1355, 2009.

8. Fjelstad AB, Hommelstad J, Sorteberg A: Infections Related to intrathecal baclofen therapy in children and adults: frequency and risk factors. *J Neurosurg Pediatr* 4(5):487-493, 2009.

9. Fan-Havard P, Nahata MC: Treatment and prevention of infections of cerebrospinal fluid shunts. *Clin Pharmacol* 6:866-880, 1987.

10. Langley JM, LeBlanc JC, Drake J, Milner R: Efficacy of antimicrobial prophylaxis in placement of cerebrospinal fluid shunts: meta-analysis. *Clin Infect Dis* 17:98-103, 1993.

11. Choux M, Genitori L, Lang D, Lena G: Shunt implantation: reducing the incidence of shunt infection. *J Neurosurg* 77:875-880, 1992.

12. Follett KA, Boortz-Marx RL, Drake JM, et al: Prevention and management of intrathecal drug delivery and spinal cord stimulation system infections. *Anesthesiology* 100(6):158-194, 2004.

13. Naumann C, Erdine S, Koulousakis A, et al: Drug adverse events and system complications of intrathecal opioid delivery for pain: origins, detection, manifestations, and management. *Neuromodulation* 2(2):92-107, 1999.

14. Murphy NA, Irwin N, Hoff C: Intrathecal baclofen therapy in children with cerebral palsy: efficacy and complications. *Arch Phys Med Rehabil* 83:1721-1725, 2002.

15. Albright AL, Turner M, Pattisapu JV: Best-practice surgical techniques for intrathecal baclofen therapy. *J Neurosurg* 104(4 suppl):233-239, 2006.

16. Kopell BH, Sala D, Doyle WK, et al: Subfascial implantation of intrathecal baclofen pumps in children: technical note. *Neurosurgery* 49:753-757, 2001.

17. Mangram AJ, Horan TC, Pearson ML, et al: Guideline for prevention of surgical site infection, 1999. Hospital Infection Control Practices Advisory Committee. *Infect Control Hosp Epidemiology* 20:250-280, 1999.

18. Burgher AH, Barnett CF, Obray JB, et al: Introduction of infection control measures to reduce infection associated with implantable pain therapy devices. *Pain Pract* 7(3):279-284, 2007.

19. Kulkarni AV, Drake JM, Lamberti-Pasculli M: Cerebrospinal fluid shunt infection: a prospective study of risk factors. *J Neurosurg* 94:195-201, 2001.

20. Shrestha NK, Banbury MK, Weber M, et al: Safety of targeted perioperative mupirocin treatment for preventing infections after cardiac surgery. *Ann Thorac Surg* 81:2183-2188, 2006.

21. van Rijen MML, Bonten M, Wenzel RP, Kluytmans JAJW: Intranasal mupirocin for reduction of *Staphylococcus aureus* infections in surgical patients with nasal carriage: a systematic review. *J Antimicrob Chemother* 61:254-261, 2008.

22. Krames ES: Intraspinal opioid therapy for chronic nonmalignant pain: current practise and clinical guidelines. *J Pain Symptom Manage* 11:333-352, 1996.

23. Krames ES: Intrathecal Infusion therapies for intractable pain: pain management guidelines. *J Pain Symptom Manage* 8:36-46, 1993.

24. Paice JA, Winkelmuller W, Burchiel K, et al: Clinical realities and economic considerations: efficacy of intrathecal pain therapy. *J Pain Symptom Manage* 14(suppl):14-26, 1997.

25. Koulousakis A, Imdahl M, Weber M: *Continuous intrathecal application of morphine in cancer pain.* Proceedings of the 8th World Congress, Vancouver, Canada, 1998.

26. Choi A, Laurito CE, Cunningham FE: Pharmacological management of postdural puncture headaches. *Ann Pharmacother* 30:831-839, 1996.

27. Sechzer PH, Abel L: Post-spinal anesthesia headache treated with caffeine. Part I. Evaluation with demand method. *Curr Ther Res* 24:307-312, 1978.

28. Jarvis AP, Grenawalt JW, Fagraeus L: Intravenous caffeine for postdural puncture headaches. *Anesth Analg* 65:316-317, 1986.

29. Feuerstein TJ, Zeides A: Theophylline relieves headaches following lumbar puncture: placebo-controlled, double-blind pilot study. *Klin Wochenschr* 64:216-218, 1986.

30. Carp H, Singh PJ, Vadhera R, et al: Effects of Serotonin-receptor agonist sumatriptan on postdural puncture headache: report of six cases. *Anesth Analg* 79:180-182, 1994.

31. Prager JP: *Complications of implantation, diagnosis and management.* Presented at Interventional Therapies Workshop, Dannemiller Memorial Educational Foundation, Memphis TN, September 22, 1996.

32. Faillace WJ: A no-touch technique protocol to diminish cerebrospinal fluid shunt infection. *Surg Neurol* 43:344-350, 1995.

33. Yaksh TL, Hassenbusch S, Burchiel K, et al: Inflammatory masses associated with IT drug infusion: a review of preclinical evidence and human data. *Pain Med* 3:300-312, 2002.

34. Toombs JD, Follett KA, Rosenquist RW, et al: IT catheter tip inflammatory mass: a failure of clonidine to protect. *Anesthesiology* 102:687-690, 2005.

35. Horais K, Hruby V, Rossi S, et al: Effects of chronic IT infusion of a partial differential opioid agonist in dogs. *Toxicol Sci* 71:263-275, 2003.

36. North RB, Cutchis PN, Epstein JA, et al: Spinal cord compression complicating subarachnoid infusion of morphine: case report and laboratory experience. *Neurosurgery* 29:778-784, 1991.

37. Hassenbusch S, Burchiel K, Coffey RJ, et al: Management of IT catheter-tip inflammatory masses: a consensus statement. *Pain Med* 3:313-323, 2002.

38. Deer T, Krames ES, Hassenbusch S, et al: Management of intrathecal catheter-tip inflammatory masses: an updated 2007 consensus statement from an expert panel. *Neuromodulation* 11(2):77-91, 2008.

39. Yaksh TL, Hassenbusch S, Burkiel K, et al: Inflammatory masses associated with intrathecal drug infusion: a review of preclinical evidence and human data. *Pain Med* 3:300-313, 2002.

40. Dickson D: Risks and benefits of long-term intrathecal analgesia. *Anaesthesia* 59:633-635, 2004.

41. Miele VJ, Price KO, Bloomfield S, et al: A review of IT morphine therapy related granulomas. *Eur J Pain* 10:251-261, 2006.

42. Deer TR: A prospective analysis of IT granuloma in chronic pain patients: a review of the literature and report of a surveillance study. *Pain Physician* 7:225-228, 2004.

43. Chaney MA: Side effects of intrathecal and epidural opioids. *Can J Anaesth* 42:891-903, 1995.

44. Wang SC, Borison HL: The vomiting center. *Archives of Neurology and Psychiatry* 63:928-941, 1950.

45. Simoneau Il, Hamza MS, Mata HP, et al: The cannabinoid agonist WIN55,212-2 suppresses opioid-induced emesis in ferrets. *Anesthesiology* 94:882-887, 2001.

46. Anderson VC, Burchiel KJ: A prospective study of long-term intrathecal morphine in the management of chronic nonmalignant pain. *Congress of Neurological Surgeons* 44(2):289-300, Feb 1999.

47. Loper KA, Ready LB, Dorman BH: Prophylactic transdermal scopolamine patches reduce nausea in postoperative patients receiving epidural morphine. *Anesth Analg* 68:144-146, 1989.

48. Wattwil M: Postoperative pain relief and gastrointestinal mobility. *Acta Chir Scand* 550:140-145, 1988.

49. Raffaeli W, Marconi G, Fanelli G: Opioid-related side-effects after intrathecal morphine: a prospective, randomized, double-blind dose-response study. *Eur J Anaesth* 23:605-610, 2006.

50. Holtsman M, Fishman SM: Opioid receptors. In Benton HT, Raja N, Molloy, RE, Liu S, et al, editors: *Essentials of Pain Medicine and Regional Anesthesia*, ed 2, Chapter 10:2005, pp 87-91.

51. Raj PR: 2000 Common analgesic side effects and treatment, *Practical Management of Pain*, ed 3, Appendix D 1025-1026.

52. Ballantyne JC, Loach AB, Carr DB: Itching after epidural and spinal opiates. *Pain* 33:149-160, 1988.

53. Hu JW, Dostrovsky JO, Sessie BJ: Functional properties of neurons in cat trigeminal subnucleus caudalis (medullary dorsal horn). I. Response to oral-facial noxious and non-noxious stimuli and projections to thalamus and subnucleus oralis. *J Neurophysiol* 45:173-192, 1981.

54. Scott PV, Fischer HBJ: Intraspinal opiates and itching: a new reflex? *BMJ* 284:1015-1016, 1998

55. Winkelmuller M, Winkelmuller W: Long-term effects of continuous intrathecal opioid treatment in chronic pain of non-malignant etiology. *J Neurosurg* 85:458-467, 1996.

56. Bailey PL, Rhondeau S, Schafer PG, et al: Dose-response pharmacology of intrathecal morphine in human volunteers. *Anesthesiology* 79:49-59, 1993.

57. Drenger B, Magora F, Evron S, et al: The action of intrathecal morphine and methadone on the lower urinary tract in the dog. *J Urol* 135:852-855, 1986.

58. Practice guidelines for cancer pain management: A report by the American Society Task Force on Pain Management, Cancer Pain Section. *Anesthesiology* 84:1243-1257, 1996.

59. Porreca F, Filla A, Burks TF: Spinal cord mediated opiate effects on gastrointestinal transit in mice. *Eur J Pharmacol* 86:135-136, 1983.

60. Thoren T, Wattwil M: Effects on gastric emptying of thoracic epidural analgesia with morphine or bupivacaine. *Anesth Analg* 67:687-694, 1988.

61. Harris JD, Kotob F: Management of opioid-related side effects. In De Leon-Casasola OA, editor: *Cancer Pain*, Chapter 18:2006, Saunders, pp 212-230.

62. Liu M, Wittbrodt E: Low-dose oral naloxone reverses opioid-induced constipation and analgesia. *J Pain Symptom Manage* 23:48-53, 2002.

63. Jacox A, Carr DB, Payne R, et al: Management of Cancer Pain. Clinical Practice Guideline no, 9. Rockville, Md: Agency for Health Care Policy and Research; US Dept of Health and Human Services, 1994 Public Health Service; AHCPR publication 94-0592.

64. Cherny NI: Opioid analgesics: comparative features and prescribing guidelines. *Drugs* 51:713-737, 1996.

65. Paice JA, Penn RD, Ryan WG: Altered sexual function and decreased testosterone in patients receiving intraspinal opioids. *J Pain Symptom Manage* 9:126-131, 1994.

66. Coffey RJ, Edgar TS, Francisco GE, et al: Abrupt withdrawal from intrathecal baclofen: Recognition and management of a potentially life-threatening syndrome. *Arch Phys Med Rehabil* 83:735-741, 2002.

67. Eisenach JC, DeKock M, Klimscha W: Alpha (2)-adrenergic agonists for regional anesthesia: a clinical review of clonidine (1984-1995). *Anesthesiology* 85(3):655-674, 1996.

68. Albright GA: Cardiac arrest following regional anesthesia with etidocaine or bupivacaine. *Anesthesiology* 51(4):285-287, 1979.

69. Huang YF, Pryor ME, Mather LE, et al: Cardiovascular and central nervous system effects of intravenous levobupivacaine and bupivacaine in sheep. *Anesth Analg* 86(4):797-804, 1998.

SECTION

III Evidence-Based Practice

Chapter 15 Management of Intrathecal Drug Delivery Systems in Patients with Co-Morbidities

Chapter 16 Cost-Effectiveness of Implanted Drug Delivery Systems

Chapter 17 Neuroaugmentation by Stimulation versus Intrathecal Drug Delivery Systems

Chapter 18 Anticoagulation Guidelines and Intrathecal Drug Delivery Systems

Chapter 19 Intrathecal Therapy for Malignant Pain

15 Management of Intrathecal Drug Delivery Systems in Patients with Co-Morbidities

Kenneth D. Candido

CHAPTER OVERVIEW

Chapter Synopsis: Intrathecal drug delivery systems (IDDS) for chronic pain can be a safe and effective procedure in properly selected patients. But patients with certain co-morbidities may be contraindicated for IDDS even if deemed otherwise appropriate. This chapter considers some of the issues that require critical attention to prevent adverse outcomes and increase the chances for successful treatment in these patients. Patients receiving antiplatelet and antithrombotic medications should refer to guidelines for neuraxial analgesia. For immunocompromised patients, including those with human immunodeficiency virus (HIV) and cancer, extra vigilance should be used to avoid the risk of perioperative infection. In patients with diabetes, rigid adherence to controlled glucose levels promotes proper healing after implantation. Obese patients may be at greater risk for the side effects of opioid drugs, which should be considered in treatment.

Important Points:
- Although specific guidelines do not exist per se on the implantation of IDDS in individuals acutely or chronically receiving antiplatelet and antithrombotic medications, the American Society of Regional Anesthesia (ASRA) Practice Advisory Guidelines pertaining to neuraxial analgesia and anesthesia are the closest available evidence for planning primary or revision surgery and management in patients otherwise deemed appropriate candidates for IDDS.
- Immunocompromised patients, including those with HIV and cancer, are at higher than average risk for developing perioperative superficial and deep infections. The rigid adherence to infection prevention, sterilization of the surgical site, pre-procedure administration of prophylactic antibiotics, and obsessive attention to wound care and management cannot be overemphasized.
- It appears that maintaining tight blood glucose control (serum glucose ≤125 mg/dL) in patients with diabetes is paramount to minimizing the development of delayed wound healing and postsurgical infectious complications. A high index of suspicion must be maintained in this patient group when dealing with insidious or delayed onset of symptomatology.
- Obesity predisposes patients to obstructive sleep apnea, among other co-morbidities, and should provide pause for concern in determining initiation doses of opioids and other respiratory depressant medications.
- Recovering addicts comprise a special population that demands intense scrutiny when determining both suitability for implantation as well as structuring follow-up visits, scheduling random supervised urine toxicologies, and eliminating conduct and personality issues that might sabotage otherwise superb surgical placement of IDDS.

Clinical Pearls:
- Patients using antiplatelet medication to prevent venous thromboembolism (VTE) should undergo an evaluation to assess their risk of clinical bleeding before undertaking IDDS therapy. Use of the ASRA guidelines for neuraxial blockade should be considered when determining suitability to proceed.
- When considering IDDS use in patients with chronic, stable infections including HIV, be prepared to use prolonged antibiotic therapy aimed at a wide spectrum of potential pathogens, including opportunistic ones.
- Maintain a high index of suspicion when dealing with diabetic patients regarding potential infections, poor wound healing, bleeding complications, and increased morbidity. Keeping serum glucose levels less than or equal to 125 mg/dL should be standard.
- Patients with a history of substance abuse including alcohol dependence present a particular challenge as concomitant depression and anxiety oftentimes undermine the best efforts at maximizing IDDS analgesia while reducing systemic use of mood-altering chemicals.

Clinical Pitfalls:
- Beware of unrecognized drug-drug interactions in individuals taking multiple NSAIDs such as aspirin in combination with COX-1 and COX-2 nonselective antiinflammatory medications or herbal medications. Although not specifically contraindicated for neuraxial blockade, such combinations may result in prolonged clinical bleeding in IDDS patients.
- Regardless of attention to detail and technique, the obese patient presents challenges that oftentimes cannot be mitigated. Obesity is an independent risk factor for development of perioperative infection and requires extended duration of vigilance in the perioperative period and beyond.
- Do not overlook the value of a pre-procedure brain imaging study in individuals undergoing implantation who have cancer, as unrecognized lesions might unfavorably influence responses to treatment.

Introduction

The placement of intrathecal drug delivery systems (IDDS) for pain and spasticity entails dealing with a group of patients having diverse needs and underlying medical conditions that demand attention either before the implantation of the IDDS or concomitant to that placement. Although it is axiomatic that proper patient selection is vital to the success of these advanced treatment modalities, predicting the effect of preexisting patient co-morbidities on outcomes often is not readily or consistently achievable. This chapter deals with the co-morbidities of these individuals and how they may potentially affect the success or lead to failure if not adequately and competently addressed. Patient optimization strategies are described to the extent that they are under control of the interventionalist. A team approach that includes seeking out consultant specialists and adhering to their recommendations is emphasized. The focus of the present discussion will include the more commonly used therapeutic agents approved by the U.S. Food and Drug Administration (FDA) for continuous intrathecal (IT) administration, morphine and baclofen, as well the more commonly encountered clinical scenarios that trigger the use of these chemicals by this delivery mechanism. Among the co-morbidities, preexisting features that may determine outcome will be discussed, and post-implantation morbidity and mortality will be featured as it potentially relates to the therapy provided. Because it is known that the most common side effects of IDDS opioid treatments include nausea or vomiting (33%), urinary retention (24%), and pruritus (26%),[1] these factors will be considered when presented with patients whose co-morbidities may not tolerate accelerated or advanced episodic or continuous side effects in those three categories.

It should be appreciated that the short- and long-term mortality in individuals receiving IDDS with opioids for *noncancer pain* management is substantially greater than a cohort of individuals not so treated.[2,3] Although it is unclear why this might be so and precisely which factors contribute to these observations, nevertheless this information is compelling in that it may reflect the underlying co-morbidities of the IDDS recipients that may be relatively undertreated or that may express themselves in the early or late post-implantation period. In the studies cited, it was found that the mortality within 3 days of implantation, at 1 month, and at 1 year were, respectively, 7.5 (confidence interval [CI], 5.7 to 9.8), 3.4 (CI, 2.9 to 3.8), and 2.7 (CI, 2.6 to 2.8) times higher than expected. The authors stated that these findings and multiple factors that contribute to them might present possible mitigation opportunities for physicians and health care facilities.[2,3]

Recommendations to reduce mortality include the algorithmic approach proposed by Deer.[4] These recommendations include using spinal cord stimulation (SCS) whenever possible in individuals with primarily neuropathic pain before considering IDDS. SCS likewise makes sense as a first-line therapy for patients with visceral pain. Peripheral nerve stimulation (PNS) should be considered as adjunctive to SCS when partial but not complete pain relief occurs after SCS placement and optimization. IDDS should be considered when SCS with or without PNS fails to provide the intended analgesic response or when SCS or PNS is not indicated.[4]

Other concomitant recommendations aimed at reducing mortality[4] include admitting patients the day of surgery for observation, regardless of whether the surgery is for a fresh implant or a revision; observing for signs of withdrawal or overdose; having the implanting physician consult with the original implanter if the two are distinct individuals for a revision; educating the patient and caregiver as to the potential consequences of evolving co-morbidities;

commencing opioid therapy with a conservative (i.e., "low") dose; and considering opioid rotation based on consultation with standard conversion tables and reducing the initial dose by 20% to account for those individuals who may be especially sensitive to the respiratory effects of novel agents.[4]

When *cancer pain* is considered, however, the use of IDDS has produced decidedly different results. In a randomized, prospective evaluation of IDDS versus comprehensive medical management for refractory cancer pain, the group receiving IDDS experienced significant reductions in fatigue, depressed level of consciousness, and reduced mortality at 6 months (53.9% alive vs. 37.2%).[5] So, it is obvious that not all patients have the same co-morbidities nor do all respond in the same manner to the treatment provided under otherwise identical therapeutic circumstances.

Co-Morbidities Affecting Intrathecal Drug Delivery System Placement and Management[6]

Use of Antiplatelet and Anticoagulant Medications

Atherosclerotic heart disease is the leading cause of morbidity and mortality in the United States and most Western countries. Coronary and cerebrovascular atherosclerosis is responsible for up to 650,000 deaths per year in the United States (more than cancer and almost six times more than accidents).[7] As such, more individuals than ever are being treated prophylactically using antiplatelet agents and anticoagulant medications to minimize the sequelae of thrombosis and infarction. Although the need for chronic anticoagulation is not considered an absolute contraindication to placement or management of IDDS,[6] care needs to be taken both in terms of the actual surgical procedure itself as well as the follow-up management of individuals so treated. It is likely that as longevity increases in westernized societies, potentially more individuals will present with pain syndromes amenable to the use of IDDS. As such, the reality of treating patients who are chronically anticoagulated must be dealt with. Oral antiplatelet drugs are a mainstay in prophylaxis of at-risk individuals because most complications result from plaque fissure or rupture with platelet activation and thrombosis. Indeed, there are rare cases not of atheroma formation but of deep venous thrombosis (DVT) associated with IT baclofen use, including one occurring ostensibly because of hypotonia in a 17-year-old patient treated for cerebral palsy who was not prophylactically receiving antiplatelet agents,[8] emphasizing that the underlying co-morbidity may influence selection of such agents in a higher risk population such as patients with cystic fibrosis. Because the incidence of neurologic dysfunction associated with hemorrhagic complications in individuals undergoing neuraxial blocks is not negligible and may be as high as 1 in 150,000 epidural catheter placements and 1 in 220,000 subarachnoid blocks under conditions not associated with the use of anticoagulant medications,[9,10] it is prudent to address the situation as it applies to individuals habitually requiring the use of agents destined to produce a thromboprophylactic effect.

In addition to DVT, other risks of IDDS include spontaneous development of subdural hematoma occurring in the face of dural puncture associated with the procedure in non-anticoagulated patients. In a case report,[10] this syndrome did not become manifest for 4 days after the surgery, emphasizing the need for heightened awareness of patients in the immediate postsurgical period up to and including the first week of instituting therapy. As the population ages and as the likelihood of encountering elderly patients in our practices becomes reality, it should be considered that the typical patient has at least four co-morbid medical problems that must be dealt with,[11,12] including those related to their atherosclerotic cardiac and cerebrovascular systems. The following summary consists of antiplatelet and anticoagulation medications in common clinical practice.

Aspirin and Nonsteroidal Antiinflammatory Drugs[9] Used by themselves, aspirin or nonsteroidal antiinflammatory drugs (NSAIDs) do not need to be discontinued before the performance of spinal or epidural neuraxial anesthesia because they do not appear to pose an added significant risk versus taking no agents that inhibit cyclooxygenase-1 (COX-1) or COX-2. Because these recommendations are exclusive to the performance of single-shot or continuous epidural catheter techniques, however, the fact remains that there are scant data to advocate either for or against the discontinuation of these drugs for the performance or maintenance of IDDS. However, it appears intuitive and inferential that the technique of IT catheter and pump placement should not impose a greater risk than those examined for spinal or catheter-epidural block (**Table 15-1**).

Clopidogrel[9] Agents such as clopidogrel, known as thienopyridine derivatives, inhibit platelet aggregation by inhibiting adenosine diphosphate–induced platelet aggregation. Used primarily to prevent cerebrovascular thromboembolism, they affect both primary and secondary platelet aggregation. They also interfere with platelet–fibrinogen binding and subsequent platelet–platelet interactions. Their use in conjunction with aspirin may increase the risk of clinical bleeding. These agents should be discontinued 7 to 10 days before the performance of the IDDS procedure and should be cautiously reinstituted, as indicated, on the day after the procedure because the full effect or steady-state level is not achieved for about 7 days from the first dose.

Unfractionated Intravenous or Subcutaneous Heparin[9] Heparin binds to antithrombin and accelerates its ability to inactivate thrombin, factor Xa and factor IXa. Subcutaneous heparin, routinely used in hospitalized patients, results in peak effect after about 2 hours. The dose administered subcutaneously is higher than that administered intravenously (IV) to compensate for the reduced bioavailability. Administration of smaller dose subcutaneous heparin (i.e., 5,000 U) for DVT prophylaxis does not prolong the activated partial thromboplastin time (aPTT) and is therefore not routinely monitored. For individuals receiving IV heparin, however, the half-life is 60 to 90 minutes, and prolongation of the aPTT of 1.5 to 2.5 times the baseline is generally sought for therapeutic effect. Alternatively, measurements of heparin levels (0.2 to 0.4 U/mL) or anti-Xa levels (0.3 to 0.7 U/mL) may reflect therapeutic effect. Reversal of IV heparin may be undertaken using protamine, in which 1 mg neutralizes 100 U of heparin. For patients who require IV heparinization in the perioperative period, it is recommended that the procedure be undertaken and the spinal catheter placed at least 1 hour before institution of heparin therapy. Because half the spinal hematomas in the literature occur during neuraxial catheter removal in heparinized patients, this should theoretically not be an issue in the case of IDDS placement. When an IT catheter would need to be removed, the recommendation is that this be undertaken after discontinuation of the heparin for a minimum of 2 to 4 hours. For subcutaneous heparin, there does not seem to be an increased risk of hematoma formation, although the previous recommendation of waiting 2 hours after the last dose before proceeding may not be prudent because this corresponds to the peak effect of the drug.

Warfarin[9] Warfarin interferes with the synthesis of vitamin K–dependent clotting factors, factors II (thrombin), VII, IX, and X.

Table 15-1: Use of Anticoagulation Medications and Intrathecal Drug Delivery System Placement and Removal[9]

NSAIDs; antiplatelet medications	No contraindications with ASA; NSAIDs; clopidogrel (Plavix) should be discontinued 7 days, and ticlopidine (Ticlid) should be discontinued 14 days before the procedure, respectively.
GP IIb/IIIa inhibitors	Tirofiban (Aggrastat) and eptifibatide (Integrilin) should be discontinued 8 hours before the procedure; for Abciximab (ReoPro), 24 to 48 hours.
Unfractionated SQ heparin	If the total daily dose is <10,000 U, there are no contraindications to proceeding. For doses >10,000 U, manage as per IV heparin guidelines.
Warfarin	Discontinue chronic warfarin therapy 4 to 5 days before procedure and assess INR. INR should be within normal range at time of IDDS placement to ensure adequate levels of all vitamin K–dependent factors (II, VII, IX, X). For removal of IDDS, ensure INR <1.5.
LMWH	Delay IDDS at least 12 hours from last dose of thromboprophylaxis with LMWH. For BID dosing, wait at least 24 hours from the last dose. Delay instituting LMWH for at least 24 hours after IDDS placement. Best use of LMWH after the procedure is once-daily dosing and no additional NSAIDs or other antithrombotic medications.
Unfractionated IV heparin	Delay IDDS placement for 2 to 4 hours after last dose. Check aPTT. Begin IV heparin 1 hour after placement. Monitor neurological status at a minimum of every 2 hours.
Herbal agents	No firm evidence, but caution is suggested when implanting IDDS.
Thrombolytics and fibrinolytics	Follow fibrinogen level and perform frequent neurological assessments. No safe interval data have been recognized from use and IDDS placement or removal.

aPTT, activated partial thromboplastin time; ASA, acetylsalicylic acid; BID, twice a day; GP, glycoprotein; IDDS, intrathecal drug delivery systems; INR, international normalized ratio; IV, intravenous; LMWH, low-molecular-weight heparin; NSAID, nonsteroidal antiinflammatory drug; SQ, subcutaneous.

The half-lives of each of these respective factors range from 6 to 8 hours for factor VII to up to 50 to 80 hours for factor II. A factor activity level of about 40% for *each factor* is adequate for normal hemostasis. An international normalized ratio (INR) greater than 1.4 may signify that factor VII activity is below 40% and may put patients at risk for bleeding. The prothrombin time (PT) is most sensitive to factors VII and X, reflecting primarily reduction in VII, which has a half-life of 6 hours. In urgent situations, which would not typify the placement of IDDS, the effects of warfarin might be reversed by oral or IV vitamin K or transfusion with fresh-frozen plasma. It is recommended that, in the face of warfarin therapy, the INR be maintained at less than 1.4 before proceeding with the implantation procedure.

Herbal Agents[9] Garlic inhibits platelet aggregation in a dose-dependent and probably irreversible manner while enhancing the effects of other antiplatelet agents as well. Ginkgo appears to inhibit platelet-activating factor. Ginseng prolongs both thrombin time and aPTT in rats. Data concerning the relative risk of perioperative herbal use in terms of association with spinal hematoma formation are anecdotal, and there is no firm evidence that such agents need to be discontinued before surgical IDDS implantation or management.

For recommendations concerning the use of low-molecular-weight heparins, thrombin inhibitors, fondaparinux, and other agents not specified above, readers are referred to Murphy[8] for a comprehensive review and analysis of the relative risks of proceeding with surgical implantation of IDDS, which is largely an extrapolation of the guidelines as they exist for neuraxial anesthesia and analgesia.

Immunocompromised Patients[6]

Immunodeficiency disorders increase the risk of infection (**Table 15-2**). This might seem to pose a significant potential problem for individuals for whom the risk-to-benefit ratio favors the implantation of a chronic IDDS. Secondary immunodeficiency disorders are more common than primary and include such entities as diabetes (see below), human immunodeficiency virus (HIV) infection, malnutrition, and chemo- or radiation-therapy recipients; elderly and critically ill patients may also be categorized as having immunocompromised states, as may those having severe prolonged illnesses.[7]

Primary immunodeficiencies include those of B-cell lineage (or Ig) (50% to 60% of all cases), T cells (5% to 10% of cases), natural killer cells, phagocytic cells, or complement proteins.

HIV infection results from one of two similar retroviruses (HIV-1 and HIV-2) that destroy $CD4^+$ lymphocytes and impair cell-mediated immunity, resulting in increased risk of infections and cancers. Subsequent manifestations are related and proportional to the level of $CD4^+$ lymphocytes. Manifestations range from asymptomatic to full-blown development of the acquired immune deficiency syndrome (AIDS). More than 40 million people are infected worldwide. Of the 3 million deaths annually and 14,000 daily new infections, 50% occur in women and one-seventh occur in children younger than 15 years old.[7]

AIDS is associated with neuropathy, and HIV disease is associated with neuropathic pain, primarily in those of advancing age, lower $CD4^+$ counts, and current combination antiretroviral therapy (CART) and in those formerly treated with dideoxynucleoside analog medications.[13] Up to 57% of HIV-positive individuals from a large multicenter study of 1539 patients experienced neuropathic pain, typically manifest as diminished vibration or sharp sensation in the legs and feet and reduced ankle reflexes, often along with burning dysesthesias.[13] It is probable that neuromodulation and IDDS are being increasingly used to manage the pain of HIV diseases that is resistant to conventional medical management.

The use of IDDS in immunocompromised patients demands careful consideration because of the potential for infectious complications.[14,15] It appears that the infection and failure rate of IDDS in HIV-positive and AIDS patients is similar to individuals not infected, however, and makes the withholding of this treatment likely unnecessary when the risk-to-benefit ratio favors proceeding to implantation.[16] It is just as logical that no patient should undergo implantation until all remote infections are identified and treated,

Table 15-2: Selected Medical Conditions: Implications for Intrathecal Drug Delivery Systems	
Medical Condition	**Implications for IDDS**
Immunocompromised states: primary and secondary	Potentially at increased risk for infectious complications, although risk has not been demonstrated, prospectively, to be higher than non-affected cohorts. May have attenuated inflammatory response that may diminish the clinical signs and symptoms associated with infection, potentially leading to delay in diagnosis. Much broader range of microorganisms causing infection, including atypical and opportunistic pathogens. Consultation with infectious disease specialist is prudent at early suspicion of infection. Prolonged antibiotic therapy likely attributable to persistent immunologic deficiencies. Prevention of infection critical because eradication after it is established may be difficult. Follow CDC guidelines concerning conduct of surgical management.
Diabetes: types 1 and 2	Expect poor or delayed wound healing. Appropriate dosing and timing of antibiotics are essential. Diabetes is the most commonly cited factor in spontaneously developing epidural abscess, and a high index of suspicion for infection must be maintained in this patient population. Vertebral osteomyelitis is also more common in this group. Diabetes is an independent risk factor in spine surgery patients for the development of superficial infections, transfusion requirements, pneumonia, in-hospital mortality, and non-routine discharge. Serum glucose levels >125 mg/dL appear to predispose patients to potential complications.
Obesity	Expect OSA as a possible risk factor with opioid infusions. Bacterial and fungal infections are possible with latent organisms residing in skin folds. Obesity is an independent risk factor for development of perioperative infection. Development of neuropathic pain should be considered. Increased vigilance and respiratory monitoring likely are essential in the early stages after implementation of opioid infusion therapy.
Substance abuse	High scores on the SOAPP (version 1) may predict the likelihood of future aberrant drug-related behaviors. Expect higher rates of cigarette smoking (with delayed wound healing and impaired blood flow), alcohol use, higher benzodiazepine use, and greater levels of anxiety and depression in recovering patients being considered for implantation.
Cancer	The possibility of hemorrhagic complications should be considered and education provided to the patient and primary caregiver. Consider pre-implant brain imaging. Surgical site infections are increased in those previously irradiated for metastatic disease.

CDC, Centers for Disease Control; IDDS, intrathecal drug delivery systems; OSA, obstructive sleep apnea; SOAPP, Screener and Opioid Assessment for Patients with Pain.

as per Centers for Disease Control (CDC) guidelines concerning conduct of elective surgical cases.[16]

Diabetes Mellitus[6]

Diabetes mellitus (DM) is impaired insulin secretion and varying degrees of resistance to insulin in the periphery, resulting in hyperglycemia.[7] Late complications of diabetes include vascular disease, peripheral neuropathy, and predisposition to infection. In type 1 diabetes, insulin production is absent because of autoimmune pancreatic β-cell destruction wherein insulin production is no longer adequate to control blood glucose levels. In type 2 diabetes, insulin secretion is inadequate, occasionally irrespective of the finding that insulin levels are very high, signifying peripheral insulin resistance and increased hepatic glucose production. The diagnosis of diabetes includes the findings of a fasting blood glucose of 126 mg/dL or above or plasma glucose of 200 mg/dL or above 2 hours after a 75-g oral glucose load (glucose tolerance test) or a glycated hemoglobin (Hgb A1C) level of 6.5% or above.

Diabetes rates in North America have been increasing substantially. In 2008, there were about 24 million people with diabetes in the United States, and among those, 5.7 million people remain undiagnosed. Another 57 million people are estimated to have prediabetes. Both types 1 and 2 are associated with patients developing neuropathy and neuropathic pain, often resistant to conventional neuropathic pain-relieving medication implementation. Neuropathy associated with diabetes affects up to 60% to 70% and results from nerve ischemia caused by microvascular disease, the direct effect of glucose on neurons, and intracellular metabolic changes that impair nerve functioning. Neuropathy is typically distal and symmetrical, and both large and small nerve fibers may be involved. In the distal hands and feet, symptoms include paresthesias; dysesthesias; and painless loss of sense of touch, vibration, proprioception, or temperature. Sixty percent of a group of 993 patients with diabetes indicated that they experience chronic daily pain, and many of those noted lack of efficacy of their pain medications to manage their symptoms.[17] The autonomic nervous system may be involved with findings of orthostatic hypotension, exercise intolerance, resting tachycardia, and nausea and vomiting, among others.

IDDS placement in diabetics, both those with types 1 and 2, should be undertaken with care and consideration (**Table 15-2**). Poor or delayed wound healing and infection are notoriously prevalent in people with diabetes. The appropriate precautions undertaken for all patients should be rigorously adhered to, and the attention to detail in the patients with diabetes may require advanced vigilance. Because the spontaneous development of both deep and superficial infection is a hallmark of diabetes,[18-23] documentation must be clear and precise in terms of the appropriate antibiotic administration and the timing of such, as well the perioperative preparation that was used to minimize extraneous sources of contamination.

In a review of 46 patients with spinal epidural abscess (with or without spinal instrumentation or injection), 46% had underlying diabetes.[18] Concurrent diabetes or other chronic illness was noted in 62% of a group of 24 patients presenting with spinal epidural abscess who did not have prior spine surgery or injections for pain management.[19]

In addition to spinal epidural abscess formation, patients with diabetes may develop infections into the retroperitoneal space,[20] intradural space,[21] the entire length of the vertebral column,[22] or into the psoas muscle.[23] Vertebral osteomyelitis is also quite common in patients with diabetes, and diabetes is the most common co-morbidity identified in a meta-analysis of 1008 patients with this disease.[24] Osteomyelitis occurs regardless of whether patients have type 1 or type 2 diabetes.[25] In addition to osteomyelitis, septic arthritis of the facet joint may occur in patients with diabetes and presents a peculiar diagnostic challenge when managing patients with chronic low back pain in addition to neuropathic pain from diabetic neuropathy.[26] For spinal surgical patients with diabetes, results have been observed that may have meaning for IDDS patients. In a major review of 197,461 spinal fusion patients of which there were 11,000 patients with diabetes (5.6%), diabetes was an independent risk factor for the development of infection, need for transfusion, pneumonia, in-hospital mortality, and nonroutine discharge.[27] Diabetes was an independent risk factor for surgical site infection in a retrospective study of 273 patients undergoing orthopedic spine operations (odds ratio [OR], 3.5) as was blood glucose above 125 mg/dL preoperatively (OR, 3.3) or above 200 mg/dL postoperatively (OR, 3.3). Obesity was also a significant risk factor (OR, 2.2; see below).[28] Surgical site infection rates were highest among risk factors in patients with diabetes undergoing posterior instrumented lumbar arthrodesis with an adjusted relative risk of 4.1.[29] Multiple additional studies in many thousands of lumbar spinal surgical patients have all noted the same phenomenon, that is, that diabetes is an independent risk factor for severe perioperative morbidity, including both deep and superficial wound infections as well as perioperative mortality.[30-35] For cervical spine procedures, the rate of recovery from cervical laminoplasty was delayed in patients with diabetes but not in smokers (OR, 2.9).[36]

In summary, patients with diabetes demand careful preoperative and perioperative care and management as well as meticulous attention to detail. Expectations must be realistic in this patient population, and a high index of suspicion for infection and a low trigger for explantation must be maintained when dealing with postoperative wound abnormalities.

Obesity[6]

Obesity is defined as a body mass index (BMI) above 30 kg/m^2 and morbid obesity as a BMI above 40 kg/m^2. Morbid obesity is associated with an average 10-year reduction in life expectancy. The prevalence of obesity in the United States is high and is increasing. Age-adjusted prevalence of obesity was 22.9% from 1988 to 1994, 30.5% from 1999 to 2000, and above 35% in 2005.[7] The prevalence among black and white men is not significantly different, but it is higher in black women compared with white women. Obesity and its complications result in up to 300,000 premature deaths per year in the United States, making it second to cigarette smoking as a cause of death. Insulin resistance (see above), dyslipidemias, and hypertension are prevalent in obese individuals. Obesity also predisposes individuals to obstructive sleep apnea (OSA), a concern when acute or chronic opioid use is instituted or if concomitant respiratory depressant medications such as benzodiazepines are added to a treatment regimen. In the obesity-hypoventilation syndrome (Pickwickian syndrome), impaired breathing results in CO_2 retention, reduced sensitivity to CO_2 as a respiratory stimulant, hypoxemia, and cor pulmonale with a risk of premature death.[7] Increased perspiration, trapped in skin folds, is conducive to fungal and bacterial growth, placing these individuals at increased risk of developing perioperative infections.

Obesity is an independent risk factor for the development of surgical site infections related to spinal surgery,[28,30,33,34] with OR of 2.2 (95% CI, 1.1, 4.7).[28] A retrospective review of 332 patients undergoing elective thoracic and lumbar spine surgery cases at a single institution performed by a single surgeon found that 71.4% had BMIs of 25 or greater; logistic regression revealed that the probability of a significant complication was related to BMI ($P <$ 0.04), including wound infections and perioperative nerve palsies and development of neuropathic pain.[37] A prospective observational cohort study[38] of 87 consecutive patients undergoing elective surgery noted that 40.8% were obese and 11.5% were morbidly obese. The overall complication incidence was 67%, but in this prospective analysis, BMI was not a positive predictor of either minor or major complications.[38] However, in a nationwide study from Canada of 244,170 patients undergoing thoracolumbar or lumbar spine fusion, higher BMI and especially morbid obesity were associated with increased overall morbidity, including wound infections, but were not associated with higher mortality.[39] Although implantation of IDDS is certainly more of a "peripheral" procedure than a laminectomy or major spinal reconstructive procedure, the one commonality is the manipulation and trespass of the central neuraxis exclusive to both types of interventions; therefore the use of spinal surgery data likely represents a "worst case scenario" when statistics are unavailable for IDDS cases.[40] A more realistic appraisal of the effects of obesity on spinal interventions may be that noted in a recent prospective analysis of 110 patients undergoing minimally invasive transforaminal lumbar interbody fusion at a single institution. In that report, BMI did not appear to have a statistically significant influence of adverse outcomes or morbidity.[41]

OSA comprises episodes of partial or complete upper airway closure (or both) that last longer than 10 seconds (**Table 15-2**). Diagnosis is based on a sleep history and polysomnography. Treatment is with continuous positive airway pressure; oral appliances; and surgery, which is reserved for refractory cases. Daytime hypersomnolence may lead to accident proneness. Hypertension, heart failure, injury, and sudden death are increased in individuals with this malady. The prevalence of OSA is 2% to 4% in developed countries with a male-to-female ratio of 4:1. Obesity and sedative use are prominent risk factors for the development of OSA.[7] Chronic opioid use in patients with OSA may be associated with a high risk of respiratory depression.[42] Volunteers administered continuous infusions of short-term opioids (remifentanil) during sleep were noted to have markedly increased episodes of central apneas.[43] OSA may be found in more than 35% of opioid-dependent patients treated with methadone for chronic maintenance.[44]

Acute but not typically chronic IT opioid (ITO) administration may be associated with respiratory insufficiency, including and up to respiratory arrest, but it is unclear what role OSA plays in influencing the development of this complication. For example, in a group of 1915 women who received 150 μg of morphine as ITO after cesarean section, 0.26% (five) developed bradypnea, but only one required naloxone administration. OSA diagnosis was not associated with increased risk of bradypnea in this retrospective review.[45] When polysomnography was performed in a pain clinic population consisting of 147 patients taking chronic oral opioids, 75% were noted to have abnormal apnea-hypopnea indices, including 39% with OSA,[46] and BMI was found to be inversely related to apnea-hypopnea index severity in an opioid using group.[47]

The American Society of Anesthesiologists (ASA) has guidelines concerning the use of neuraxial opioids in high-risk individuals, including those potentially at risk for respiratory depression.[48] Although these recommendations pertain to the use of opioids to mange acute pain, they should be read by all interventionalists who intend on implanting IDDS in OSA patients. The specific recommendations regarding OSA include increased vigilance in the first 12 hours after ITO, monitoring ventilation, oxygenation, and level of consciousness at least hourly; for the next 12 hours, monitoring should be a minimum of once every 2 hours. Extended monitoring should be done every 4 hours for the next 48 hours because it is known that initiation of therapy, especially ITO therapy, may be associated with delayed respiratory depression onset, particularly caused by the delay from pump initiation until the drug reaches the catheter tip.[49]

Following these guidelines, it appears that patients with OSA may be viable candidates for IDDS therapy and indeed may actually improve when they are liberated from the effects of higher dose systemic oral or patch opioid analgesic therapies.[6]

Substance Abuse

Chronic pain and addiction often overlap. It is almost inconsequential which issue preceded the other; the end result is that the treatment approaches to individuals either with a history of substance misuse or an ongoing abuse represents a serious challenge to even the most astute clinician. The decision to proceed toward opioid therapy for chronic pain in the recovering addict must be undertaken with great care and consideration. Eventually, a decision might be made to proceed toward implantation of an IDDS. The optimal methods to predict risk of aberrant drug-related behaviors both before as well as after initiation of opioid therapy are uncertain.[50] High scores on the Screener and Opioid Assessment for Patients with Pain (SOAPP) (version 1) weakly increased the likelihood for future aberrant drug-related behaviors[50] (**Table 15-2**). Part of the problem is that definitions for aberrant drug-related behaviors are not standardized across studies examined.[50] In one prospective study of 253 patients with chronic pain, the incidence of addiction ranged from 14.4% to 19.3% depending on which criteria were used for assessment.[51] Those classified as addicted smoked more cigarettes, drank more alcohol, used higher doses of opioids and benzodiazepines, and had higher levels of depression than those not so classified.[51] Although obvious red flags do exist among addicted patients, such as doctor shopping, losing prescriptions, frequent attendance at a pain center, and requests for early refills, many addicts are quite savvy to the mechanisms that may be used to thwart the most sophisticated attempts aimed at detection and intervention.[52]

In addition to the obvious health concerns when considering opioids for chronic nonmalignant pain, there are legal constraints as well, which include the fear of prescriber regulation and oversight and medical malpractice claims that arise when adverse outcomes result from prescription medication problems. In the ASA Closed Claims Database, medication management comprised 17% of 295 chronic noncancer pain claims from 2005 to 2008.[53] Medication management patients tended to be younger men with low back pain, and 94% of claimants were prescribed opioids with 58% having additional psychoactive drug prescriptions as well.[53] Death was the most common outcome (57%), and inappropriate medication management by physicians was identified in 59% of cases.[53]

IDDS would, on the surface, seem to be the ideal therapy for someone with a history of addiction because the reliance on oral or cutaneous opioids might be minimized. However, there are no strong data to suggest that the reliance on opioids by other routes of administration or the concomitant use of other mood-altering chemicals is curtailed to any extent when using IDDS in recovering addicts. Indeed, there have been reports of clever attempts to bypass the primary rationale for pump insertion—that of providing analgesia while minimizing systemic opioid-related side effects. In one case report, an incarcerated male back pain patient with an existing morphine pump was found to have a cloudy fluid in the pump aspirate at the time of refill that exceeded the anticipated amount of residual drug. In addition to opiates, phencyclidine, methamphetamine, and propoxyphene were also identified in the aspirate. The pump and catheter were removed to limit the potential for self-abuse in this individual.[54] Another case report of the death of a 36-year-old man exemplifies a related phenomenon—instead of adding adulterants to the pump, in this case, the patient withdrew morphine for self-injection, resulting in a massive overdose of morphine and respiratory arrest.[55] A postmortem assessment of the residual morphine dose revealed only 230 mg instead of the expected 488 mg, and serum toxicological evaluation corroborated the likelihood of morphine self-intoxication.[55]

Identifying presently addicted individuals is a significant challenge, but when it is accomplished, it suggests that therapy proceed to IDDS in accordance with the guidance and recommendations of an addictionologist.[6] Such patients frequently manifest personality disorders and can be manipulative, demanding, passive-aggressive and noncompliant, as attested to by the aforementioned case reports.

Cancer

Cancer pain is one of the most frequently encountered pain syndromes, occurring in up to 75% of patients.[56] By applying the World Health Organization analgesic ladder, adequate analgesia may be attained in 75% to 90% of patients.[57] The remainder may benefit from IDDS. Using IDDS decreases pain intensity and reduces opioid-related side effects. According to the 2007 Polyanalgesic Consensus Conference, first-line therapies include morphine, ziconotide, and hydromorphone, but only morphine and ziconotide are approved by the U.S. FDA for IT therapy.[58] More IDDS patients achieved success (defined as ≥20% reduction in pain and toxicity) and had enhanced survival than those managed medically for cancer pain.[58] In a prospective evaluation of 55 patients treated with IDDS for cancer, the most frequent indication for using this route of opioid administration was the presence of adverse effects and poor pain control on systemic drugs. Statistical differences in pain intensity and decreases in intensity of drowsiness and confusion were noted, as was the ability to reduce systemic opioid intake.[59]

Although it is true that IDDS are useful in cancer pain, these patients are uniquely predisposed to certain side effects and complications (**Table 15-2**). Among these, pontine hemorrhage has been described in a 70-year-old woman with metastatic breast cancer who developed mental status and gait changes 2 days after implantation. This emphasizes the need to consider pre-implant imaging of the brain in patients with widely metastatic malignancies.[60] Spinal irradiation is another consideration before implanting patients who have cancer. Surgical site infections are up to 30 times higher in patients undergoing spinal surgery who had previous irradiation than in those who have not, providing some pause before accepting the challenge of using this intervention for this group of patients.[61]

Chronic Low Back Pain and Failed Back Surgery Syndrome

Chronic low back pain and failed back surgery syndrome (FBSS) are two indications for advanced therapies including SCS and, at times, IDDS. In FBSS, IDDS has been shown to be cost-effective compared with medical management. In a group of 67 FBSS patients wherein 23 had IDDS therapy who were followed for 5 years, the actual cumulative cost for IDDS was $29,410 versus $38,000 for conventional pain therapy.[62] Furthermore, the Oswestry Disability Index showed a 27% improvement compared with 12% favoring IDDS.[62] A separate analysis in FBSS patients found the 5-year costs of IDDS to average $82,893 when calculated in patients having "good to excellent pain relief."[63] Similar cost-effective findings have been noted in chronic low pain patients who have not undergone previous spinal surgery.[64] More than 65% of implanted low back pain patients reduced their Oswestry scores by at least one level at 1-year follow-up compared with baseline.[65]

Although IDDS is effective in these populations for reducing pain symptoms, in the FBSS group, it may be that work interruption and the effect of pain on their sex lives did not change in one retrospective review of 36 patients.[66] Another important consideration is attempting to reconcile new-onset symptoms in this patient population. In a case report, a patient developed new-onset, intractable radicular pain 3 months after implantation of a one-piece catheter into the lumbar subarachnoid space. Subsequent computed tomography revealed the catheter in the intervertebral foramen, and repositioning of the catheter alleviated the symptoms.[67] If this IDDS had been performed in an individual with low back pain or FBSS, it might have been misconstrued as a recurrence of the underlying disease process, thereby delaying implementation of a timely intervention to rescue the device.

Miscellaneous Co-Morbidities

IDDS may be used in individuals with multiple health issues not described above, including those with chronic kidney or liver disease, elderly patients, and patients with neurological conditions. Chronic hemodialysis predisposes patients to infections, including those of the central nervous system (CNS). It is crucial that new or worsening pain complaints in these patients be investigated thoroughly to rule out the possibility of space-occupying lesions in the CNS in those receiving IDDS.[68] Likewise advanced liver disease may predispose patients to spinal infections, even absent IDDS, and these infections are frequently associated with neurological deficits requiring urgent attention.[69,70] The same concerns hold true for those of advance age, who are as well predisposed to acute and chronic spinal infections up to and including epidural abscess and osteomyelitis, even without an implanted device.[71]

Conclusions

IDDS is uniquely suited to aid individuals with chronic pain or spasticity. Efficacy and safety have been well documented for a multitude of medical conditions associated with a cost savings that is significant and calculable. Interventionalists are cautioned to evaluate patients thoroughly to avoid the pitfalls associated with underestimating or undervaluing the co-morbidities that can lead to catastrophic results in the face of otherwise uncomplicated technical catheter and system placement.

References

1. Turner J, Sears J, Loeser J: Programmable intrathecal opioid delivery systems for chronic noncancer pain: a systematic review of effectiveness and complications. *Clin J Pain* 23:180-195, 2007.
2. Coffey R, Owens M, Broste S, et al: Medical practice perspective: identification and mitigation of risk factors for mortality associated with intrathecal opioids for non-cancer pain. *Pain Med* 11:1001-1009, 2010.
3. Coffey R, Owens M, Broste S, et al: Mortality associated with implantation and management of intrathecal opioid drug infusion systems to treat noncancer pain. *Anesthesiology* 111:881-891, 2009.
4. Deer T: A critical time for practice change in the pain treatment continuum: we need to reconsider the role of pumps in the patient care algorithm. *Pain Med* 11:987-989, 2010.
5. Smith T, Staats P, Deer T, et al: Randomized clinical trial of an implantable drug delivery system compared with comprehensive medical

management for refractory cancer pain: impact on pain, drug-related toxicity, and survival. *J Clin Oncol* 20:4040-4049, 2002.

6. Deer T, Smith H, Cousins M, et al: Consensus guidelines for the selection and implantation of patients with noncancer pain for intrathecal drug delivery. *Pain Physician* 13:175-213, 2010.

7. Merck Research Laboratories: *The Merck manual of diagnosis and therapy*, ed 18, Whitehouse Station, NJ, 2006, Merck Research Laboratories.

8. Murphy N: Deep venous thrombosis as a result of hypotonia secondary to intrathecal baclofen therapy: a case report. *Arch Phys Med Rehabil* 83:1311-1312, 2002.

9. Horlocker T, Wedel D, Rowlingson J, et al: Regional anesthesia in the patient receiving antithrombotic or thrombolytic therapy. ASRA Practice Advisory. *Reg Anesth Pain Med* 35:64-61-1, 2010.

10. Velarde C, Zuniga R, Leon R, Abram S: Cranial nerve palsy and intracranial subdural hematoma following implantation of intrathecal drug delivery device. *Reg Anesth Pain Med* 25:76-78, 2000.

11. DiBari M, Virgillo A, Matteuzzi D, et al: Predictive validity of measures of comorbidity in older community dwellers: the Insufficienza Cardiaca negli Anziani Residenti a Dicomano Study. *J Am Geriatr Soc* 54:210-216, 2006.

12. Rozzini R, Frisoni G, Ferrucci L, et al: Geriatric index of comorbidity: validation and comparison with other measures of comorbidity. *Age Ageing* 31:277-285, 2002.

13. Ellis R, Rosario D, Clifford D, et al: Continued high prevalence and adverse clinical impact of human immunodeficiency virus-associated sensory neuropathy in the era of combination antiretroviral therapy: the CHARTER study. *Arch Neurol* 67:552-558, 2010.

14. Staats P, Yearwood T, Charapata S, et al: Intrathecal ziconotide in the treatment of refractory pain in patients with cancer or AIDS: a randomized control trial. *JAMA* 291:63-70, 2004.

15. Risdahl J, Khanna K, Peterson P, Molitor T: Opioids and infection. *J Neuroimmunol* 83:4-18, 1998.

16. Follett K, Boortz-Marx R, Drake J, et al: Prevention and management of intrathecal drug delivery and spinal cord stimulation system infections. *Anesthesiology* 100:1582-1594, 2004.

17. Krein S, Heisler M, Piette J, et al: The effect of chronic pain on diabetes patients' self-management. *Diabetes Care* 28:65-70, 2005.

18. Tang H, Lin H, Liu Y, Li C: Spinal epidural abscess: experience with 46 patients and evaluation of prognostic factors. *J Infect* 45:76-81, 2002.

19. Pereira C, Lynch J: Spinal epidural abscess: an analysis of 24 cases. *Surg Neurol* 63(suppl 1):S26-S29, 2005.

20. Grabysa R, Moczulksa B: Spinal epidural abscess penetrating into the retroperitoneal space in patient with diabetes mellitus type 2: early diagnosis and treatment requirement. *Pol Arch Med Wewn* 118:68-72, 2008.

21. Nadkarni T, Shah A, Kansal R, Goel A: An intradural-extramedullary gas-forming spinal abscess in a patient with diabetes mellitus. *J Clin Neurosci* 17:263-265, 2010.

22. Elsamaloty H, Elzawawi M, Abduljabar A: A rare case of extensive spinal epidural abscess in a diabetic patient. *Spine* 35:E53-E56, 2010.

23. Oblak M, Oblak C, Stankovic S: Psoas and spinal epidural abscess in a diabetic patient: case report. *Diabetes Res Clin Pract* 68:274-277, 2005.

24. Mylona E, Samarkos M, Kakalou E, et al: Pyogenic vertebral osteomyelitis: a systematic review of clinical characteristics. *Semin Arthritis Rheum* 39:10-17, 2009.

25. Isobe Z, Utsugi T, Ohyama Y, et al: Recurrent pyogenic vertebral osteomyelitis associated with type 2 diabetes mellitus. *J Int Med Res* 29:445-450, 2001.

26. Michel-Batot C, Dintinger H, Blum A, et al: A particular form of septic arthritis: septic arthritis of facet joint. *Joint Bone Spine* 75:78-83, 2008.

27. Browne J, Cook C, Pietrobon R, et al: Diabetes and early postoperative outcomes following lumbar fusion. *Spine* 32:2214-2219, 2007.

28. Olsen M, Nepple J, Riew K, et al: Risk factors for surgical site infection following orthopaedic spinal operations. *J Bone J Surg Am* 90:62-69, 2008.

29. Chen S, Anderson M, Cheng W, Wongworawat M: Diabetes associated with increased surgical site infections in spinal arthrodesis. *Clin Orthop Relat Res* 467:1670-1673, 2009.

30. Pull ter Gunne A, Cohen D: Incidence, prevalence, and analysis of risk factors for surgical site infection following adult spinal surgery. *Spine* 34:1422-1428, 2009.

31. Veeravagu A, Patil C, Lad S, Boakye M: Risk factors for postoperative spinal wound infections after spinal decompression and fusion surgeries. *Spine* 34:1869-1872, 2009.

32. Watanabe M, Sakai D, Matsuyama D, et al: Risk factors for surgical site infection following spine surgery: efficacy of intraoperative saline irrigation. *J Neurosurg Spine* 12:540-546, 2010.

33. Schuster J, Rechtine G, Norvell D, Dettori J: The influence of perioperative risk factors and therapeutic interventions on infection rates after spine surgery: a systematic review. *Spine* 35(suppl):S125-S137, 2010.

34. Fang A, Hu S, Endres N, Bradford D: Risk factors for infection after spinal surgery. *Spine* 30:1460-1465, 2005.

35. Glassman S, Alegre G, Carreon L, et al: Perioperative complications of lumbar instrumentation and fusion in patients with diabetes mellitus. *Spine J* 3:496-501, 2003.

36. Kim H, Moon S, Kim H, et al: Diabetes and smoking as prognostic factors after cervical laminoplasty. *J Bone Joint Surg Br* 90:1468-1472, 2008.

37. Patel N, Bagan B, Vadera S, et al: Obesity and spine surgery: relation to perioperative complications. *J Neurosurg Spine* 6:291-297, 2007.

38. Yadia S, Malone J, Campbell P, et al: Obesity and spine surgery: reassessment based on a prospective evaluation of perioperative complications in elective degenerative thoracolumbar procedures. *Spine J* 10:581-587, 2010.

39. Shamji M, Parker S, Cook C, et al: Impact of body habitus on perioperative morbidity associated with fusion of the thoracolumbar and lumbar spine. *Neurosurgery* 65:490-498, 2009.

40. Vaidya R, Carp J, Bartol S, et al: Lumbar spine fusion in obese and morbidly obese patients. *Spine* 34:495-500, 2009.

41. Rosen D, Ferguson S, Ogden A, et al: Obesity and self-reported outcome after minimally invasive lumbar spinal fusion surgery. *Neurosurgery* 63:956-960, 2008.

42. Farney R, Walker J, Cloward T, Rhondeau S: Sleep-disordered breathing associated with long-term opioid therapy. *Chest* 123:632-639, 2003.

43. Bernards C, Knowlton S, Schmidt D, et al: Respiratory and sleep effects of Remifentanil in volunteers with moderate obstructive sleep apnea. *Anesthesiology* 110:41-499, 2010.

44. Sharkey K, Kurth M, Anderson B, et al: Obstructive sleep apnea is more common than central sleep apnea in methadone maintenance patients with subjective sleep complaints. *Drug Alcohol Depend* 108:77-783, 2010.

45. Kato R, Shimamoto H, Terui K, et al: Delayed respiratory depression associated with 0.15 mg intrathecal morphine for cesarean section: a review of 1915 cases. *J Anesth* 22:112-116, 2008.

46. Webster L, Choi Y, Desai H, et al: Sleep-disordered breathing and chronic opioid therapy. *Pain Med* 9:425-432, 2008.

47. Walker J, Farney R, Rhondeau S, et al: Chronic opioid use is a risk factor for the development of central sleep apnea and ataxic breathing. *J Clin Sleep Med* 15:455-461, 2007.

48. Horlocker T, Burton A, Connis R, et al: Practice guidelines for the prevention, detection, and management of respiratory depression associated with neuraxial opioid administration. *Anesthesiology* 110:218-230, 2009.

49. Rathmell J, Miller M: Death after initiation of intrathecal drug therapy for chronic pain. *Anesthesiology* 111:706-708, 2009.

50. Chou R, Fanciullo G, Fine P, et al: Opioids for chronic noncancer pain: prediction and identification of aberrant drug-related behaviors: a review of the evidence for an American pain society and American academy of pain medicine clinical practice guideline. *J Pain* 10:131-146, 2009.

51. Højsted J, Nielsen P, Guldstrand S, et al: Classification and identification of opioid addiction in chronic pain patients. *Eur J Pain* 14(10):1014-1020, 2010.

52. Baldacchino A, Gilchrist G, Fleming R, Bannister J: Guilty until proven innocent: a qualitative study of the management of chronic non-cancer pain among patients with a history or substance abuse. *Addict Behav* 35:270-272, 2010.

53. Fitzgibbon D, Rathmell J, Michna E, et al: Malpractice claims associated with medication management for chronic pain. *Anesthesiology* 112:948-956, 2010.

54. Burton A, Conroy B, Garcia E, et al: Illicit substance abuse via an implanted intrathecal pump. *Anesthesiology* 89:1264-1267, 1998.

55. Gock S, Wong S, Stormo K, Jentzen J: Self-intoxication with morphine obtained from an infusion pump. *J Anal Toxicol* 23:130-133, 1999.

56. Fitzgibbon D: Interventional procedures for cancer pain management: selecting the right procedure at the right time. *J Support Oncol* 8:60-61, 2010.

57. Pasutharnchat K, Tan K-H, Hadi M, Ho K-Y: Intrathecal analgesia in patients with cancer pain-An audit in a tertiary institution. *Ann Acad Med Singapore* 38:943-946, 2009.

58. Lawson E, Wallace M: Current developments in intraspinal agents for cancer and noncancer pain. *Curr Pain Headache Rep* 14:8-16, 2010.

59. Mercadante S, Intravaia G, Villari P, et al: Intrathecal treatment in cancer patients unresponsive to multiple trials of systemic opioids. *Clin J Pain* 23:793-798, 2007.

60. Rosenfeld D, Trentman T, Patel N: Pontine hemorrhage following a recently implanted intrathecal drug delivery system. *Pain Pract* 9:312-316, 2009.

61. Demura S, Kawahara N, Murakami H, et al: Surgical site infection in spinal metastasis: risk factors and countermeasures. *Spine* 15:635-639, 2009.

62. Kumar K, Hunter G, Demeria D: Treatment of chronic pain by using intrathecal drug therapy compared with conventional pain therapies: a cost-effectiveness analysis. *J Neurosurg* 97:803-810, 2002.

63. de Lissovoy G, Brown R, Halpern M, et al: Cost-effectiveness of long-term intrathecal morphine therapy for pain associated with failed back surgery syndrome. *Clin Ther* 19:96-112, 1997.

64. Rainov N, Heidecke V: Management of chronic back and leg pain by intrathecal drug delivery. *Acta Neurochir Suppl* 97:49-56, 2007.

65. Deer T, Chapple I, Classen A, et al: Intrathecal drug delivery for treatment of chronic low back pain: report from the national outcomes registry for low back pain. *Pain Med* 5:6-13, 2004.

66. Raphael J, Southall j, Gnanadurai T, et al: Long-term experience with implanted intrathecal drug administration systems for failed back syndrome and chronic mechanical low back pain. *BMC Musculoskeletal Disord* 3:1-8, 2002.

67. Ko V, Ferrante F: New onset lumbar radicular pain after implantation of an intrathecal drug delivery system: imaging catheter migration. *Reg Anesth Pain Med* 31:363-367, 2006.

68. Gezici A, Ergun R: Cervical epidural abscess in haemodialysis patients by catheter related infection: report of two cases. *J Korean Med Sci* 25:176-179, 2010.

69. Cross R, Howell C: Two cases of spontaneous epidural abscess in patients with cirrhosis. *South Med J* 96:291-293, 2003.

70. Urrutia J, Bono C, Mery P, et al: Chronic liver failure and concomitant distant infections are associated with high rates of neurological involvement in pyogenic spinal infections. *Spine* 34:E240-E244, 2009.

71. Cunha B: Osteomyelitis in elderly patients. *Clin Infect Dis* 35:287-293, 2002.

CHAPTER

16 Cost-Effectiveness of Implanted Drug Delivery Systems

Steven M. Rosen

CHAPTER OVERVIEW

Chapter Synopsis: As with any chronic implantation procedure, intrathecal drug delivery systems (IDDS) present high upfront costs that can be recovered over some period of usage. Chapter 16 presents an overview of the procedure's cost-effectiveness. Typically, the costs of the intrathecal drug delivery device are recuperated between 18 months and 3 years after implantation. As long-term use of the device continues, further savings accrue. Issues that could improve the cost-effectiveness of IDDS include longer battery lifetime, proper pre-implantation patient trialing, and more effective drugs and drug combinations.

Important Points:
- Cost-effectiveness data will greatly influence future intrathecal drug device and medication utilization.
- There is a paucity of long-term data concerning IDDS.
- As with all implanted devices, there are high upfront costs associated with down-the-road cost savings.
- All studies show long-term cost savings with implanted drug devices. The cross-over point occurs between 18 months and 3 years.
- The interval to the cross-over point can be reduced by minimizing upfront costs and complication rates.
- Standardizing trialing techniques and maximizing trialing efficiency are essential to improving results and cost-effectiveness.
- Increasing battery life will minimize replacement costs.
- More effective intrathecal medications and drug combinations will allow better pain relief and allow IDDS to better compete with alternate pain-relieving techniques.
- Recent studies have shown the cost benefits of IDDS in a more rigorous manner.

Introduction

Intrathecal (IT) infusions through implanted drug delivery systems have been used since 1981 to treat patients with chronic intractable pain. There is extensive medical literature showing benefit, especially with decreased pain and disability. No studies have demonstrated a lack of benefit from IT infusion therapy compared with conventional medical pain management. However, most of the literature consists of case series and retrospective reviews, and there is a paucity of randomized controlled trials (RCTs).

Cost–benefit analyses are increasingly being used to determine whether new technology should be reimbursed or if older technology will continue to be reimbursed. It is difficult to determine the cost–benefit profile of implanted spinal drug delivery systems because the primary clinical endpoint is improved quality of life (QoL). It is easier to measure pain reduction and pump accuracy, which are the endpoints for studies approved by the U.S. Food and Drug Administration (FDA). In addition, other treatments may decrease pain and improve QoL. Behavioral therapies, physical therapy, pain medications, injections, spine surgery, and spinal cord stimulation (SCS) also treat patients with chronic noncancer pain and must be considered in a comprehensive cost–benefit analysis. There are much better data concerning the cost benefits of spinal stimulation than for IT drug delivery systems (IDDS), and a landmark randomized cross-over study has showed cost benefits for spinal stimulation compared with redo spine surgery.[1] Cancer pain may also be treated (and life expectancy possibly improved) with IT drug infusions[2] as well as with radiation therapy, chemotherapy, surgery, or combinations of all these techniques. The American Recovery and Reinvestment Act will provide more than $1 billion to Comparative-Effectiveness Research. If fully funded and implemented, the results of these studies will have a great influence over how we are able to treat patients with chronic pain in the future.[3]

Stakeholders will compete for influence. Governments and insurance companies will try to decrease costs. Medical device companies will attempt to increase sales and develop new products. The Washington State Health Care Authority commissioned an analysis by the ECRI Institute[4] to determine the cost implications for implantable infusion pumps. This was used to deny coverage for implanted drug delivery systems by state-funded programs in Washington. Medtronic, Inc. commissioned an analysis by Guillemette et al[5] to ascertain the costs associated with spinal pump implantation and management and to compare this with the cost of standard medical pain management. This was recently updated. Abroad, the National Health Service in Great Britain uses value-based purchasing, which greatly restricts the use of implantable drug delivery devices to treat chronic pain. The political and economic landscape in the United States is changing so that patient benefit may no longer be the primary deciding factor in the reimbursement of new or existing medical technologies.

This chapter reviews the available medical literature concerning the cost benefits of IT infusions for pain relief. Suggestions are made to maximize the cost-effectiveness of spinal infusion pumps so we may continue to use this therapy to decrease pain and maximize QoL in our patients with severe chronic pain who have failed conventional pain management.

The Problem

IT infusions have been used since 1981[6] to optimize pain control, first in cancer patients and more recently in patients with severe, chronic, noncancer pain. Almost all studies have been retrospective. Cost-effectiveness analysis must assess whether the technology actually decreases chronic pain and then the incidence and severity of complications before one can determine what cost is necessary to obtain benefit.

Several studies have attempted to use control groups to compare patients with spinal infusion pumps to patients without spinal infusion pumps. Doleys et al[7] compared a group of 50 pump patients with a group of 40 patients using oral opioids as well as with a group of 40 patients that had completed a residential pain treatment program. Effectiveness was evaluated at 3 years. Pain, measured by the Numeric Pain Rating scale, decreased by 35.5% in the pump group. It decreased by 8% in the rehabilitation group and 8.5% in the oral opioid group. However, there was no change in physical function. No tabulation of complications was performed. Whereas 10% of the oral opioid group was working at follow-up, 26% of the pump group and 23% of the rehabilitation group were working at 3 years. Thimineur et al[8] compared 38 patients who had an implanted spinal pump with 31 who failed a pump trial and then compared them with a control group of 41 newly referred patients. Pain and anxiety decreased in the pump group. Pain decreased by 27% in the pump group (Visual Analogue Scale) and increased by 7% in the group that failed the pump trial. Disability scores decreased in the pump group, but physical function did not improve. Two large prospective trials have recently been published. Deer et al[9] described a multicenter prospective trial in 2004. All patients had back pain; the great majority had previous spine surgery. At 12 months, back pain decreased by 48 percent and leg pain by 32%. Disability scores decreased. Rauck et al[10] published the results from the Prometra drug delivery pump trial in 2010. This was a multicenter, prospective trial. Pain, measured by Visual Analogue Scales, decreased by 2 at 1 month, and this was maintained at 1 year. Disability scores, measured by the Oswestry Disability Index, decreased by 12 at 1 month and were maintained at 1 year. Anderson and Burchiel[11] reported that 36% of patients had greater than 50% pain reduction at 2 years. A total of 47% of patients were disabled pre-implant versus 35% afterward. The percentage of patients using systemic opioids decreased from 93% to 30% at 2 years. Recently, Patel et al[12] published a systematic review of IT infusion devices for the treatment of chronic noncancer pain. The quality of evidence was rated as level II-3 or III for treatment of noncancer pain. Level II-3 evidence is obtained from multiple case series, and level III evidence includes those of respected authorities and clinical descriptive studies as well as case reports from expert committees. Level I evidence comes from at least one RCT.

In addition to pain relief, complication rates are essential to a cost–benefit analysis. Complication rates vary and imply differences in surgical technique. Adverse events requiring reoperation have been reported between 12% and 40% (Table 16-1). The high complication rates imply variable implant techniques that may be improved with standardization of surgical protocols. Although

Table 16-1: Complications Requiring Reoperation

Author	Year	Ratio	Percentage
Deer et al[9]	2004	21/154	14%
Rauck et al[10]	2010	13/110	12%
Raphael et al[13]	2002	10/56	28%
Kumar[14]	2001	4/25	16%
Roberts et al[15]	2001	32/81	40%
Anderson and Burchiel[11]	1995	5/25	20%

significant, the cost of revision or repeated operations in patients with spinal pumps must be compared with the need for repeated operations in patients who have had previous back surgery, especially those who may require fusions, and with the need for further palliative treatment in patients with intractable pain after back surgery. North et al[16] showed better results and cost benefits in patients who had spinal stimulators placed after laminectomy and discectomy compared with those who had further spine surgery. The risk of granuloma formation is approximately 0.5%. Unfortunately, the risk is highest with IT morphine. Morphine is the only opioid approved for IT administration, and it will be difficult to obtain FDA approval for any study that does not use an FDA-approved drug for pain relief.

There is a paucity of data on pump survival. Medtronic[17] reports a 1% technical failure rate per year. In addition to technical complications, pumps may need to be explanted because of death, infection, intolerable side effects, or persistent granuloma formation. The Prometra study[10] included nine deaths from natural causes in 2 years, resulting in a 4% drop-off per year. Pump survival as well as patient survival data are crucial to a proper cost-effectiveness analysis.

Cost–Benefit Studies

The First Cost Study

Bedder et al[18] compared five patients who were treated with epidural infusions with 15 patients who were treated with IT pump therapy. The results were reported in 1991. The epidural infusions were performed through an implanted du Pen catheter. In 1991, both implanted pumps and tunneled du Pen catheters were being used for chronic pain control, especially in cancer patients. The actual costs were estimated for 1 year. The cost for the IT drug device was $21,368 per year. The cost of the epidural infusion was $34,938 per year. The initial cost was higher with the implanted drug pump, but the cost of both systems was equal at 3 months, and the implanted drug delivery device was cost beneficial after that. The high initial cost of the IT drug device was explained by the cost of the pump versus a tunneled epidural catheter. This study has limited applicability in 2010, but it was the first to show a high up-front cost for IT drug devices that decreased with time associated with a cross-over point at which the IT drug device becomes cost beneficial. This study compared implanted drug pumps with epidural infusions through external pumps. All other studies compared IDDS with conventional medical pain management.

A Computer Simulation

A more in-depth analysis was published by de Lissovoy et al[19] in 1997. A computer model was used to estimate the cost of IT drug devices versus medical pain management measured in 1994 dollars.

All patients had prior back surgery with persistent pain. Treatment costs were simulated. The cost of therapies was estimated using a detailed analysis of billing data from two practices, statewide hospital discharge diagnoses in Florida and Medicare maximum allowable charges per procedure. Drug prices were derived from wholesale prices. The cost of medical management was estimated using the case histories of representative patients. Adverse event probabilities were estimated using expert judgment from previously published data. Elective pump removal was estimated at 3% annually. All patients had back surgery but with persistent pain. Treatment costs were simulated. The IT pump life was estimated at 48 months. The alternative treatment was pain medications. No cost allowance was made for further back surgery in the non-pump group. Pump failure rates were estimated using actuarial data from Medtronic, Inc. and a higher failure rate was assigned to model a worst-case scenario. Higher surgical complication rates and costs were used to model a worst-case scenario.

The expected 60-month total cost per patient with an implanted drug device was $82,893. The best-case costs were $53,488, and the worst-case costs were $125,100 for patients with implanted drug devices. The expected costs were $82,893. The 60-month total cost for medical pain management was $85,186. The best-case scenario showed cost benefits for IT drug devices at 11 months. The base-case analysis showed cost benefit at 22 months. The worst-case scenario showed no cost benefit at any time with a possible loss of $40,000 over a 6-year period (**Fig. 16-1**). The cost benefit of IT drug devices began to decrease at 48 months as replacement costs began to mount. Again, alternative medical treatment did not include a cross-over for surgery, which would increase the competitive advantage of the IT drug device over alternative medical care.

This study was reviewed by Mueller-Schwefe[20] in 1999, but clinical correlates were added such as the increasing cost benefits in long-term patients and the potential to further add to the cost benefit of IT pumps when polyanalgesia is used, assuming that the use of combinations of spinal analgesics in addition to opioids provides additional benefit and decreases the costs of oral pain medications.

A Canadian Study

Kumar et al[21] analyzed actual costs in patients with failed back surgery who were referred to a regional pain center in Canada. Four hundred patients were referred for SCS. Eighty-eight patients failed the spinal stimulator trial. The remaining patients were divided into two groups. One group received a spinal infusion pump trial, and 23 patients were implanted and followed for 5 years. The control group consisted of 44 patients who were not treated with IT drug pumps. The group that failed the pump trial was excluded from the study. Both groups were followed for 5 years.

This study illustrates the difficulty in conducting an ethical economic study in chronic pain patients. The fact that the 21 patients who failed the pump trial were excluded from the study may bias the results toward responders who received a pump implant. Furthermore, the control group (which did not receive a pump trial) may have included difficult-to-treat patients who would require more expensive treatments compared with the patients who responded to pump therapy. On the other hand, it would be morally unacceptable to implant pain pumps in patients who failed the pump trial. Pumps were replaced at 5-year intervals.

Kumar et al[21] estimated the best- and worst-case scenarios for the pump treatment groups. Of 23 patients, nine had no complications in the 5-year follow-up period. The other 14 patients had one or more complications and were included in the worst-case analysis. Overall, pump patients showed decreased pain scores and improvement in disability scores at 5 years. The cost of conventional pain management was $56,727 at the end of 5 years. Conventional pain management patients required more hospital admissions, emergency department (ED) visits for breakthrough pain, and physical therapy. The Oswestry Disability Index decreased by 27% in the pump group compared to 12% in the control group. The best-case analysis showed a cost of $41,811 with an implanted spinal pump. These patients had no complications after pump implantation. Worst-case analysis showed a cost of $46,052. These were the pump patients who had post-implant complications. Not surprisingly, initial costs were higher in the IT drug therapy group. The cross-over point where IT drug therapy became cost-effective

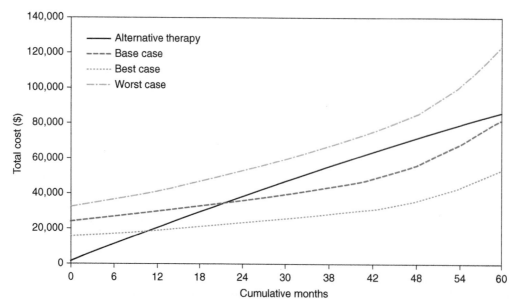

Fig. 16-1 Cumulative expenditure for intrathecal morphine therapy (IMT) over 60 months compared with that for alternative therapy. IMT is characterized by a relatively substantial initial cost for implant surgery, whereas a constant monthly cost is assumed for alternative therapy (medical management).

was at 26 months in the best-case scenario and 30 months in the worst-case scenario. Under no scenario was the 5-year cost of the implanted drug device group higher than the group receiving conventional pain management (**Fig. 16-2**). Kumar et al[21] estimated that IT drug devices would be cost beneficial even if the pump cost increased by 50%. If complication rates rose by 50%, the break-even period would be increased to 26 months. If battery life increased, the cross-over point would not change, but the cost benefit of IT drug therapy would increase even more with time.

A Randomized Trial of Trialing

Anderson et al[22] compared the cost benefit of two different screening methods for IT pump therapy. Patients were screened using either an epidural infusion or single-shot IT injections. Multiple measures, including a pain relief threshold of 50%, were required to proceed with a permanent implant. Twelve of 18 patients responded to IT trial injections. Fifteen of 19 patients responded to screening with an epidural infusion. Patients were followed for 6 months. Screening costs were lower in the IT group likely secondary to decreased operating room costs because the epidural catheters were placed in the operating room. Successful pain relief was reported in 60% to 65% of patients. There were no differences in outcomes between groups. Screening costs were lower in the IT group. The cost of IT screening was $1862. The cost of the epidural screening was $4762. The cost of the permanent pump implant was approximately $20,000. Overall costs were decreased by 15% using IT rather than epidural screening. This study shows that cost savings can be obtained while still providing optimal care.

The Actuarial Study

Guillemette et al's[5] analysis was commissioned by Medtronic, Inc. but performed by an independent third party. The analysis was created specifically for the Washington State Department of Labor and Industry as part of its value-based purchasing initiative. However, the results are applicable throughout the United States. The analysis included all patients who received implanted IDDS who were in the Ingenix database. Ingenix Consulting is a wholly owned subsidiary of United Health, Inc., and is privy to all pharmacy, laboratory, and utilization data of all United Health Care

enrollees. Claims data were used to evaluate the economic effects of IT drug delivery on outcomes and costs of care before and after implantation. All patients who had pumps were included so that all diagnoses were included, and complications, including the need for reoperation, were included in the data. Data were stratified to include noncancer pain, cancer pain, and spasticity patients. Patients implanted with an IDDS between January 2006 and January 2009 were eligible. This included 1408 pain and spasticity patients. Patient costs were aligned to the implant month and then repriced to a standardized national pricing schedule over a 6-year cycle. This included data 3 years before implantation, the month of the implant, and then 3 years after implantation. Pre-implant costs were assumed to accrue at the same slope. This simulated conventional pain treatment in the absence of IT drug implantation.

Conclusions were that IT drug delivery was less expensive than conventional pain treatments for noncancer and cancer pain as well as spasticity (**Fig. 16-3**). The financial break-even point occurred in the second year for malignant and nonmalignant pain and in the third year for spasticity patients. Reductions in ED visits and pain-relieving injections were documented. The longitudinal analysis could be modified using assumptions as to the cost of the implant, duration of battery life, and estimated future medical costs. The time to cost neutrality was between 18 months and 3 years. As with all previous analyses, there was a high upfront cost followed by decreasing long-term costs. Additional costs after 1 year for all patients were $13,740, but by year 2, savings were $4048, and by year 3, cost savings were $13,612. Additional costs for nonmalignant pain patients were $11,423 in year 1 and $8453 in year 2, but by year 3, there was $3809 in savings, which increased over time (**Table 16-2**). There was a dip in cost savings in year 6 and seven presumably secondary to replacement costs. Battery life did not change the time to cost neutrality, but an assumed battery life of 6 years increased the long-term cost savings compared with a battery life of 3 years by decreasing replacement costs. Decreasing the cost of pumps and catheters would decrease the time to cost neutrality and increase long-term savings. Additional cost savings would accrue every time a pump was replaced. At this time, the data have not been stratified to determine how much benefit would

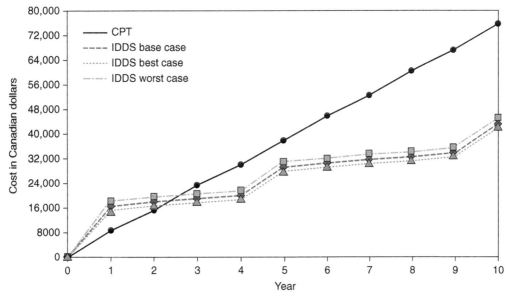

Fig. 16-2 Line graph illustrating cumulative costs of IDDS compared with conventional pain therapies (CPT) projected for a 10-year period.

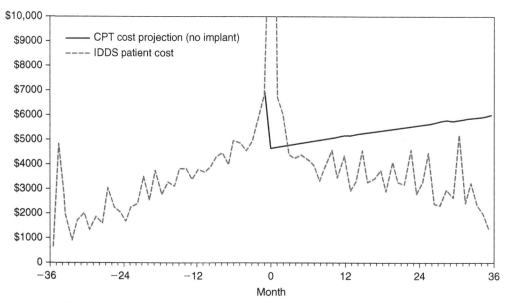

Fig. 16-3 Intrathecal drug delivery system (IDDS) cost projection. The average claim cost experience of an IDDS implant patient (*green*) is shown relative to the simulated conventional pain therapies (CPT) cost (*purple*) based on an actuarial projection of pre-implant costs.

Table 16-2: Additional Costs/Savings in Nonmalignant Pain Patients with Implanted Drug Delivery Systems (IDDS) Compared with Conventional Pain Therapies (CPT)

	CPT Cost Projection with No Implant ($)	IDDS Patient Cost ($)	Additional Costs/ (Savings) ($)	Additional Costs/ (Savings) per Year ($)
Month of implant	2993	14,416	11,423	11,423
1 year after implant	40,503	48,957	8453	8453
2 years after implant	80,248	76,438	(3809)	(1905)
3 years after implant	121,781	107,323	(14,458)	(4819)
4 years after implant	164,579	144,365	(20,214)	(5053)
5 years after implant	208,059	190,129	(17,930)	(3586)
6 years after implant	251,944	246,405	(5,539)	(923)
7 years after implant	296,237	288,692	(7,545)	(1078)
8 years after implant	340,942	320,816	(20,125)	(2516)
9 years after implant	386,062	359,613	(26,449)	(2939)
10 years after implant	431,602	399,029	(32,574)	(3257)
15 years after implant	665,737	626,572	(39,165)	(2611)
20 years after implant	910,964	865,423	(45,541)	(2277)
30 years after implant	1,436,825	1,381,098	(55,727)	(1858)

occur if implants occurred in an outpatient surgical center versus a hospital setting. Outpatient implants would decrease upfront costs and decrease the time to cost neutrality as well as accrue further savings every time the pump was replaced. This analysis was originally commissioned by Medtronic to estimate future budget costs for Washington State. However, the Ingenix data were collected nationally and as such represent cost estimates for the whole United States. Actual costs for 3 years before and for 3 years after pump implantation were estimated using the Ingenix database but not specifically tabulated per patient. Every data analysis showed varying degrees of cost savings for implantable drug delivery devices compared with other treatment options. After 18

months, no scenarios showed increased costs for implantable drug delivery systems compared with other treatments.

The Nihilistic View

This ECRI analysis[4] was commissioned by the Washington State Health Care Authority and reviewed the medical literature as well as the previously described actuarial analysis commissioned by Medtronic, Inc.[5] The report is available online. The overall conclusion was that the analytical evidence is insufficient to determine whether the long-term costs of implantable infusion pumps are different from those of non-pump treatments in the management of chronic noncancer pain. This report was used by the Washington

State Health Care authority to recommend against coverage of IDDS. Thirteen case series were used to determine efficacy, effectiveness, and harms and cost issues associated with implantable infusion pumps. Seven case studies were used to evaluate efficacy and effectiveness (**Fig. 16-4**). Three case reports[19-21] and the actuarial study by Guillemette et al[5] were reviewed to determine the cost implications and cost-effectiveness for implantable infusion pumps. Despite all case reports showing some benefit from IT infusion pump therapy, the evidence was deemed to be too weak to draw a conclusion. The de Lissovoy et al[19] analysis was dismissed because it was 11 years old. It was also dismissed because the wide range of costs ($53,000 to $125,000) implied that the results were not very robust. The Kumar et al[21] analysis was dismissed because Canadian cost structures were dissimilar to those in the United States and because the control group (nonresponders to the temporary trial) may not have been comparable to the study group (those that responded to the temporary trial). The analysis by Guillemette et al[5] was dismissed because it was funded by Medtronic, Inc. and because the estimate for the non-pump treatment was said to have been based on the costs during the month before implantation. This would artificially raise the costs of non-pump treatment and bias the results toward the use of IDDS compared with conventional pain therapies. The primary author (Guillemette) has confirmed that pre-pump costs were based on estimate of the average costs during the 3 years before the pump implant rather than on the first month before implantation.

The Recent Abstract

The Larsen et al[23] abstract from the 2010 American Academy of Pain Medicine Annual Meeting retrospectively calculated the cost of systemic medications 3 months before implant compared with the costs of IT plus systemic medications 1 year after implant. Systemic medications included opioids, nonopioids, benzodiazepines, muscle relaxants, antidepressants (selective serotonin reuptake inhibitors and serotonin–norepinephrine reuptake inhibitors), and hypnotics. Forty-eight pumps were implanted. The average

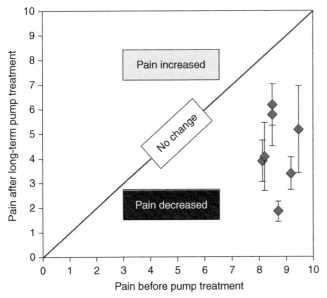

Fig. 16-4 Average pain scores before and after treatment with implantable infusion pump for each included study. (Adapted from ECRI Institute: *HTA final report: implanted infusion pumps for chronic non cancer pain.* Washington State Health Care Authority, accessed July 18, 2008, from http://www.hta.hca.wa.gov.)

pre-pump medication cost was $2134.41 per month. The average post-pump medication cost was $1602.85 per month. Average drug costs decreased by 24.9% at 1 year. This abstract did not report trial and implant costs, and all pumps were still in use after 1 year.

Ziconotide in the United Kingdom

Dewilde et al's[24] report evaluates the cost-effectiveness of ziconotide for use in the United Kingdom. The study was funded by Eisai Europe Ltd., the makers of ziconotide. The quality-adjusted life year (QALY) is the preferred measure to evaluate cost-effectiveness in the United Kingdom. The QALY is the number of years that would be added by an intervention. A cost of 20,000 to 30,000 pounds per year QALY is acceptable for a new technology to be approved. Data, including Visual Analog Scale (VAS) scores, were taken from the pivotal ziconotide study.[25] Best supportive care (BSC) was taken from the placebo arm of the study. Patients were assumed to have a preexisting pump. The ziconotide dose was 0.26 μ/hr.

The base-case analysis showed the cost of ziconotide treatment to be 112,598 British pounds compared with a cost of 94,734 for BSC. The incremental cost-effectiveness ratio with a 95% confidence interval was 27,443 pounds per QALY.

Data were constrained by the fact that only 20.5% of patients had a greater than 30% reduction in VAS. Because ziconotide is expensive and has a narrow therapeutic window, higher doses than 0.26 μ/hr had substantial and negative effects on the cost-effectiveness results. This study illustrates the difficulty in determining cost utility when pain reduction occurs in subgroups that may not be easy to define.

Conclusions

Implantable IT drug devices have been used for almost 30 years to treat patients with severe chronic and incapacitating pain. Outcome data are sparse and difficult to compare among studies. It is difficult to design an ethical controlled spinal infusion pump study because the placebo arm requires implanting a nonfunctioning pump, and surgical implantation entails uncommon but significant risks. It is important to realize that patients who fail a pump trial may not be an adequate control group compared with those who proceed with a permanent implant. An appropriate study would include a cross-over option. It would likely be similar to North and associates'[16] study, which compared spinal stimulation with further spine surgery. In the United States, the largest group of potential patients would have failed back surgery with predominant axial pain showing opioid responsiveness. It is difficult for one center to obtain enough patients to perform a statistically significant study. Also, trialing and implant techniques as well as outcome and outcomes measurements vary among centers. Standardized trialing and implant protocols as well as outcome measurements would have to be used. That said, as of 2010, all studies to date have shown varying degrees of pain relief and reductions in disability. A fair and balanced review of the medical literature shows that implanted drug delivery systems provide pain relief with a real but low incidence of side effects in an otherwise extremely difficult-to-treat group of patients.

The cost–benefit studies reviewed in this chapter allow some general conclusions. The studies of Bedder et al,[18] de Lissovoy et al,[19] and Kumar et al[21] all show a cross-over point where IT infusions become cost-effective. This occurs between 18 and 36 months when IT infusion therapies are compared with conventional pain therapies. The study by Anderson and associates[22] shows that cost benefits can also be obtained during trialing without impacting proper patient selection and decreasing long-term benefit. The Guillemette et al[5] analysis shows the cross-over points occur between 18 months and 3 years for all types of pain and shows decreased pharmacy usage, ED visits, and further procedural interventions. The recent abstract by Larsen et al[23] confirms pharmacy savings after pump implant. Extrapolation of the Ingenix data shows that increased battery life and decreased complications increase the cost benefits of implanted drug delivery systems.

How can the neuromodulation community work to improve cost-effectiveness? Improvements in technology have increased the interval between battery changes, which will reduce long-term costs. Standardization of catheter insertion and pump implant techniques will decrease complication rates and improve cost-effectiveness over time. There is still no consensus as to catheter positioning in the spinal canal for various pain conditions. It has been shown that an IT bolus trial is less expensive than an epidural infusion trial and does not change outcomes. Trialing techniques are variable, and decreasing false-positive trials and the costs of those trials will enhance cost-effectiveness. However, this probably will not decrease overall pain management costs because these costs will be shifted into non-pump treatment categories. Improved training in fellowships and postgraduate courses will decrease complication rates and thus improve cost-effectiveness over time. Because adverse drug events, including granulomas, are likely dose related, reliable dose-response studies will allow us to minimize drug dosing. This will allow us to minimize adverse drug events, improve outcomes, decrease complications, and reduce excess drug costs. There are no studies showing improved outcomes from IT polyanalgesia. Using drug combinations validated for IT delivery will enhance effectiveness and minimize complications as well as excess pharmacy costs. Improved sterility and stability data will allow refill intervals to be extended, which will also minimize long-term costs. Simple manipulation of Guillemette et al's[5] data shows that increased battery life decreases long-term costs but not the interval to cost neutrality. However, decreased complication rates will decrease the interval to the cross-over point as well as increase long-term cost-effectiveness.

In the end, it is important to recognize that it is impossible to assess the value of pain reduction in a strictly monetary sense. To a large extent, our treatment of patients with pain and disability defines who we are as a society. A small but real decrease in pain may be invaluable to an individual patient. A cost–benefit analysis only measures costs as outcomes. It is difficult to measure cost-effectiveness when most case series measure different outcome measures. Physicians have a primary responsibility to patients and a secondary responsibility to payers. A review of outcomes literature shows a consistent trend toward positive results with IDDS, and there are no published cost analysis studies showing a lack of benefit with IT drug delivery. Clearly, further study is needed to confirm these conclusions, but it seems that at the minimum, the cost benefits between IDDS and conventional pain management favors IT drug delivery except in the short-term and worst-case scenarios.

References

1. North RB, Shipley J, Taylor RS: The cost-effectiveness of spinal cord stimulation. In Krames E, Peckham PH, Rezai AR, editors: *Neuromodulation*, 2009, pp 355-376.
2. Smith TJ, Staats PS, Deer T, et al: Randomized clinical trial of an implantable drug delivery system compared with comprehensive medical management for refractory cancer pain: impact on pain, drug-related toxicity, and survival. *J Clin Oncol* 20(19):4040-4049, 2002.
3. Selker HP, Wood AJ: Industry influence on comparative-effectiveness research funded through health care reform. *N Engl J Med* 361:2595-2597, 2009.
4. ECRI Institute: HTA final report: implanted infusion pumps for chronic non cancer pain. Washington State Health Care Authority, accessed July 18, 2008, from http://www.hta.hca.wa.gov.
5. Guillemette S, Wudi S, Leier J, et al: Medical cost impact of intrathecal drug delivery. AAPM 2010 annual meeting abstracts. *Pain Med* 11(2):290, 2010.
6. Onofrio BM, Yaksh TL, Arnold PG: Continuous low-dose intrathecal morphine administration in the treatment of chronic pain of malignant origin. *Mayo Clin Proc* 56:516-520, 1981.
7. Doleys DM, Brown JL, Ness T: Multidimensional outcomes analysis of intrathecal, oral opioid, and behavioral-functional restoration therapy for failed back surgery syndrome: a retrospective study with 4 years follow-up. *Neuromodulation* 9:270-283, 2006.
8. Thimineur MA, Kravitz E, Vodapally MS: Intrathecal opioid treatment for chronic non-malignant pain: a 3-year prospective study. *Pain* 109:242-249, 2004.
9. Deer T, Chapple I, Classen A et al: Intrathecal drug delivery for treatment of chronic low back pain: report from the National Outcomes Registry for Low Back Pain. *Pain Med* 5(1):6-13, 2004.
10. Rauck R, Deer T, Rosen S, et al: Accuracy and efficacy of administration of intrathecal morphine sulfate for treatment of intractable pain using the Prometra Programmable Pump. *Neuromodulation* 2010, in press.
11. Anderson VC, Burchiel KJ: A prospective study of long-term intrathecal morphine in the management on non malignant pain. *Neurosurgery* 44:289-300, 1999.
12. Patel V, Manchikanti L, Singh V, et al: Systemic review of intrathecal infusion systems for long-term management of chronic non-cancer pain. *Pain Physician* 12:345-360, 2009.
13. Raphael JH, Southall JL, Gnanadurai TV, et al: Long-term experience with implanted intrathecal drug administration systems for failed back syndrome and chronic mechanical low back pain. *BMC Musculoskelet Disord* 20:17, 2002.
14. Kumar K, Kelly M, Pirlot T: Continuous intrathecal morphine treatment for chronic pain of nonmalignant etiology: long-term benefits and efficacy. *Surg Neurol* 55:79-86, 2001.
15. Roberts LJ, Finch PM, Goucke CR, et al: Outcome of intrathecal opioids in chronic non-cancer pain. *Eur J Pain* 5:353-361, 2001.
16. North RB, Kidd DH, Farrokhi F, et al: Spinal cord stimulation versus repeated lumbosacral spine surgery for chronic pain: a randomized, controlled trial. *Neurosurgery* 56(1):98-106, discussion 106-107, 2005.
17. Medtronic: *July 2009 Model 86637 Synchromed II Battery performance-pump survival, Synchromed II Product Advisory*, Minn, MN, 2009, Medtronic.
18. Bedder MD, Burchiel K, Larson A: Cost analysis of two implantable narcotic delivery systems. *J Pain Symptom Manage* 6:368-373, 1991.
19. de Lissovoy G, Brown R, Halpern M, et al: Cost-effectiveness of long-term intrathecal morphine therapy for pain associated with failed back surgery syndrome. *Clin Ther* 19(1):96-112, 1997.
20. Mueller-Schwefe G, Hassenbusch SJ, Reig E: Cost-effectiveness of intrathecal therapy for pain. *Neuromodulation* 2(2):77-87, 1999.
21. Kumar K, Hunter G, Demeria D: Treatment of chronic pain by using intrathecal drug therapy compared with conventional pain therapies: a cost-effectiveness analysis. *J Neurosurg* 97:803-810, 2002.
22. Anderson V, Burchiel K, Cooke B: A prospective, randomized trial of intrathecal injection vs. epidural infusion in the selection of patients for continuous intrathecal opioid therapy. *Neuromodulation* 6(3):142-152, 2003.
23. Larsen C, Webster L, Fakata K: Costs of pain medications pre-IT pump implantation compared to post-IT pump implantation: a retrospective analysis [abstract]. *Pain Med* 11(2):295-296, 2010.
24. Dewilde S, Verdian L, MacLaine GDH: Cost-effectiveness of ziconotide in intrathecal pain management for severe chronic pain patients in the UK. *Curr Med Res Opin* 25(8):2007-2019, 2009.
25. Rauck RI, Wallace MS, Leong MS, et al: A randomized double-blind, placebo-controlled study of intrathecal ziconotide in adults with sever chronic pain. *J Pain Symptom Manage* 31:393-406, 2006.

17 Neuroaugmentation by Stimulation versus Intrathecal Drug Delivery Systems

Corey W. Hunter, Sudhir Diwan, and Timothy R. Deer

CHAPTER OVERVIEW

Chapter Synopsis: Chronic pain presents many challenges to both pain physicians and patients. In addition to drug-based approaches, interventional therapies available include neuroaugmentation (i.e., spinal cord stimulation with an implantable device), intrathecal drug delivery systems (IDDS), and neurodestructive procedures. Careful attention to each patient's particular situation provides the key to attaining the best course of treatment. Efficacy, risks, and other considerations of each treatment can vary dramatically with the type and origin of pain. For example, cancer pain is best treated more aggressively, so IDDS might be used more readily than in noncancer chronic pain patients. Patients with visceral or somatic nociceptive pain might respond better to IDDS than those with neuropathic pain. In contrast, spinal cord stimulation has proven a more successful treatment course for those experiencing failed back surgery syndrome (FBSS) and sympathetically driven pain such as complex regional pain syndrome. This efficacy may arise in part from the treatment's involvement of the peripheral nervous system, often improving vascularization. This chapter considers many of the issues facing pain clinicians in weighing these various interventional approaches to treating patients with many different types of chronic pain.

Important Points:
- Before deciding to proceed with one implantable modality over another, astute pain physicians need to account for not only the potential risks involved but also the cause of the pain and the presenting pattern.
- Both neuroaugmentation and IDDS have a unique utility in patients with FBSS; however, careful consideration should be given when choosing the appropriate methodology to ensure success. The development of new spinal cord stimulation and peripheral nerve stimulation systems have changed this paradigm and led clinicians to consider stimulation before using IDDS.

Clinical Pearls:
- Neuroaugmentation utilizes a lead placed in the epidural space, whereas IDDS has a catheter placed through the dura and lies intrathecally.
- The mechanism of action for IDDS is known and is relative to the drugs delivered directly to receptors, while that of neuroaugmentation remains relatively unknown.
- Whereas neuroaugmentation is preferred for neuropathic pain, ischemic pain, visceral pain, and sympathetically driven pain, IDDS is favored for nociceptive and cancer pain.

Clinical Pitfalls:
- Neuroaugmentation requires precise lead placement at all times, which may necessitate revision if migration occurs.
- Drug-related side effect with IDDS can occur during the maintenance phase as well as during the perioperative period.
- Granuloma formation with IDDS, though rare, is a devastating complication.
- While some overlap is present in the indications for each system, there are other pain etiologies that are specifically treated by either IDDS or neuroaugmentation. If the wrong one is chosen, the patient's complaints will be ineffectively managed.

Introduction

Although the armamentarium for physicians involved in the management of patients with chronic pain is extensive, significant portions of patients do not respond to the traditional treatments and methods available, leaving diligent practitioners to search for better and more creative solutions. Concurrently, when a given method appears to be efficacious but the side effects seem intolerable or unsafe to the patient, assiduous practitioners must return to the drawing board to discover ways to maintain the mechanism at hand while circumventing the unwanted. These ideals led to the discovery and implementation of implantable devices for the management of chronic and intractable pain. These devices have gained increasing popularity over the past two decades because of improved technology and patient selection. The options described in this chapter are often the key to avoiding the failure to provide acceptable relief in complex pain patients.

Although the theories inherent to neurostimulation and intrathecal drug delivery systems (IDDS) are dichotomous at face value and seem to provide different views in the approach of the attending physician, they are united in the simple idea of providing pain relief at a centralized source while attempting to avoid many of the side effects inherent to the treatment of chronic pain. Oral medications such as nonsteroidal antiinflammatory drugs, opiates, and anticonvulsants all have well-documented efficacies in treating pain, but when combined with patients requiring long-term care and escalating doses, one becomes confronted with potentially disastrous complications such as gastric ulcers, respiratory depression, constipation, and overdose. The issues of drug abuse, diversion, and addiction have also become major public health problems in recent years throughout the United States. The fine balance in offering effective treatment while skirting unwelcome problems is not always available.

Algorithms have been designed for the stepwise treatment of pain to allow physicians a standardized roadmap in specific pain syndromes. The intent is to prevent one from becoming trapped in one methodology and to protect the patient by progressing to appropriate therapies based on a risk-to-benefit ratio. Krames[1] described a "pain treatment continuum" for nonmalignant pain, which outlined the order in which treatments such as exercise programs, over-the-counter medications, adjunct medications, nerve blocking, and oral opioids should be used compared with one another (**Fig. 17-1**). Using the KISS principle, "keep it sweet and simple," the decision making for choosing one therapy over another was based on invasiveness and initial cost. Some therapies could be used in series or in parallel while abandoning those that do not work in favor of more invasive and costly therapies. As such, the final three steps of his continuum are described as neuroaugmentation (spinal cord stimulation [SCS]), IDDS, and neurodestructive procedures. Krames[2] stated that "because there are multiple choices, both interventional and noninterventional for the management of pain, the treating physician should choose one therapy over another in a rational manner. ..." However, the rationality of the time stemmed from limited research regarding implantable devices and their efficacy compared with those deemed "early-line therapy."

No two patient populations are alike, which negates the idea of a panacea formula. For example, patients with cancer pain or other end-of-life conditions may have different requirements in their pain control, and because of the potentially time-sensitive nature of their conditions, it may be advisable to move through the treatment algorithm at a more aggressive pace. The treatment of these complex pain states led to the evolution of the World Health Organization's three-step analgesic ladder for cancer pain in 1996 and ultimately a revision in 1997. This algorithm outlined a more aggressive approach, which starts with medication and progresses to IDDS much sooner than with noncancer patients.[3,4]

With the idea of evolving pain models in mind, as well as the present availability of information to mine for decision making, Krames and colleagues[5,6] revised his algorithm of pain care into

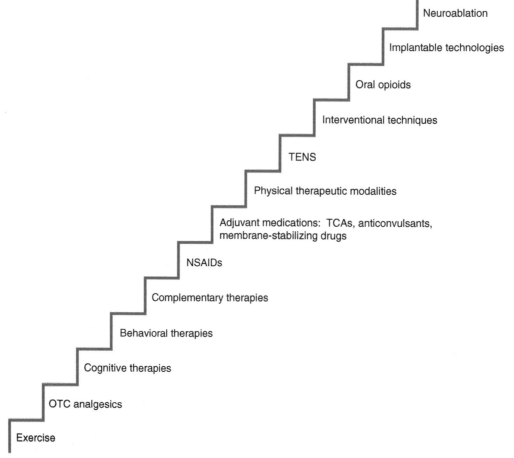

Fig. 17-1 Based on the KISS ("keep it sweet and simple") principle, it was suggested that efficacious therapies deemed cheaper and less invasive be used before those also proven to be efficacious yet more costly and possessing greater penchant for harm. As each successive therapy is tried and failed, it is discarded, and the next step up is taken.[2] NSAID, nonsteroidal antiinflammatory drug; OTC, over-the-counter; TENS, transcutaneous electrical nerve stimulation; TCA, tricyclic antidepressant.

what he referred to as the SAFE principles, or safety, appropriateness, fiscal neutrality, and efficacy (**Fig. 17-2**). Since the time of his initial philosophy, long-term data became available for patient improvement as well as cost comparisons to the less invasive therapies he advised to attempt first. It was previously surmised that it may be in the interest of the patient or even third-party payers to wait until all less costly and less invasive treatment options have failed before attempting interventions such as neuroaugmentation or IDDS; upon review of the current literature, this ideal no longer held true. Recent studies have suggested that implantable devices such as SCS might be more efficacious than conservative approaches such as oral opioids, costly rehabilitation programs, and polypharmacy administration and that is less costly over the lifetime of the patient.[5,7] Given these findings, it is best to reconsider the position of neurostimulation and IDDS as only last-line interventions.

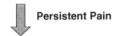

Step 1: Less costly and efficacious therapies in parallel

- Exercise
- OTC analgesics and weak opioid therapies
- Injection therapies to reduce inflammation (e.g., epidural lysis of adhesions, epidural depot steroid)
- Physical restoration, including movement therapies and postural training
- Cognitive and behavioral therapies to improve coping, reduce stress, and improve self locus of control

Persistent Pain

Choosing three costly and efficacious therapies when all below have failed to provide long-lasting relief of pain

- Long-term opioid maintenance with membrane stabilization
- Another reoperation, or
- SCS, PNFS, or both

STEP 2: SAFE principles analysis

- SCS, PNFS, or both
- Long-term opioid and membrane stabilization maintenance or IDDS
- Another reoperation

Fig. 17-2 An example of how to use the safety, appropriateness, fiscal neutrality, and efficacy (SAFE) principles for a patient with failed back surgery syndrome. The principle starts with safe, efficacious, and less costly therapies in parallel in a judicious manner, moving past therapies that are either ineffective or work with limited efficacy. Evaluation of initial cost and cost-over-time are evaluated using these principles. When using such principles, invasive therapies such as neuroaugmentation and intrathecal drug delivery systems (IDDS) will be appropriately positioned and not arbitrary at the end of the algorithm. OTC, over-the-counter; PNFS, peripheral nerve field stimulation.

Intrathecal Drug Delivery Systems

The infusion of opioids intraspinally is directly linked to the 1970s discovery of μ receptors in both the spinal cord and brain.[8] Direct administration of morphine to the spinal cord of rats produced a measurable analgesia, which eventually led to intraspinal injections in humans and produced equally effective analgesia.[9] Several years later, the initial work describing the continuous infusion of intrathecal (IT) morphine in patients with pain secondary to malignancy was published.[10] Wang et al[11] demonstrated that bolus injections of morphine into the IT space produced pain relief in patients with cancer.

Since the late 1980s, the treatment of patients with chronic pain refractory to conventional therapies via IT infusions of opioids and other analgesia medications has been steadily increasing.[12] IDDS uses the aforementioned concept of direct application of very low-dose opioids or other analgesics directly into the IT space via an implantable drug infusion system.[10,13] The growing popularity stemmed from using implantable technology, which created the ability to provide continuous infusion, thereby forging a stable cerebrospinal concentration of the desired opioid and in doing so avoiding the fluctuations in pain relief known to be inherent to either multiple bolus injections or oral administration.[14] Recent technological advances in IDDS have allowed for increased safety and reliability, which has created the opportunity to conduct further clinical testing of established medications, mixtures, and new analgesic compounds for use in IT administration. Most importantly, the field of IT administration via IDDS has expanded its utility to patients with nonmalignant causes for their pain, such as failed back surgery syndrome (FBSS).

Mechanism of Action

Opioid analgesics administered intraspinally are dosed at a fraction of that required for systemic administration. They primarily affect the presynaptic and postsynaptic receptors of the substantia gelatinosa of the posterior horn of the spinal cord (**Fig. 17-3**). The advantage of IT delivery is that potent analgesia can be obtained without interfering with sensations of touch, motor function, or sympathetic reflexes.[11] IT opioid delivery is additionally advantageous over systemic administration because of the continuous levels of pain relief and avoidance of the peaks and troughs as mentioned above as well as the ability to use lower doses and reduced risk of overall side effects. Because the IT dose of morphine can be fractionated to as little as one 300th of the oral morphine equivalent, fewer central nervous system (CNS) and systemic side effects are experienced.[15]

When attempting to use an IDDS, the two most important factors to account for are the drug(s) to be used and the type of pain to be treated (the latter is discussed in the next section). The safe and effective utilization of intraspinal infusions and ultimately IT delivery lies in the knowledge of the pharmacology of the drugs delivered and the pharmacodynamics of the drugs in the intraspinal space. The distribution and absorption of a particular drug placed IT is based on several mitigating factors; most important are the drug characteristics.[16,17] Upon IT injection, there is rostral diffusion, and the final cisternal concentration is dictated by the lipophilic nature of the substance. Other factors to take into account are cerebrospinal fluid (CSF) factors such as specific gravity, baricity, and CSF flow. With this in mind, the physician can tailor a treatment to the specific needs of the patient by adjusting the "cocktail" of medications available in the pump at each subsequent follow-up by merely making adjustments during the refill visits.

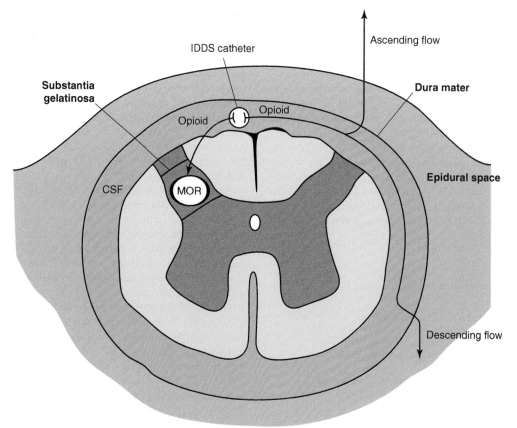

Fig. 17-3 Schematic of intrathecal drug delivery systems (IDDS) in a cross section of the spinal cord via an opioid substrate. The catheter tip lies beneath the dura mater in the intrathecal (IT) space. The opioid is released into the IT space and acts on the μ-opioid receptors (MOR) located in the substantia gelatinosa of the dorsal horn of the spinal cord, also known as lamina II. There is also suspected flow within the IT space as the opioid mixes with the cerebrospinal fluid (CSF) and is therefore subjected to potential rostral and caudal spread, as represented by the *ascending* and *descending* arrows.

Currently, morphine is one of only three medications approved by the Food and Drug Administration for use in IDDS; the others are ziconotide and baclofen. Because of its hydrophilic properties and potent receptor affinity, morphine was labeled the "gold standard" for the treatment of chronic pain. Its hydrophilic nature also prevents it from readily crossing the blood–brain barrier and creates higher CSF concentrations. Baclofen is approved for use in patients with spasticity and neuromuscular diseases and is not a primary agent used for pain.

Efficacy

IDDS of opioids is widely accepted for the treatment of cancer pain and has gained increasing popularity in cases of chronic nonmalignant pain. At the International Consensus Conference in Brussels in 1998, it was recommended that IDDS should be used in patients with chronic nonmalignant pain as long as the patients were appropriately selected according to specific criteria.[18]

In patients with pain secondary to cancer, oral or subcutaneous administration of morphine can provide effective analgesia in approximately 80% of patients.[15] When more invasive therapies such as IDDS are used, an additional 10% to 15% of patients can be provided with pain relief. Systemic administration of opioids should still be preferred as long as function is not impaired; however, because of the occasionally high requirements of some cancer patients, treatment with oral or intravenous (IV) opioids can make them incoherent, depress respiratory function, cause fatigue, decrease libido, change hormonal levels, cause urinary

retention, and reduce quality of life. In these cases, IDDS should be considered an appropriate step to offer appropriate pain relief.[19] Patient selection is paramount when considering IDDS because careful screening offers the best chance of successful treatment outcome. The following essential criteria should be adhered to when selecting a patient for an IDDS:

1. Failed treatment with oral opioids because of an inability to tolerate side effects or achieve acceptable relief. This rule may not apply to those trialed for ziconotide because it is not in the opioid classification.
2. Life expectancy of at least 3 months. This criterion is difficult to predict because many patients experience improved survival with improved pain relief and reduction of oral opioids.
3. The patient should have no occlusion to flow or mechanical exclusion to implant such as hardware in the area of implant, localized infection, tumor occlusion of the spinal cord or IT sac, or systemic infection. It is critical to have acceptable CSF circulation.[15]

As with many treatments in the field of pain, some pain syndromes are more responsive to IDDS. Pelvic cancer, pancreatic cancer, and cancer with metastasis to bone are the most responsive to IDDS. Further characterization with the type of pain can provide additional prognostication for potential success. For example, patients with visceral pain and somatic nociceptive pain respond quite well, but those with neuropathic characteristics do not respond as well. The use of novel agents and a combination of

Table 17-1: Indications for Use

Neurostimulation	Intrathecal Drug Delivery System
Neuropathic pain and peripheral neuropathy	Cancer pain
Visceral pain	Nociceptive pain
Ischemic pain	Nerve root injury
Sympathetically-driven pain	Deafferentation pain
Peripheral vascular disease	Spinal cord injury pain
Multiple sclerosis	
Postherpetic neuralgia	
FBSS	
Arachnoiditis	
CRPS (RSD and causalgia)	

CRPS, complex regional pain syndrome; FBSS, failed back surgery syndrome; RSD, reflex sympathetic dystrophy.

agents such as a local anesthetic with an opioid or an opioid with ziconotide may result in better outcomes in challenging pain settings (**Table 17-1**).[20]

By comparison, nonmalignant pain models should be treated with more prudence before considering IDDS (e.g., casual therapies have been exhausted, failure of less-invasive therapies) but should nonetheless be considered in the right patient. In 2004, Deer et al[21] collected data from the National Outcomes Registry for Low Back Pain and found that the most common conditions treated with IDDS were FBSS (66.2%), degenerative disc disease (36.8%), and radicular leg pain (28.7%). Those patients that received IDDS reported a statistically significant improvement in pain from their baselines at 6 and 12 months ($P < 0.001$). The reduction in pain at 12 months was 32% to 48%, and there was a 66% improvement in functionality.

As with cancer pain, visceral and somatic nociceptive pain seems to respond better that neuropathic pain. Additionally psychological factors are more likely to play a role in potential success. Patients with major psychiatric disorders such as active psychosis and severe depression should be treated before implantation when identified. Caution should also be used in those with opioid tolerance leading to dose escalation and potential psychological dependence.[15] Another major difference in this patient population is the type of drugs to be used because these patients tend to have a lesser response to systemic opioids and may require more complex management over time. Moreover, the dose titration should be more conservative.

Neuroaugmentation by Stimulation

Neuroaugmentation via the use of SCS has been used for more than 30 years for the treatment of refractory chronic pain, most notably FBSS and complex regional pain syndrome (CRPS). The introduction of this methodology was seeded in the well-heralded work on the "gate-theory" by Melzack and Wall[22] in 1965, although the exact mechanism of SCS has never been proven. Compared with IDDS, in which a specific receptor and site of action is the accepted premise, neuroaugmentation's ability to function is shrouded in speculation. The idea that stimulation to large fibers "closes the gate" in the dorsal horn, which in turn prevents the small fibers from accomplishing their intention to communicate pain, is surmised by the "gate theory" and predominates the school of thought for those looking to explain how it works. Although electrical stimulation therapies inspired by the gate control theory

have succeeded, it is still a source of debate and controversy because it predicts that all types of pain should be inhibited when, in fact, they are not. It stands to reason that both acute and chronic pain, as well as nociceptive and neuropathic pain, could be effectively treated as long as large fibers were stimulated; however, this has not proven to be the case. Many patients have mixed pain syndromes and have responses to SCS when the treating physician believes the chances are less than ideal of achieving a good outcome. This consideration makes it imperative to trial those patients who may have a neuropathic component to their pain.

Mechanism of Action

As already stated, there are no definitive explanations as to why neuroaugmentation works. Although the gate control theory continues to dominate most discussions, there are other consistent findings beyond that explained by gate control, which may provide insight and beg interjection into the proposed mechanism of action. When implanting an SCS, one applies a lead over the dorsal column in the epidural space. The conductivity of the intraspinal elements in relation to the lead placement dictates the electrical stimulation provided. For example, a neuron will depolarize and create an action potential when it is made more positive; this is created by applying a negatively charged external cathode. Conversely, a negatively charged neuron will hyperpolarize and reduce its ability to propagate an action potential, which is accomplished through the placement of a positively charged, external anode. Therefore the active electrode to produce stimulation is derived from the cathode, and the anode serves to shield nearby structures from the effects of the stimulation. This allows the physician to direct the area of stimulation.[23]

Conductivity of stimulation to the desired area is paramount to neuroaugmentation. This draws comparison to IDDS because both rely on delivery of the catalyst to the spinal cord in a specific region, and any factor that interferes with this could compromise the potential success. However, IDDS relies on a drug to reach a general region of the spinal cord, which corresponds to the patient's complaints of pain, but SCS requires a more specific and elegant method of exactness. This implies that neuroaugmentation requires proper patient selection, as well as precise lead placement, but IDDS requires only proper patient selection and careful follow-up.

The classic goal of SCS is to produce a field of paresthesias directly over the patient's pain complaints by stimulating the relevant spinal cord structures without stimulating the nearby nerve root.[24] Without the appropriate coverage of paresthesias, neuroaugmentation will be unsuccessful in providing successful pain relief. The relatively low threshold of dorsal root sensory fibers requires the implanting physician to place the lead sufficiently in the midline to prevent dorsal root involvement with currently available technology. Specific devices to stimulate the dorsal root ganglion are now in development and may modify the way we approach these complicated pain syndromes. Contrast this with IDDS, in which the catheter tip need not be placed with the same degree of precision. The application of varying drugs with different grades of hydrophilic versus lipophilic nature can allow a more directed approach to only the wanted regions of the cord. Although there is a certain degree of guesswork involved, IDDS can suffer minor changes in tip placement without major interruptions in relief, but the slightest lead migration might change the coverage entirely and thus create intermittent failures in pain control. As mentioned previously, the interchangeable use of anodes and cathodes allows not only for accuracy in coverage but also for evolving treatment to account for the ever-changing patient and the occasional lead migration. By creating a cathodal field, one can produce a technique known as "guarding" to prevent unwanted areas to be stimulated, simultaneously creating better penetration in the spinal cord and thereby increasing the efficacy. The use of two cathodes in the "double-guarded" array surrounded on each end by an anode that has been described by Deer et al[21] has led to increased coverage and when used crossing the midline. In many cases, this has led to coverage of both legs, the axial spine, and all dermatomes below L2.

Again, the exact mechanisms of neuroaugmentation remain somewhat enigmatic; however, there are many recorded findings that provide some insight. There does not appear to be any reversal of the effects of SCS by administration of naloxone, so one could conclude there is no relationship between stimulation and the release of endogenous opioid pain-relieving mechanisms.[23] However, there does appear to be an effect of SCS on the neurochemistry of the spinal cord, more specifically in the dorsal horn. Administration of SCS in normal rats has shown an increase in γ-aminobutyric acid (GABA) in the dorsal horn after stimulation, more specifically in rats showing a positive response to the stimulation. Moreover, rats not responding show no increase.[25] This finding is further compounded by the discovery that SCS-induced inhibition of the spinothalamic tract can potentiated by the addition of GABA agonist and negated by the administration of GABA antagonists (**Fig. 17-4**).[26,27]

From a neurophysiologic perspective, it has been found in animal models that neuroaugmentation acts predominantly on

A-β fibers, not C-fibers, and acts to decrease the spontaneous activity of wide-dynamic range neurons.[23,28] There is, of course, the effect of orthodromic activation of the dorsal columns, which leads to supraspinal effects as well as a "closing the gate" by antidromic activation of large-diameter fibers. This suggests a vast difference from IDDS because the effects of neuroaugmentation impact the peripheral nervous system as well as the CNS. The largest effect to neuroaugmentation to draw comparison against IDDS lies in the ability to impact the sympathetic nervous system. SCS antianginal and anti-ischemic effects are well documented because the former represents the single largest application of SCS in Europe. SCS results in vasodilation and increased flow rates in the extremities through the afferent inhibition and antidromic activation of the sympathetic nervous system.[23]

Efficacy

In a study published by Kumar in 1998 representing patients over a 15-year span, it was reported that the five most common indications for treatment with SCS were FBSS, peripheral vascular disease, peripheral neuropathy, multiple sclerosis, and CRPS, previously known as reflex sympathetic dystrophy. In his study, he reported an overall success rate of establishing acceptable pain relief in 59% of patients; of patients deemed successful, 43% reported excellent pain relief. In a literature search documented within, an average success rate of 54% was seen across 16 reported studies. The largest percentage of successful response to SCS was noted in peripheral

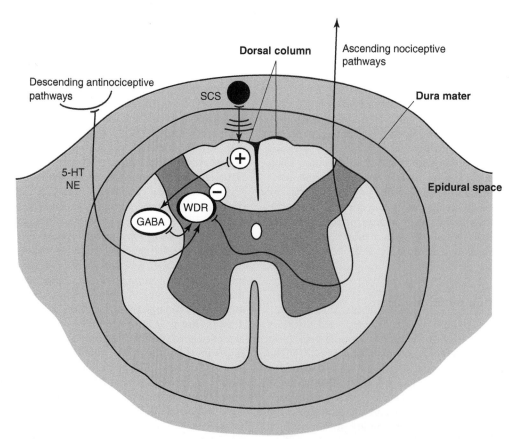

Fig. 17-4 Schematic of the proposed mechanism of neuroaugmentation via spinal cord stimulation (SCS) in a cross section of the spinal cord. The SCS lead is placed over the dura mater in the epidural space. A signal is transmitted toward the spinal cord, which stimulates the dorsal column. This leads to up-regulation of γ-aminobutyric acid GABA, which in turn suppresses the wide-dynamic range (WDR) neurons. This suppression is surmised to "close the gate" and thereby prevent pain transmission along the ascending nociceptive pathways. There is also a resulting descending, antinociceptive response, which functions via serotonergic (5-HT) and noradrenergic (NE) pathways and serves to further suppress the WDR neurons.

neuropathy (73.7% or 14 of 19 patients) and reflex sympathetic dystrophy (100% or 13 of 13 patients).[29] FBSS had a success rate of 52%, and in a similar literature search, it was found to be successful in 53% of patients across 10 studies. Kumar went on to describe that patients without surgical procedures before implant respond better, and if surgery was present in the history, having a shorter transition time to implant improved the outcome. He concluded that pain etiologies such as cauda equina syndrome, primary bone and joint pain, and paraplegic pain do not respond well (which, in contrast, do seem to respond to IDDS) (**Table 17-1**).

The findings that neurostimulation has preferential success for some pain types (neuropathic) and likely failure in others (nociceptive) has been seen in several studies. It has been proposed that SCS is most lucrative in neuropathic or sympathetically-driven pain states, with success rates approaching 70%,[30] likely in no small part because of its ability to directly affect the sympathetic nervous system.[23] North et al[31,32] reported that SCS was successful in producing pain relief that exceeded 50% for patients in follow-up as long as 20 years and accomplishing 60% relief in arachnoiditis.[33] North and Wetzel[34] proposed that SCS had success rates reported as high as 88% in FBSS, suggesting it may even be superior to reoperation; however, it was still ineffective in the treatment of nociceptive pain. They found that it was most successful in intractable angina and ischemic pain (because of changes in blood flow by direct affect to the sympathetic nervous system), as well as CRPS and neuropathic pain after spinal surgery.

More recently, in 2004 Turner et al[7] published a systematic review with findings suggesting that SCS is effective in treating both FBSS and CRPS; however, it was limited in patients with mixed leg and back pain. Meglio et al[35] reported in 1989 that SCS was most effective in vasculopathic pain, low back pain, and neuropathic pain (postherpetic neuralgia) and was the least effective in cancer pain and deafferentation models. These findings are worthy of comparison with IDDS, in which the most successful patients are those with nociceptive pain and cancer pain, with the lowest success rate in patients with neuropathic pain. Both IDDS and neuroaugmentation do possess overlap in their ability to treat FBSS, as noted previously; IDDS, however, does not seem to be limited by mixed pain pictures such as the inclusion of the back with the lower extremities, which may suggest some superiority by comparison. These assessments, as well as the uniqueness of each method, must be carefully calculated before deciding which methodology to implement (**Table 17-2**).

Comparison of Complications

Any surgical procedure carries inherent risks and complications. Bleeding is an obvious risk, which can occur either intraoperatively or postoperatively in both neuroaugmentation and IDDS. This is a relatively rare complication because these procedures do not require extensive surgery, and the areas involved are not particularly vascular. Most instances of bleeding are associated with implantation and are seen either from inadequate hemostasis or in the subcutaneous tissue from pocket formation. Wound hematoma or seroma and epidural hematoma are also particularly worrisome, but again, their incidence is not overwhelming as long as standard precautions and stringent hemostasis are achieved. The risk of infection is relatively low in these patients because one is dealing with a clean, surgical wound. Moreover, manufacturers recommend prophylactic administration of IV antibiotics, which serves to further decrease an already low complication rate.

Although both neurostimulation and IDDS carry common risks intrinsic to the obvious similarities between the two, there are

Table 17-2: Direct Comparison Between Neuroaugmentation and Intrathecal Drug Delivery Systems

	Neurostimulation	Intrathecal Drug Delivery Systems
Anatomy	Epidural placement	Intrathecal placement
Mechanism	Unknown	Drug-specific actions
Maintenance	Variable; occasional reprogramming	Regular refills
Trial	Can go home same day	Requires hospital stay
Ease of use	Requires specific coverage of paresthesias; extremely dependent on anatomy and precise placement of electrode on correct area; external programmer allows patient to account for momentary changes and office-based reprogramming for more permanent changes in coverage over time	Catheter need only be in the relative region of the spinal cord corresponding to comparative dermatome but requires sufficient knowledge of pharmacology and pharmacokinetics
Mortality	1.4:1	7.5:1
Complications	Lead migration, lead fracture, infection	Overdose, drug-related side effects, granuloma, infection

distinctions in the potential complication rate as well as the particular risks and complications that each carry individually. The overall complication rate in SCS implantation ranges from 34% to 41%.[7,29] Although this may seem high, the regularly irreversible nature of the procedure, lack of reporting of any long-term complications ever being noted, and the fact that most complications were not life threatening, neuroaugmentation has been gaining overwhelming support and popularity.[36] The most common complication reported across all studies is lead migration with rates ranging from 23.1% to 27%.[7,29,30,34] In 1989, Racz et al[37] reported lead migration rates as high as 69%; however, in a follow-up, North et al[32] reported that lead migration was steadily declining, attributing this trend toward improving technical efficiency. Although lead migration by itself is not a serious complication and does not even potentially put the patient at particular risk, it does change the coverage pattern of stimulation and potentiate the patient toward reporting failure of pain control. Revision of lead placement typically follows, with the goal of placing the lead back in the original place or attempting to recreate the pattern that provided previous success. Revision does require bringing the patient back to the operating room and reexposing him or her to all of the initial risks of intervention for an additional time. Advances in anchoring systems and progressive attention toward averting lead migration have allowed for this preventable complication to be minimized, thus increasing the already potent success rates of neuromodulation. In addition to lead migration, lead breakage has been reported in 3.4% to 9.1% of cases. This is a more taxing complication because it requires a more extensive revision such that the leads must be removed and replaced. If the leads have fractured within the epidural space, neurosurgical intervention may be required.

Infection carries a relatively low risk compared with lead migration or fracture with a reported rate of 3.4% to 4.6%.[7,29] Other complications such as CSF leak and hardware malfunction or even more rare outcomes such as micturition inhibition and spinal cord compression have been reported.[38,39] However, the unpredictable and seemingly unpreventable nature of these should not enter into the equation when deciding on the appropriateness of neuroaugmentation.

IDDS requires a surgical technique that is virtually identical in nature except for an intentional dural puncture and placement of a catheter into the IT space rather than the epidural space. The unique risks associated with IDDS are accounted for by the drug component involved. As previously mentioned, a particular appeal of IDDS is the ability to circumvent many of the unwanted side effects of systemic opioid usage. In a systematic review by Turner et al[40] in 2007, the most commonly reported drug-related side effects were nausea or vomiting (33%), urinary retention (26%), and pruritus (26%).[41-44] Other noted side effects were provocation of asthma, insomnia, dry mouth, myoclonic jerk, spasm, dizziness, loss of appetite, diarrhea, and headache. Deer et al[21] reported that the most common adverse effect over 12 months was reaction to the medication (5.1%). Hardware complications were reported commonly; 18% reported catheter-related complications after implant, 19% had catheter obstruction or occlusion, and 12% had catheter migration.[38] The need for surgical revision appears to be less with IDDS than with SCS, but no comparative study has been performed in a prospective fashion.

Another potentially troubling problem is the development of an IT granuloma or inflammatory mass at the tip of the IT catheter. This is a serious complication that can result in spinal cord damage and irreversible neurological dysfunction if not promptly recognized. Because IDDS patients must return regularly for refills, diligent physicians are afforded the opportunity of frequent follow-up; therefore any changes on physical examination that would suggest the presence of such a granuloma can be immediately addressed. On the basis of preclinical data, it was found that high concentrations and high daily doses of morphine are more likely to cause granuloma formation at the catheter tip.[45,46] It is more difficult to predict the overall incidence in humans compared with animals; however, the incidence is around 1.16% after 6 years.[47]

A particular concern one should have when deciding whether or not to initiate IDDS is the potential associated mortality, especially if neurostimulation is simultaneously being considered. There is a 7.5% increase in mortality over the first 3 days after an IDDS-related procedure in noncancer patients (which includes pump refill and reprogramming) compared with a 1.4% increase in SCS implant. Of note, although the relative risk is greatest immediately after the implant, the largest number of deaths occurred during therapy maintenance; this could be potentially attributed to human error in reprogramming or careless disregard during refill maintenance.[48,49] In 2006, concerned by a cluster of three opioid-related deaths concerning IDDS, Coffey et al[48,49] published an extensive review. They concluded that there is an increased mortality with IDDS compared with neuroaugmentation. These authors went on to report that although data are available to support the continued use in cancer pain, more data were required to support a safe comparison in noncancer patients even though noncancer patients currently comprise the majority of patients with IDDS. Coffey et al[48,49] found that drug overdose (28.4%) and cardiac events (15.8%) were the top two reasons for reported causes of death in noncancer patients. It was not concluded by any means that IDDS ceased to have a safe utility in noncancer patients, but a warning for conscientiousness use was implied (as the post-implant mortality may be secondary to human error), and the authors suggested that further data were needed for a sufficient

	Neurostimulation	Intrathecal Drug Delivery System
Pros	• Decreased mortality • Less frequent follow-up • Changes in pain patterns can be accounted for by reprogramming • No dosing or medication involved	• Catheter tip placement need not be exact • Tip can move somewhat without compromising relief • Pain relief can be tailored by changing medication in pump
Cons	• Requires correct coverage by paresthesias at all times • Lead migration can require re-intervention • No effect on acute pain or nociceptive pain	• Increased mortality • Regular follow-up and refills • Drug-related side effects • Minimal effect on neuropathic pain

Table 17-3: Advantages and Disadvantages of Each Modality to Consider

evaluation to be made. By using accepted standards and safeguards regarding medication management, one can minimize the potentially hazardous risks associated with the IT delivery of opioids while reaping the benefits in the right patients.

Discussion

The use of both neurostimulation and IDDS are critical parts of the current pain treatment continuum. Both have documented safety and efficacy for patients with pain patterns that are refractory to conventional or less invasive techniques. However, when discussing safety and potential risk outcome, neuroaugmentation has an edge over IDDS in that the mortality and possibility of serious complications is higher in the latter. In appropriate patients, IDDS is the appropriate choice despite the risks, and the overall success appears to outweigh the complications when considering the co-morbidities of untreated pain.

As reported previously, there are striking differences in indication for both; IDDS has more use in patients with nociceptive and cancer pain, and neurostimulation has carved out a niche with visceral, neuropathic, and ischemic pain. With the obvious overlap in the area of FBSS and the like, one needs to make a decision as to which therapy he or she will propose to the patient and pursue (Table 17-3). A new treatment algorithm should be considered when confronted with this dilemma.

1. SCS should always be considered in patients with neuropathic pain before placing a pump.
2. SCS should be considered as an alternative to IDDS for visceral pain syndromes when appropriate.
3. Peripheral nerve stimulation (PNS) should be considered as an adjuvant to SCS when the latter therapy gives partial but incomplete coverage pattern. This may allow treatment without a pump.
4. IDDS should be considered in the algorithm when SCS with or without PNS fails or is not appropriate. In patients undergoing IT drug delivery, new precautions should be followed.[50]

References

1. Krames ES: Intraspinal opioid therapy for chronic nonmalignant pain: current practice and clinical guidelines. *J Pain Symptom Manage* 11(6):333-352, 1996.

2. Krames ES: Interventional pain management appropriate when less invasive therapies fail to provide adequate analgesia. *Med Clin Am* 83(3):787-808, 1999.

3. World Health Organization Expert Committee: Cancer pain relief and palliative care. *World Health Organization Technical Report Series* 804:1-73, 1990.

4. Catala E: *Intrathecal administration of opiates in cancer patients.* Paper presented at satellite symposium of the European Federation of IASP Chapters Second Congress, Barcelona, Spain, September 22-23, 1997.

5. Krames E, Poree L, Deer T. Levy R: Implementing the SAFE principles for the development of pain medicine therapeutic algorithms that include neuromodulation techniques. *Neuromodulation* 12(2):104-113, 2009.

6. Krames E, Poree L, Deer T, Levy R: Rethinking algorithms of pain care: the use of the S.A.F.E principles. *Pain Med* 10(1):1-5, 2009.

7. Turner JA, Loeser JD, Deyo RA, Sanders SB: Spinal cord stimulation for patients with failed back surgery syndrome or complex regional pain syndrome: a systematic review of effectiveness and complications. *Pain* 108:137-147, 2004.

8. LaMonte C, Pert CB, Snyder SH: Opiate receptor binding in primate spinal cord: distribution an changes after dorsal root section. *Brain Res* 112:407-412, 1976.

9. Yaksh T, Rudy TA: Analgesia mediated by a direct spinal action of narcotics. *Science* 192:1357-1358, 1976.

10. Onofrio BM, Yaksh TL, Arnold PG: Continuous low-dose intrathecal morphine administration in the treatment of chronic pain of malignant origin. *Mayo Clin Proc* 56:516-520, 1981.

11. Wang JF, Nauss LA, Thomas JE: Pain relief by intrathecally applied morphine in man. *Anesthesiology* 50:149-151, 1979.

12. Deer T, Krames ES, Hassenbusch SJ, et al: Polyanalgesic Consensus Conference 2007: recommendations for the management of pain by intrathecal (intraspinal) drug delivery: report of an interdisciplinary expert panel. *Neuromodulation* 10(4):300-328, 2007.

13. Coombs DW, Saunders RL, Gaylor MS, et al: Continuous epidural analgesia via implanted morphine reservoir. *Lancet* 2:425-426, 1981.

14. Kwan JW: Use of infusion devices for epidural or intrathecal administration of spinal opioids. *Am J Hosp Pharm* 47(suppl 1):S18-S23, 1990.

15. Deer T, Winkelmuller W, Erdine S, et al: Intrathecal therapy for cancer and nonmalignant pain: patient selection and patient management. *Neuromodulation* 2(2):55-66, 1999.

16. Payne R: CSF distribution of opioids in animals and man. *Acta Anesthesiol Scan Suppl* 1:38-46, 1987.

17. Kroin JS, Ali A, York M et al: The distribution of medication along the spinal canal after chronic intrathecal administration. *Neurosurgery* 33:226-230, 1993.

18. Task Force of the European Federation of IASP Chapters, (EFIC): Neuromodulation of pain: a consensus statement prepared in Brussels 16-18 January. *Eur J Pain* 2:203-209, 1998.

19. Lamer TJ: Treatment of cancer-related pain: when orally administered medications fail. *Mayo Clin Proc* 69:473-480, 1994.

20. Portenoy RK: Cancer pain: pathophysiology and syndromes. *Lancet* 339:1026-1031, 1992.

21. Deer T, Chapple I, Classen A, et al: Intrathecal drug delivery for treatment of chronic low back pain: report from the national outcomes registry for low back pain. *Pain Med* 5(1):6-13, 2004.

22. Melzack R, Wall PD: Pain mechanisms: a new theory. *Science* 150:971-979, 1965.

23. Oakely JC, Prager JP: Spinal cord stimulation: mechanisms of action. *Spine* 27(22):2574-2583, 2002.

24. Barolat G, Massaro F, He J, et al: Mapping of sensory responses to epidural stimulation of the intraspinal neural structures in man. *J Neurosurg* 78:233-239, 1993.

25. Stiller C-O, Cui J-G, O'Connor WT, et al: Release of GABA in the dorsal horn and suppression of tactile allodynia by spinal cord stimulation in mononeuropathic rats. *Neurosurgery* 39:367-375, 1996.

26. Cui J-G, Meyerson BA, Sollevi A, et al: Effects of spinal cord stimulation on tactile hypersensitivity in mononeuropathic rats is potentiated by GABAB and adenosine receptor activation. *Neurosci Lett* 247:183-186, 1998.

27. Duggan AW, Fong FW: Bicuculline and spinal inhibition produced by dorsal column stimulation in the cat. *Pain* 22:249-259, 1985.

28. Linderoth B, Foreman R: Physiology of spinal cord stimulation: review and update. *Neuromodulation* 2(3):150-164, 1999.

29. Kumar K, Toth C, Nath RK, Laing P: Epidural spinal cord stimulation for treatment of chronic pain—some predictors of success. A 15-year experience. *Surg Neurol* 50:110-121, 1998.

30. Henderson JM, Schade CM, Sasaki J, et al: Prevention of mechanical failures in implanted spinal cord stimulation systems. *Neuromodulation* 9(3):183-191, 2006.

31. North RB, Ewend MG, Lawton MT, et al: Spinal cord stimulation for chronic, intractable pain: superiority of "multichannel" devices. *Pain* 44:119-130, 1991.

32. North RB, Kidd DH, Zahurak M, et al: Spinal cord stimulation for chronic, intractable pain: two decades' experience. *Neurosurgery* 32:384-395, 1993.

33. Dela Porte C, Seigfried J: Lumbosacral spinal fibrosis spinal arachnoiditis: its diagnosis and treatment by spinal cord stimulation. *Spine* 8:593-603, 1983.

34. North RB, Wetzel FT: Spinal cord stimulation for chronic pain of spinal origin: a valuable long-term solution. *Spine* 27(22):2584-2591, 2002.

35. Meglio M, Cioni B, Rossi GF: Spinal cord stimulation in management of chronic pain, a 9-year experience. *J Neurosurg* 70:519-524, 1989.

36. Cameron T: Safety and efficacy of spinal cord stimulation for the treatment of chronic pain: a 20-year literature review. *J Neurosurg* 100:254-267, 2004.

37. Racz GB, McCarron RF, Talboys P: Percutaneous dorsal column stimulation for chronic pain control. *Spine* 14:1-4, 1989.

38. Grua ML, Michelagnoli G: Rare adverse effect of spinal cord stimulation: micturition inhibition. *Clin J Pain* 26(5):433-434, 2010.

39. Lennarson PJ, Guillen BS: Spinal cord compression from a foreign body reaction to spinal cord stimulation: a previously unreported complication. *Spine* 35(25):E1516-E1519, 2010.

40. Turner JA, Sears JM, Loeser JD: Programmable intrathecal opioid delivery systems for chronic noncancer pain: a systematic review of effectiveness and complications. *Clin J Pain* 23(2):180-195, 2007.

41. Hassenbusch SJ, Stanton-Hicks M, Covington, et al: Long-term intraspinal infusions of opioids in the treatment on neuropathic pain. *J Pain Symptom Manage* 10:527-543, 1995.

42. Angel IF, Gould HJ, Jr, Carey ME: Intrathecal morphine pump as a treatment option in chronic pain of nonmalignant origin. *Surg Neurol* 49:92-98, 1998.

43. Tutak U, Doleys DM: Intrathecal infusion systems for treatment of chronic low back pain and leg pain of noncancer origin. *South Med J* 89:295-300, 1996.

44. Willis KD, Doleys DM: The effects of long-term intraspinal infusion therapy with noncancer pain patients: evaluation of patient, significant-other, and clinical staff appraisals. *Neuromodulation* 2:241-253, 1999.

45. Deer T, Krames ES, Hassenbusch SJ, et al: Management of intrathecal catheter-tip inflammatory masses: an updated 2007 consensus statement from an expert panel. *Neuromodulation* 11:77-91, 2008.

46. Allen JW, Horais KA, Tozier NA, et al: Time course and role of morphine dose and concentration in intrathecal granuloma formation in dogs: a combined magnetic resonance imaging and histopathology investigation. *Anesthesiology* 105:581-589, 2006.

47. Fishman SM, Ballantyne JC, Rathmell JP: *Bonica's management of pain*, ed 4, Baltimore, 2010, Lippincott, Williams & Wilkins.

48. Coffey RJ, Owens ML, Broste SK, et al: Mortality associated with implantation and management of intrathecal opioid drug infusion systems to treat noncancer pain. *Anesthesiology* 111(4):881-891, 2009.

49. Coffey RJ, Owens ML, Broste SK, et al: Medical practice and perspective: identification and mitigation of risk factors for mortality associated with intrathecal opioids for non-cancer pain. *Pain Med* 11:1001-1009, 2010.

50. Deer TR: A critical time for practice change in the pain treatment continuum: we need to reconsider the role of pumps in the patient care algorithm. *Pain Med* 11:987-989, 2010.

18 Anticoagulation Guidelines and Intrathecal Drug Delivery Systems

Sukdeb Datta

CHAPTER OVERVIEW

Chapter Synopsis: Implantation of a device that delivers intrathecal analgesic drugs is an intrinsically invasive procedure. As with any surgical procedure, special consideration must be given to patients with increased or complicated risks of surgical bleeding. Such patients include those with systematic diseases such as von Willebrand disease, renal disease, and other conditions that include therapeutic use of antithrombotic medications. Although underlying conditions must be cared for, the risk of increased neuraxial bleeding with medications such as warfarin must be considered. This chapter includes many of the issues that deserve attention in this patient population when undergoing intrathecal drug delivery systems (IDDS) implantation surgery.

Important Points:
- Development of standards for perioperative venous thromboembolism and use of potent antithrombotics may lead to implications regarding heightened risk of neuraxial bleeding.
- Systematic diseases such as von Willebrand disease, advanced liver disease, renal disease, or patients taking warfarin need special risk stratification.
- Both drug- and patient-related factors need to be evaluated.
- For patients taking warfarin, bridging therapy is recommended for high-risk patients.
- Fibrinolytics and thrombolytics: With streptokinase, bleeding risk is increased for 24 hours after administration; for alteplase, interventions can be performed 6 hours after the last administration; and for reteplase, interventions can be performed 24 hours after the last administration.
- For unfractionated intravenous and subcutaneous heparin, the activated partial thromboplastin time should be monitored; effects may be neutralized with protamine.
- For low-molecular-weight heparin (LMWH), the bleeding risk can be increased up to 12 hours after injection.
- For nonsteroidal antiinflammatory drugs, the drug-free interval should be at least 12 hours to up to 2 weeks for certain drugs (piroxicam, tenoxicam).
- A consensus panel recommends a white blood cell count of at least 2×10^9/L or an absolute neutrophil count of greater than 1000/μL. If the platelet count is less than 20×10^3/μL, the risk versus benefit of implantation should be carefully considered.

Clinical Pearls:
- Risk stratification is essential and includes proper identification of patient, procedure, and drug-related factors.
- Abnormal renal function, advanced age, and concomitant NSAID use enhance effects of LMWH.
- Relative risk of neuraxial procedures has been estimated. There is no increased risk in the presence of aspirin therapy. Traumatic insertion increases the relative risk to 11. Aspirin and intravenous heparin increase the risk to 26. Timing of heparinization can influence the risk of bleeding. If heparinization is started within 1 hour of a neuraxial block, the risk is 25. If heparinization is delayed more than 1 hour, the risk drops to 2.
- Technique-specific factors may influence the risk or consequence of bleeding. These factors depend on whether the target structure is near a major vascular or neurological structure or a confined space, type of needle used, number of passes, caliber of needle, use of fluoroscopy and contrast, and use of aspiration.

Clinical Pitfalls:
- In patients receiving anticoagulants, risk stratification for development of blood clots and pulmonary emboli dictates treatment. It is essential that consultation be multidisciplinary to avoid conflicts in management goals.
- A majority of the risk is during catheter placement.
- No consensus exists in management of intrathecal pumps and anticoagulation. It is best to consider recommendations for regional anesthetic techniques before intrathecal implants.

Introduction

The development of standards for the prevention of perioperative venous thromboembolism (VTE) as well as introduction of increasingly more potent antithrombotic medications have resulted in concerns regarding the heightened risk of neuraxial bleeding. In response to these patient issues, the American Society of Regional Anesthesia and Pain Medicine (ASRA) published its Third Edition Guidelines on regional anesthesia in the patient receiving antithrombotic or thrombolytic therapy in 2010.[1] In 2010, the Nordic guidelines for neuraxial blocks in disturbed hemostasis from the Scandinavian Society of Anesthesiology and Intensive Care Medicine was published.[2] No such guidelines exist, however, for intrathecal (IT) pump implants. Considering that IT implants use similar principles, it may be appropriate to consider guidelines in the context of guidelines published for neuraxial blocks.

von Willebrand Factor and Bleeding Complications

von Willebrand factor (vWF) is a multimeric and multivalent adhesive protein that is essential for platelet adhesion to the subendothelium and for stabilization of factor VIII procoagulant activity in circulation. The quantitative measurement of vWF involves essentially two different approaches. The first is based on interaction between vWf and glycoprotein (GP) Ib of the platelet membrane in the presence of ristocetin (ristocetin cofactor activity, Ricof) and depends not only on the amount of factor but also on its ability to bring about this interaction, large multimers being more active. The second approach involves the immunological quantitation of vWf (vWf:Ag) by its interaction with specific polyclonal or monoclonal antibodies.[3]

Bleeding Complications and Interventional Pain Management

Epidural catheterization and regional blocks have been successfully carried out in patients with hemophilia A when factor VIII replacement was carried out.[4-6] Epidural catheterization has been successfully performed in patients with von Willebrand disease when vWf:Ag and Ricof levels reached certain thresholds.[7,8] Advanced liver disease, with associated portal hypertension and hypersplenism, poses a unique risk for procedure-related bleeding. Epidural hematomas after catheterization have been reported in patients with mild liver disease.[9] In renal disease, a delayed epidural hematoma has been reported. In this patient, coagulation studies and bleeding history were normal.[10]

Anticoagulation increases the risk of bleeding. Spontaneous bleeding occurs in 3% to 7% of patients receiving warfarin.[11] Bleeding occurs in fewer than 3% of patients receiving fractionated or unfractionated heparin.[11] Thrombolytics present the greatest risk of bleeding with a 6% to 30% incidence.[11]

Thus, considering the severe nature of complication, there is a need for anticoagulation guidelines for intrathecal drug delivery systems (IDDS). Any such guidelines should be based on clear rationale and primarily depend on drug- and patient-related factors.

The recommended time limits from the last dose of a drug to the implant are generally based on the plasma half-life of the drug. After the implant is placed, the time to the next dose of the drug is based on the time from intake of the drug to its peak effect or maximum plasma concentrations, taking into account that it takes at least 8 hours for a platelet plug to solidify into a stable clot.[12]

Warfarin

Long-term anticoagulation with warfarin is often indicated for patients with a history of VTE, mechanical heart valves, and atrial

Table 18-1: Half-Lives of Factors

Factor	Half-Life (hr)
VII	6-8
IX	24
X	25-60
II	50-80

fibrillation. In addition, patients with bare metal or drug-eluting coronary stents require antiplatelet therapy with aspirin or thienopyridine derivatives (e.g., clopidogrel) for varying durations. Risk stratification is essential. Evidence-based guidelines for the perioperative management of antithrombotic therapy has been recently established by the American College of Chest Physicians (ACCP).[13] In general, for patients with moderate to high risk of thromboembolism, bridging therapy is recommended (and the prevention of thromboembolism is valued over the potential for increased surgical bleeding). Conversely, no bridging therapy is recommended for patients at low risk for thromboembolism. Although recommendations for management are relatively simple, complexity arises in the determination of who is at "high risk." This evaluation is perhaps best performed within an integrated multidisciplinary clinic by thrombophilia experts.[14]

Warfarin exerts anticoagulant activity by an indirect mechanism by interfering with the synthesis of vitamin K–dependent clotting factors, factors II (thrombin), VII, IX, and X. The effects of warfarin are not apparent until a significant amount of biologically inactive factors are synthesized and are dependent on factor half-life (**Table 18-1**).[15]

An understanding of the correlation between the various vitamin K–dependent factor levels and the prothrombin time (PT) is critical to safe practice of spinal interventions. Calculation of the international normalized ratio (INR) allows for the standardization or comparison of PT values among laboratories. Importantly, the INR is based on the values from patients who were taking stable anticoagulant doses for at least 6 weeks. Therefore, the INR is less reliable early in the course of warfarin therapy.[15]

Clinical experience with patients who are congenitally deficient in factors II, IX, and X suggests that a factor activity level of 40% for each factor is adequate for normal or near normal hemostasis.[16] Bleeding may occur if the level of any clotting factor is decreased 20% to 40% of baseline. The PT is the most sensitive to the activities of factors VII and X and is relatively insensitive to factor II. During the first few days of therapy, the PT reflects primarily a reduction of factor VII, the half-life of which is approximately 6 hours. After a single dose of warfarin, marked prolongation of INR may occur, although factor levels are still present. However, with additional doses, an INR greater than 1.4 is typically associated with factor VII activity of less than 40%. The reduction in factor X and II also contributes to the PT prolongation as therapy continues.

Risk Factors Associated with Warfarin Therapy
Several other factors are necessary to evaluate risk factors with warfarin therapy. Age, female sex, and preexisting medical conditions (lower patient weight; liver, cardiac, and renal disease) are associated with enhanced response to warfarin. Asian patients require lower doses than white patients. Multiple drug interactions exist.

- **Fibrinolytic and thrombolytic therapy:** The fibrinolytic system dissolves intravascular clots as a result of the action of plasmin.

Plasmin is produced by the cleavage of a single peptide bond of the inactive precursor, plasminogen. The resulting compound is a nonspecific protease capable of dissolving fibrin clots and other plasma proteins, including several coagulation factors. Exogenous plasminogen activators such as streptokinase and urokinase not only dissolve thrombus but also affect circulating plasminogen. Endogenous tissue plasminogen activators such as alteplase and tenecteplase are more fibrin selective and have less effect on circulating plasminogen. Clot lysis leads to elevation of fibrin degradation products, which have an anticoagulant effect by inhibiting platelet aggregation.

- **Streptokinase:** Streptokinase has relatively long-lasting effects, and the risk of bleeding is increased for 24 hours after its administration.
- **Alteplase:** Alteplase is a recombinant human plasminogen activator with a high affinity for fibrin. It is relatively inactive in the systemic circulation. It has a fast onset and is eliminated rapidly; no more than 10% is left in the plasma 20 minutes after discontinuation of the infusion. It is recommended that no less than 6 hours is allowed to elapse before a procedure.[2]
- **Reteplase:** Reteplase is a recombinant human plasminogen activator with a high affinity to fibrin. However, its elimination is rather slow, similar to that of streptokinase. It is recommended that no less than 24 hours is allowed to elapse before an interventional pain procedure.[2]
- **Unfractionated intravenous (IV) and subcutaneous heparin (UFH):** The major anticoagulant effect of heparin is attributable to a unique pentasaccharide that binds to antithrombin (AT) with high affinity and is present in approximately one-third of heparin molecules. Binding of this heparin pentasaccharide to AT accelerates its ability to inactivate thrombin (factor IIa), factor Xa, and factor IXa. Anticoagulant activities of UFH depend on both the number of heparin molecules with the pentasaccharide chain and the size of the molecules containing the pentasaccharide sequence. Larger molecular-weight heparins catalyze the inhibition of both factor IIa and Xa. Smaller molecular-weight heparins catalyze inhibition of only factor Xa.[17,18] Whereas IV injection results in immediate anticoagulant activity, subcutaneous injection results in a 1- to 2-hour delay. The anticoagulant effect of heparin is both dose- and molecular-size-dependent and is not linear but increases disproportionately with increasing doses. For example, the biologic half-life of heparin increases from 30 minutes after 25 U/kg IV to 60 minutes with 100 U/kg IV to 150 minutes with a bolus of 400 U/kg(18).

When given in therapeutic doses, the anticoagulant effect of heparin is typically monitored with the activated partial thromboplastin time (aPTT). Adequate therapeutic effects (in patients with VTE or unstable angina) is achieved with a prolongation of the aPTT to between 1.5 and 2.5 times the baseline value,[19] heparin level between 0.2 and 0.4 U/mL, or anti-Xa between 0.3 and 0.7 U/mL.[19] Administration of small-dose (5000 U) subcutaneous heparin for prophylaxis of DVT generally does not prolong aPTT and is typically not monitored. However, it can result in unpredictable (10-fold variability) and therapeutic blood concentrations of heparin in some patients 2 hours after administration.[20]

One of the advantages of heparin anticoagulation is that its effect may be rapidly reversed with protamine. Each milligram of protamine can neutralize 100 U of heparin. Because the half-life of IV heparin is 60 to 90 minutes, only heparin given in immediately preceding hours need to be considered when calculating the protamine dose. For example, a patient receiving a continuous infusion of 1200 U/hr requires approximately 25 mg of protamine. Neutralization of subcutaneously administered heparin may require a prolonged infusion of protamine owing to the continued absorption.[17]

Low-Molecular-Weight Heparin

The biochemical and pharmacologic properties of low-molecular-weight heparin (LMWH) differ from that of UFH.[17,21-24] LMWH activity cannot be monitored by anti-Xa levels; it has a prolonged half-life and cannot be reversed by protamine. For example, the elimination half-life of LMWH, which is 3 to 6 hours after subcutaneous injection, is dose-independent. Anti-Xa levels peak 3 to 5 hours after administration. However, because the half-life is three to four times that of UFH, significant anti-Xa activity is still present 12 hours after injection.

Prolonged LMWH therapy may be associated with an accumulation of anti-Xa activity and fibrinolysis.[25] The plasma half-life of LMWH also increases in patients with renal failure.[26] The anticoagulant effects of standard heparin are neutralized by an equimolar dose of protamine. Because of reduced protamine binding to LMWH fractions, only the anti-IIa activity of LMWH is completely reversed, but the anti-Xa activity is not fully neutralized. Both anti-IIa and anti-Xa activity may return up to 3 hours after protamine reversal, possibly because of release of additional LMWH from the subcutaneous depot. The clinical significance of the residual anti-Xa effect is unknown.[21]

Nonsteroidal Antiinflammatory Medications

Nonsteroidal antiinflammatory drugs (NSAIDs) inhibit platelet cyclooxygenase (COX) and prevent the synthesis of thromboxane A2. Platelets from patients who have been taking these medications have normal platelet adherence to subendothelium and normal primary hemostatic plug formation. Depending on the drug administered, aspirin and other NSAIDs may produce opposing effects on hemostatic mechanisms. For example, platelet COX is inhibited by low-dose aspirin (60 to 325 mg/dL), but larger doses (1.5 to 2 g/day) also inhibit prostacyclin (a potent vasodilator and platelet aggregation inhibitor) by vascular endothelial cells, resulting in paradoxic thrombogenic effects.[27,28] As a result, low-dose aspirin (81 to 335 mg/dL) is theoretically a greater risk factor for bleeding than higher doses.

It has been suggested that bleeding time is the most reliable predictor of abnormal bleeding in patients receiving antiplatelet drugs. However, there is no evidence to suggest that bleeding time can predict hemostatic compromise.[29,30] Platelet function is affected for the life of the platelet after aspirin ingestion; other nonsteroidal analgesics (naproxen, piroxicam, ibuprofen) produce a short-term defect that normalizes within 3 days.[31]

Celecoxib (Celebrex) is an antiinflammatory agent that primarily inhibits COX-2, an inducible enzyme that is not expressed in platelets and thus does not cause platelet dysfunction.[32] After single and multidosing, there have not been findings of significant disruption of platelet aggregation, and there is no history of undesirable bleeding events.

The antiplatelet effect of the thienopyridine derivatives ticlopidine and clopidogrel results from the inhibition of adenosine diphosphate induced platelet aggregation. These antiplatelet agents, used in prevention of cerebrovascular thromboembolic events, affect both primary *and* secondary platelet aggregation. Ticlopidine (Ticlid) and clopidogrel (Plavix) also interfere with platelet-fibrinogen binding and subsequent platelet–platelet interactions.[33] Thienopyridine derivatives demonstrate both time- and dose-dependent effects; steady state is achieved within 7 days for clopidogrel and 14 to 21 days for ticlopidine, although this may be achieved with higher loading doses (e.g., 300 mg of clopidogrel). For example, steady-state levels of clopidogrel are reached within 2 to 15 hours with 300- to 600-mg loading doses.[29] Although often administered in combination with aspirin, the concomitant use of clopidogrel or ticlopidine and aspirin may be associated with increased risk of hemorrhagic events. Serious hematological adverse reactions, including agranulocytosis, thrombotic, thrombocytopenic purpura, and aplastic anemia, have resulted in placement of a black box warning on ticlopidine. The ACCP recommends discontinuation of clopidogrel for 7 to 10 days,[34] but in patients with high risk of recurrent angina, discontinuation for 5 days has been suggested.[35] Although it is possible to assess residual clopidogrel effect using assays of platelet function (e.g., PFAII, P2Y12 assay), only a normal result would be reassuring, and the clinical applicability of these tests remains undetermined at the present time.[36] The potency of these medications is demonstrated by recent reports of spontaneous spinal hematoma during clopidogrel therapy.[37-39] Recently, the Nordic guidelines[2] for NSAIDs recommended the following:

- In patients treated with an NSAID, the treatment should be discontinued before a central neuraxial block. The drug-free interval should be no less that those outlined in **Table 18-2**.
- In patients planned for central neuraxial block, the guidelines recommend that a nonselective NSAID is replaced by another analgesic (e.g., celecoxib) in the immediate perioperative period (recommendation grade D; evidence category IV).
- The same intervals as in **Table 18-2** should be applied before manipulation or removal of an epidural or spinal catheter. NSAID can be started or restarted about 1 hour after central neuraxial block.

Guidelines for Prevention of Spinal Complications

A comparison of the Belgian Association for Regional Anesthesia with those of the German Society of Anesthesiology and Intensive Care[40] and the ASRA guidelines reveal several similarities as well as differences. The management of patients receiving thrombolytics, UFH, and antiplatelet therapy is remarkably similar. The ASRA guidelines for LMWH are much more conservative than the corresponding European statements owing to the large number of hematomas in North America. It is notable that an indwelling epidural catheter during single daily dosing of LMWH is still considered safe in Europe. However, if the patient is receiving antiplatelet therapy, LMWH will not be administered 24 hours before needle placement or catheter removal (e.g., in the case of an indwelling catheter for an IT pump trial).

An additional major difference is the management of patients receiving fondaparinux (**Table 18-3**). The German guidelines allow maintenance of an indwelling epidural catheter, although this is recommended against in both the Belgian and ASRA statements. Both European guidelines support neuraxial techniques (including

Table 18-2: Half-lives and Recommendations Regarding Discontinuation of Some Nonsteroidal Antiinflammatory Drugs

Drug	Half-life (hr)	Recommended Interval from Last Dose Until CNB
Diclofenac	1-2	12 hr
Ibuprofen	2	12 hr
Ketoprofen	2	12 hr
Indomethacin	4.5	24 hr
Ketorolac	4-6	24 hr
Naproxen	10-17	48 hr
Lornoxicam	4	24 hr
Piroxicam	10-70	2 wk
Tenoxicam	72	2 wk
COX-2-specific inhibitors		No effects on platelets

CNB, central neuraxial block; COX, cyclooxygenase.

Table 18-3: Properties of Some Commonly Used Antihemostatic Drugs

Drug or Class	Target Factor(s)	Time to Peak Effect	Plasma Half-life	Monitoring	Antidote	Antihemostatic Effect
Heparin (IV)	II and X (1/1)	<30 min	1-2 hr	aPTT	Protamine	Moderate or severe
LMWH (SQ)	II and X (1/3)	3-4 hr	4-7 hr	Anti-Xa activity	Protamine	Moderate or severe
Fondaparinux	X	2-3 hr	17-20 hr	Anti-Xa activity	—	Moderate or severe
ASA	Platelets (irreversible)	~1 hr	0.5 hr	Platelet function Analyzer or Multiplate	Desmopressin	Mild
NSAID	Platelets (reversible)	Variable	See Table 18-2	Platelet function Analyzer or Multiplate	Desmopressin	Mild
ADP-receptor blocker (e.g., clopidogrel)	Platelets (irreversible)	3-7 days	8 hr	Platelet function Analyzer or Multiplate	Platelets	Moderate
VKA drugs (e.g., warfarin)	II, VII, IX, and X	5 days (oral intake)	Variable	INR	Vitamin K factor concentrate / Human plasma	Moderate at INR 2-3 / Severe at INR >3

ADP, adenosine diphosphate; aPTT, activated partial thromboplastin time; ASA, aspirin; INR, international normalized ratio; LMWH, low-molecular-weight heparin; NSAID, nonsteroidal antiinflammatory drug; VKA, vitamin K antagonist.

continuous epidural analgesia) in the presence of direct thrombin inhibitors. However, this is relatively contraindicated by the ASRA guidelines owing to the prolonged half-life (particularly in patients with renal insufficiency), narrow therapeutic window, and limited available safety information. The ACCP recommendations[41] reflect a somewhat more conservative approach with warfarin (limit epidural analgesia <48 hours) and more liberal recommendations with LMWH (epidural analgesia allowed with twice-daily dosing).

Patient-Related Factors

- **Hematologic factors:** All conditions listed in **Table 18-4** increase the risk of developing a postprocedure spinal hematoma. The risk should be evaluated after consultation with a specialist.[2]
- **Renal failure:** Patients with chronic renal failure may experience hemorrhagic as well as thromboembolic complications. Platelet disorders (thrombocytopenia and platelet inhibition) and abnormal platelet–vessel wall interactions seem to be the most important causes, but anemia (altered blood rheology, especially when hematocrit decreases below 30%), erythropoietin deficiency, and abnormal production of nitric oxide have all been implicated. Hemodialysis will diminish but not eliminate the risk of bleeding. Desmopressin or conjugated estrogen may have beneficial effects on uremic bleeding.
- **Hepatic dysfunction:** Hepatic dysfunction can increase the risk of a spinal hematoma by a decreased synthesis of coagulation factors, especially those that are vitamin K–dependent (factors II, VII, IX, and X), causing an increase in INR. Many patients also have thrombocytopenia. In patients with portal hypertension, blood may be diverted to epidural veins, which are devoid of valves and therefore become dilated and prone to bleeding. Central neuraxial block is contraindicated in patients with severe hepatic dysfunction with elevated INR or platelets below 100×10^9/L (recommendation grade D; evidence category IV).[2]
- **Spinal deformities and vascular malformations:** In patients with ankylosing spondylitis or other severe spinal disorders, such as symptomatic spinal stenosis or osteoporosis, the number of attempts at central neuraxial block should be limited to three, and in the case of a bloody tap, the procedure should be abandoned (recommendation grade D; evidence category IV). In patients with known intraspinal vascular abnormalities, central neuraxial blocks should be avoided (recommendation grade D; evidence category IV).[2]
- **Gender and age:** Elderly patients, especially women, commonly have several risk factors for spinal hematoma. They have a high risk for thromboembolic complications but also a high risk for hemorrhagic complications. In the postoperative setting, a reduced dose of LMWH should be considered in patients with body weight of less than 55 kg (recommendation grade D; evidence category IV).[2]

Table 18-4: Some Conditions Associated with Increased Bleeding Tendency[2]

	Platelet Disorder	Coagulation Factor Deficiency
Start of hematoma formation	Immediate (minutes)	Delayed (hours, days)
Locus of spontaneous bleeding	Mucous membranes (nose, GI or urogenital tract), skin	Muscles, joints, skin, retroperitoneal
Manifestation	Petechiae, ecchymosis	Hematoma, hemarthrosis, ecchymosis
Inherited conditions	von Willebrand disease (1:50 to 1:500) [autosomal, recessive (mild, common) or dominant (severe, rare)]* Ehlers-Danlos syndrome (1:5000?)† Storage pool disease (rare) COX deficiency (rare) Bernard-Soulier (extremely rare) Glanzmann's thrombasthenia (extremely rare)	Factor VIII deficiency (1:5000) boys (X-linked, recessive) Factor IX deficiency (1:30,000) boys (X-linked, recessive) Factor VII deficiency (1:500,000) boys or girls (autosomal, recessive)
Acquired conditions	ITP, autoimmune diseases, amyloidosis, sepsis, drug-dependent deficiency, uremia, cancer, DIC, HIV	Hepatic disease, vitamin K deficiency, celiac disease, DIC
Drug-induced	ASA, NSAID, dipyridamole, ADP inhibitors, GP IIb/IIIa inhibitors, heparin or other drug-induced thrombocytopenia (HIT-I and HIT-II)	Vitamin K antagonists, thrombin inhibitors, UFH, LMWH, pentasaccharides

*Individuals with von Willebrand disease have normal platelets but reduced amount of von Willebrand disease factor in plasma and platelets, which affects adhesion of platelets to the injured vessel wall.
†Individuals with Ehlers-Danlos syndrome have normal platelets but have deficient collagen, leading to vessel fragility and decreased platelet function.
ADP, adenosine diphosphate; ASA, aspirin; COX, cyclooxygenase; DIC, disseminated intravascular coagulation; GP, glycoprotein; HIT, heparin-induced thrombocytopenia; HIV, human immunodeficiency virus; ITP, idiopathic thrombocytopenic purpura; LMWH, low-molecular-weight heparin; NSAID, nonsteroidal antiinflammatory drug; UFH, unfractionated heparin.

Anticoagulant Therapy Guidelines from an Expert Panel on Intrathecal Drug Delivery Systems[42]

In patients receiving anticoagulants, risk stratification for development of blood clots and pulmonary emboli dictates treatment. Patients considered at low risk can have anticoagulants stopped and proceed with trial and implantation when the INR normalizes. Oral anticoagulants may be resumed the night of surgery. In the moderate-risk group, LMWH may be administered to protect against thrombosis until the INR decreases to 1.5. LMWH should be discontinued 24 hours before the trial and pump implantation procedures and is resumed 12 hours postoperatively along with oral anticoagulants (**Table 18-5**).[42]

Hematologic Factors

The panel consensus is that a white blood cell (WBC) count of 2×10^9 or less or an absolute neutrophil count of 1000/µL or less may be a contraindication for surgical placement of an IDDS pump depending on the patient's condition. Patients with a lower WBC

Table 18-5: Summary of International Guidelines Pertinent to Neuraxial Procedures in Patients Receiving Thromboprophylaxis

	Antiplatelet Medications	UFH		LMWH
		Subcutaneous	**Intravenous**	
German Society for Anaesthesiology and Intensive-Care Medicine*	NSAIDs: no contraindication; hold LMWH, fondaparinux for 36-42 hr Thienopyridines and GP IIb/IIIa are contraindicated	Need placement 4 hr after heparin; heparin 1 hr after needle placement or catheter removal	Needle placement or catheter removal 4 hr after discontinuing heparin; heparinize 1 hr after neuraxial technique; delay bypass surgery 12 hr if traumatic	Neuraxial technique: 10-12 hr after LMWH; next dose 4 hr after needle or catheter placement Delay block for 24 hr after therapeutic dose
Belgian Association for Regional Anesthesia†	NSAIDs: no contraindication Discontinue ticlopidine 14 days, clopidogrel 7 days, and GP IIb/IIIa inhibitors 72 hr in advance	Not discussed	Heparinize 1 hr after neuraxial technique Remove catheter during normal aPTT; reheparinize 1 hr later	Neuraxial technique: 10-12 hr after LMWH; next dose 4 hr after needle or catheter placement Delay block for 24 hr after therapeutic dose
American Society of Regional Anesthesia and Pain Medicine	NSAIDs: no contraindication Discontinue ticlopidine 14 days, clopidogrel 7 days, and GP IIb/IIIa inhibitors 8-48 hr in advance	No contraindication with twice-daily dosing and total daily dose <10,000 U; consider delaying heparin until after block if technical difficulty is anticipated; the safety of neuraxial blockade in patients receiving >10,000 U of UFH daily or more than twice-daily dosing of UFH has not been established	Heparinize 1 hr after neuraxial technique; remove catheter 2-4 hr after last heparin dose; no mandatory delay if traumatic	Twice-daily dosing: LMWH 24 hr after surgery regardless of technique; remove neuraxial catheter 2 hr *before* first LMWH dose Single-daily dosing: according to European standards *but* with no additional hemostasis-altering drugs Therapeutic dose: delay block for 24 hr
American College of Chest Physicians‡	NSAIDs: no contraindication Discontinue clopidogrel 7 days before neuraxial block	Needle placement 8-12 hr after dose; subsequent dose 2 hr after block or catheter withdrawal	Needle placement delayed until anticoagulant effect is minimal	Needle placement 8-12 hr after dose; subsequent dose 2 hr after block or catheter withdrawal; indwelling catheter safe with twice-daily dosing Therapeutic dose: delay block for >18 hr

*Adapted from the German Society for Anesthesiology and Intensive Care Medicine Consensus guidelines. *Acta Anaesthesiol Scand* 54:16-41, 2010.
†Adapted from Vandermeulen E, Singelyn F, Vercauteren M, et al: Belgian guidelines concerning central neural blockade in patients with drug-induced alteration of coagulation: an update, *Acta Anaesthesiol Belg* 56:139-146, 2005.
‡Adapted from Geerts WH, Bergqvist D, Pineo GF, et al: Prevention of venous thromboembolism: American College of Chest Physicians Evidence-Based Clinical Practice Guidelines (8th edition), *Chest* 133(suppl):381S-453S, 2008.
aPTT, activated partial thromboplastin time; GP, glycoprotein; LMWH, low-molecular-weight heparin; NSAID, nonsteroidal antiinflammatory drug; UFH, unfractionated heparin.

count (e.g., $\leq 1.5 \times 10^9$/L) may undergo the procedure if growth factor treatment has been started. For patients undergoing aggressive chemotherapy associated with low WBC nadirs, coordination of schedules with an oncologist is recommended to minimize surgical infection risks and to avoid significant delays in cancer treatment.

Thrombocytopenia risk also needs to be addressed in this patient population. If the platelet count is 20×10^3/μL or less, the risk versus benefit of implantation should be carefully considered. Platelet transfusion may be an option for these patients.

References

1. Horlocker TT, Wedel DJ, Rowlingson JC, et al: Regional anesthesia in the patient receiving antithrombotic or thrombolytic therapy: American Society of Regional Anesthesia and Pain Medicine Evidence-Based Guidelines (third edition). *Reg Anesth Pain Med* 35:64-101, 2010.
2. Breivik H, Bang U, Jalonen J, et al: Nordic guidelines for neuraxial blocks in disturbed haemostasis from the Scandinavian Society of Anaesthesiology and Intensive Care Medicine. *Acta Anaesthesiol Scand* 54:16-41, 2010.
3. Rodeghiero F, Castaman G: The von Willebrand factor. *Ric Clin Lab* 20:143-153, 1990.
4. Christie-Taylor GA, McAuliffe GL: Epidural placement in a patient with undiagnosed acquired haemophilia from factor VIII inhibitor. *Anaesthesia* 54:367-371, 1999.
5. Shah RV, Kaye AD: Bleeding risk and interventional pain management. *Curr Opin Anaesthesiol* 21:433-438, 2008.
6. Kang SB, Rumball KM, Ettinger RS: Continuous axillary brachial plexus analgesia in a patient with severe hemophilia. *J Clin Anesth* 15:38-40, 2003.
7. Milaskiewicz RM, Holdcroft A, Letsky E: Epidural anaesthesia and von Willebrand's disease. *Anaesthesia* 45:462-464, 1990.
8. Stedeford JC, Pittman JA: Von Willebrand's disease and neuroaxial anaesthesia. *Anaesthesia* 55:1228-1229, 2000.

9. Dunn D, Dhopesh V, Mobini J: Spinal subdural hematoma: a possible hazard of lumbar puncture in an alcoholic. *JAMA* 241:1712-1713, 1979.

10. Grejda S, Ellis K, Arino P: Paraplegia following spinal anesthesia in a patient with chronic renal failure. *Reg Anesth* 14:155-157, 1989.

11. Levine MN, Raskob G, Landefeld S, Kearon C: Hemorrhagic complications of anticoagulant treatment. *Chest* 119(suppl):108S-121S, 2001.

12. Rosencher N, Bonnet MP, Sessler DI: Selected new antithrombotic agents and neuraxial anaesthesia for major orthopaedic surgery: management strategies. *Anaesthesia* 62:1154-1160, 2007.

13. Douketis JD, Berger PB, Dunn AS, et al: The perioperative management of antithrombotic therapy: American College of Chest Physicians Evidence-Based Clinical Practice Guidelines (8th edition). *Chest* 133(suppl):299S-339S, 2008.

14. Dowling NF, Beckman MG, Manco-Johnson M, et al: The U.S. Thrombosis and Hemostasis Centers pilot sites program. *J Thromb Thrombolysis* 23:1-7, 2007.

15. Ansell J, Hirsh J, Hylek E, et al: Pharmacology and management of the vitamin K antagonists: American College of Chest Physicians Evidence-Based Clinical Practice Guidelines (8th edition). *Chest* 133(suppl):160S-198S, 2008.

16. Xi M, Beguin S, Hemker HC: The relative importance of the factors II, VII, IX and X for the prothrombinase activity in plasma of orally anticoagulated patients. *Thromb Haemost* 62:788-791, 1989.

17. Hirsh J, Bauer KA, Donati MB, et al: Parenteral anticoagulants: American College of Chest Physicians evidence-based clinical practice guidelines (8th edition). *Chest* 133(suppl):141S-159S, 2008.

18. Hirsh J, Raschke R, Warkentin TE, et al: Heparin: mechanism of action, pharmacokinetics, dosing considerations, monitoring, efficacy, and safety. *Chest* 108(suppl):258S-275S, 1995.

19. Murray DJ, Brosnahan WJ, Pennell B, et al: Heparin detection by the activated coagulation time: a comparison of the sensitivity of coagulation tests and heparin assays. *J Cardiothorac Vasc Anesth* 11:24-28, 1997.

20. Gallus AS, Hirsh J, Tuttle RJ, et al: Small subcutaneous doses of heparin in prevention of venous thrombosis. *N Engl J Med* 288:545-551, 1973.

21. Cosmi B, Hirsh J: Low molecular weight heparins. *Curr Opin Cardiol* 9:612-618, 1994.

22. Holst J, Lindblad B, Bergqvist D, et al: Protamine neutralization of intravenous and subcutaneous low-molecular-weight heparin (tinzaparin, Logiparin). An experimental investigation in healthy volunteers. *Blood Coagul Fibrinolysis* 5:795-803, 1994.

23. Kessler CM, Esparraguera IM, Jacobs HM, et al: Monitoring the anticoagulant effects of a low molecular weight heparin preparation. Correlation of assays in orthopedic surgery patients receiving ardeparin sodium for prophylaxis of deep venous thrombosis. *Am J Clin Pathol* 103:642-648, 1995.

24. Levine MN, Planes A, Hirsh J, et al: The relationship between anti-factor Xa level and clinical outcome in patients receiving enoxaparin low molecular weight heparin to prevent deep vein thrombosis after hip replacement. *Thromb Haemost* 62:940-944, 1989.

25. Lojewski B, Bacher P, Iqbal O, et al: Evaluation of hemostatic and fibrinolytic alterations associated with daily administration of low-molecular-weight heparin for a 12-week period. *Semin Thromb Hemost* 21:228-239, 1995.

26. Tryba M: European practice guidelines: thromboembolism prophylaxis and regional anesthesia. *Reg Anesth Pain Med* 23:178-182, 1998.

27. Amezcua JL, O'Grady J, Salmon JA, Moncada S: Prolonged paradoxical effect of aspirin on platelet behaviour and bleeding time in man. *Thromb Res* 16:69-79, 1979.

28. Godal HC, Eika C, Dybdahl JH, et al: Aspirin and bleeding-time. *Lancet* 1:1236, 1979.

29. Rodgers RP, Levin J: Bleeding time: a guide to its diagnostic and clinical utility. *Arch Pathol Lab Med* 114:1187-1188, 1990.

30. Rodgers RP, Levin J: A critical reappraisal of the bleeding time. *Semin Thromb Hemost* 16:1-20, 1990.

31. Cronberg S, Wallmark E, Soderberg I: Effect on platelet aggregation of oral administration of 10 non-steroidal analgesics to humans. *Scand J Haematol* 33:155-159, 1984.

32. Leese PT, Hubbard RC, Karim A, et al: Effects of celecoxib, a novel cyclooxygenase-2 inhibitor, on platelet function in healthy adults: a randomized, controlled trial. *J Clin Pharmacol* 40:124-132, 2000.

33. Patrono C, Baigent C, Hirsh J, Roth G: Antiplatelet drugs: American College of Chest Physicians evidence-based clinical practice guidelines (8th edition). *Chest* 133(suppl):199S-233S, 2008.

34. Douketis JD, Bakhsh E: Perioperative management of antithrombotic therapy. *Pol Arch Med Wewn* 118:201-208, 2008.

35. Fox KA, Mehta SR, Peters R, et al: Benefits and risks of the combination of clopidogrel and aspirin in patients undergoing surgical revascularization for non-ST-elevation acute coronary syndrome: the Clopidogrel in Unstable angina to prevent Recurrent ischemic Events (CURE) Trial. *Circulation* 110:1202-1208, 2004.

36. Paniccia R, Antonucci E, Gori AM, et al: Different methodologies for evaluating the effect of clopidogrel on platelet function in high-risk coronary artery disease patients. *J Thromb Haemost* 5:1839-1847, 2007.

37. Karabatsou K, Sinha A, Das K, Rainov NG: Nontraumatic spinal epidural hematoma associated with clopidogrel. *Zentralbl Neurochir* 67:210-212, 2006.

38. Morales Ciancio RA, Drain O, Rillardon L, Guigui P: Acute spontaneous spinal epidural hematoma: an important differential diagnosis in patients under clopidogrel therapy. *Spine J* 8:544-547, 2008.

39. Sung JH, Hong JT, Son BC, Lee SW: Clopidogrel-induced spontaneous spinal epidural hematoma. *J Korean Med Sci* 22:577-579, 2007.

40. Vandermeulen E, Singelyn F, Vercauteren M, et al: Belgian guidelines concerning central neural blockade in patients with drug-induced alteration of coagulation: an update. *Acta Anaesthesiol Belg* 56:139-146, 2005.

41. Geerts WH, Bergqvist D, Pineo GF, et al: Prevention of venous thromboembolism: American College of Chest Physicians Evidence-Based Clinical Practice Guidelines (8th edition). *Chest* 133(suppl):381S-453S, 2008.

42. Stearns L, Boortz-Marx R, Du Pen S, et al: Intrathecal drug delivery for the management of cancer pain: a multidisciplinary consensus of best clinical practices. *J Support Oncol* 3:399-408, 2005.

19 Intrathecal Therapy for Malignant Pain

Lisa Jo Stearns

CHAPTER OVERVIEW

Chapter Synopsis: Cancer pain presents particular challenges to both patients and clinicians. Because malignant pain often accompanies a terminal illness, the cost-to-benefit analysis differs somewhat from that for patients with chronic lifelong pain conditions. An intrathecal drug delivery system (IDDS) may be considered too invasive and costly for cancer patients, but this chapter shows that an implantable pump may cost less than hospital admissions for uncontrolled pain. The chapter also considers pain that may arise secondarily to cancer treatment, including neuropathic pain or complex regional pain syndrome from nerve damage during surgeries or other therapies. Early, aggressive pain therapies can help prevent some of these outcomes when properly tailored to a patient's specific needs.

Important Points:
- Patient selection is based on uncontrolled pain, intolerable side effects of medications, and/or decreasing performance scores.
- Available intrathecal drug delivery systems include external systems and implantable, programmable systems.

Clinical Pearls:
- Malignant pain should be treated aggressively with frequent adjustments and polyanalgesia regimens adjusted as pain changes. Patient safety should always be considered. Survivorship ultimately determines the risk-benefit ratio of aggressive medication titration.
- Medication titration and infusion management in the polyanalgesic setting must consider the side effects of all medications in the infusate with programming changes. This is particularly important with the bolus option utilized in intrathecal therapy.

Clinical Pitfalls:
- Early complications of intrathecal drug delivery device implantation include postdural puncture headache, which may produce profound nausea and vomiting resulting in a subdural bleed, pocket or spine incision seroma, infection, bleeding, nerve injury, fat necrosis, or non-healing wounds secondary to effects of radiation.
- Late complications of intrathecal drug delivery device implantation include catheter migration, catheter occlusion, catheter dislodgement or fracture, pump malposition, rotor stall, pump programming errors, pump pocket fills, and catheter inflammatory mass.
- Therapy failure may be secondary to disease progression, catheter complications, pump complications, pharmacological errors, or human errors. An algorithm should be developed and executed to determine where the problem exists.

Introduction

Pain continues to be one of the major challenges patients face while fighting malignancy. Fifty percent of patients diagnosed with cancer report pain.[1] It is estimated that 10% of all cancer patients die with unrelieved pain. In others, functionality and quality of life are impacted secondary to side effects from medication directed at treating pain. Despite these statistics, many oncologists and palliative care physicians are reluctant to incorporate intrathecal (IT) therapy into their pain algorithms. IT delivery of medication is thought to be too invasive and expensive relative to the overall gains in pain control and functional status.

Oncologists rely on performance and toxicity scores to determine eligibility for clinical trials and aggressive treatment regimens. Although most patients' pain can be relieved by traditional methods, the side effect profiles of opioids, antiinflammatory drugs, antispasmodics, anticonvulsants, and antidepressants impact performance scores.[2] In the future, payers are likely to become stricter on functional and performance status qualifications for treatment. To date, there have been few prospective randomized trials assessing pain relief, functional restoration, and quality of life assessment in medical management versus IT therapy in malignancy. More studies need to be conducted assessing these points.

In 2009, Medicare spent $55 billion on physician and hospital payments for the last 8 weeks of life.[3] Uncontrolled symptoms and poor pain management lead to unnecessary hospitalizations. The cost of implanting an external intrathecal drug delivery system (IDDS) is less than $5000 or typically less than one hospital observation stay. The cost of an implanted programmable system is approximately $25,000 or just over the price of one admission for uncontrolled pain in a cancer patient.[2] In the long term, both systems may reduce hospital admissions for uncontrolled pain and complications secondary to side effects from medications.

An external or internal pump may deliver IT therapy for pain associated with malignancy. In both cases, a long-term IT catheter is placed and tunneled to the desired exit site or indwelling port or pump location site. The choice of an internal or external system is based on life expectancy, cost, and convenience to the patient and provider. Historically, if the life expectancy is longer than 3 months, an indwelling system is more cost effective. The burden of filling the implanted pump in a patient who is likely to become bedbound in the terminal stages must be considered. Home health agencies and hospice companies vary in expertise in implantable and externalized IT therapy systems. The burden of care lies with the implanter until able to pass off to a reliable resource for long-term care of the system. The pump manager should be cognizant of IT polyanalgesia, patient-controlled blousing, and complications related to the system.

Finally, cancer is becoming a chronic disease with long-term pain sequelae from treatment. Patients may develop severe neuropathic and nociceptive pain secondary to treatment. Aggressive surgical protocols may result in the development of complex regional pain syndrome (CRPS) either from direct nerve trauma or secondary to tissue injury and sympathetic sensitization. More aggressive radiation therapies lead to cutaneous and deep nerve injury. Chemotherapy regimens may result in peripheral and autonomic neuropathy. Much of this remains unrecognized until the pain becomes unresponsive to traditional treatment modalities. These patients transition from malignant pain to chronic pain patients and develop long-term disability secondary to the treatment for their malignancy and lack of early pain control.

Patient Selection

Patients whose pain remains unrelieved with conventional medical management or have untoward side effects of medications are candidates for IT delivery of medication. More aggressive chemotherapy regimens require low toxicity and high functional status scores to qualify for treatment.[4] The initiation of IT therapy in this patient population often improves functional status with improved appetite, decreased constipation, and reduced fatigue.[2]

The primary focus for patients with malignancy is improving quality of life and functional status. Idealistically, patients would be introduced to the pain service early in the disease treatment process when their symptoms can be aggressively managed and treatment options reviewed frequently. Most patients, unfortunately, are only referred when standard cancer therapeutic regimens fail and the patient refuses hospice. Many of these patients present on consultation to the pain service with anorexia and cachexia and large necrotic wounds and often have been bedbound. Poor nutritional status, pancytopenia, clotting disorders, and the presence of anasarca place these patients at risk for perioperative complications. Although surgical risk may be higher in this patient population, most patients opt for improved pain and symptom management when offered IT therapy. After the institution of IT therapy and reduction of medication side effects, many patients are able to return to an independent functional life. Furthermore, these patients may go on to qualify for clinical trials based on improved performance scores after implantation.

Trialing

Trialing for IT therapy in malignant pain is controversial. The goals of trialing are threefold: to demonstrate to the patient and patient's family the effectiveness of IT infusion before undergoing a surgical procedure, to convince the implanter or oncologist that it will be an effective therapy, and to satisfy third-party payers requirements for implantation prior authorization.

The implanter should be aware of the therapy window and possible time constraints for implantation. In patients whose cancer is metastatic and time is of the essence, a trial is not necessary or recommended. In these cases, drug selection is based on patient history and pain types at implantation. If the implanter is unsure of the patient's life expectancy or of likely functional status

improvement, a long-term catheter may be used as the trial system and converted to an internal system at a later date.

Trialing Methods

The trial may consist of a single-shot or infusion trial in the epidural or IT space. Single-shot trials are of little clinical use and are rarely predictive of clinical improvement with infusion systems but satisfy payers' requirements for hospital reimbursement. Epidural trials are often used to improve pain relief and mental status while avoiding a postdural puncture headache (PDPH). Epidural infusion trials should be avoided in patients with a history of epidural tumor spread or severe spinal stenosis in the lumbar region. These patients may develop irreversible weakness of the lower extremities with high-volume epidural infusions. IT infusion trials are the most predictive of clinical success with infusion systems and allow accurate medication selection and dosing before implant. Unfortunately, this approach has a high incidence of spinal headache. Increased nausea and vomiting secondary to a PDPH leads to escalation of anorexia and cachexia and therefore worsening performance scores. Although an epidural blood patch remains an option for headache relief, the immunocompromised status of the patient must be considered with infection risk.

Medication Selection

Drug selection for the trial is based on patient history, allergies, and pain type. Monotherapy or polyanalgesic therapy approaches may determine the success of the trial. Distinct pain types may be successfully treated with monotherapy. Complex pain, however, will likely respond to a targeted receptor approach. (For medication selection specifics, see the IDDS management section.)

Current Intrathecal Drug Delivery Technology

Current IDDS consists of external and internal delivery systems. The decision to use an externalized system is based on the duration of therapy, cost, and life expectancy of the patient. Internal systems are preferred in patients undergoing aggressive cancer treatment regimens in which infection risk is high and who are not in the terminal phase of the disease. Internal systems allow for more freedom of movement and fewer equipment-related complications (**Box 19-1**). Over time, internal systems become cost-effective as the cost of home infusion therapy maintenance increases over time.

Externalized Systems

Externalized systems are composed of a small ambulatory infusion pump connected to the IT catheter. These systems are maintained either by the physician's practice or by a home health agency. Many different types of ambulatory infusions pumps are available for rent or for sale (prices range from $300 to $5000). Compounded medications are delivered through the pump.

Some clinicians prefer the epidural route as opposed to the IT route for more regional control of pain. For diffuse pain, this route has few or no advantages over the IT space. The epidural space

---

Box 19-1: Complications Associated with Externalized Systems

Infection
Transudate weeping at the exit site
Dislodgement and or fracture of the catheter
Catheter migration
Pump programming errors
Pump failures

tends to fibrose over time, which may lead to ineffective pain relief and increased pain at the catheter-tip location. Also, the infusion requires high volume of medication for effect, making the eternal system quite heavy. Added weight of the infusion system should be considered in ambulatory patients because it may lead to falls and pathological fractures. In bedbound patients, external epidural infusions including local anesthetic may be used to create a surgical block, thereby eliminating the pain from pathological fractures or bowel obstructions when placed at the appropriate level.

These systems deliver a minimum of 0.1 mL/hr, so appropriate concentrations of medications must be considered. A 250-mL bag plus the infusion pump rarely weighs more than 5 lb and is of concern in patients with poor functional status who are trying to maintain their ambulatory status. Most insurance carriers, Medicaid, and Medicare will pay for home infusions in terminally ill patients. Skilled nursing facilities and some rehabilitation facilities do not accept patients with externalized systems. For patients under hospice care, hospice-registered nurses under the direction of a pain physician or a hospice medical director maintain the infusions. At end of life, externalized systems allow for easy titration and medication changes with minimal inconvenience to the provider or the patient.

Selection of the catheter type is based on anticipated duration of therapy. Short-term catheters (labor and delivery epidural catheters) are used when life expectancy is less than 2 weeks. Polyurethane catheters (DuPen, Algoline) are used for longer use. Some clinicians prefer to use a port system (Epidural Port-a-Cath) to minimize infection risk associated with externalized catheters. Using a radiopaque catheter is recommended to easily identify and monitor catheter-tip position radiographically. Short-term catheters with internal metal coils are not recommended for use longer than 1 month because they may prohibit future magnetic resonance imaging (MRI) diagnostic scans.

Implantable Systems: Constant-Flow and Programmable Systems

Intrathecal Pump System Components and Function
The two basic components of an implantable IDDS are the pump and the catheter.

Pumps   The infusion pump holds the drug to be delivered, which is transported through the catheter into the IT space. The pump can be either constant flow or programmed by a microprocessor. Depending on the pump size and dosing, the total drug volume in the pump could last a few days or a few months, but it must be refilled at regular intervals. The pump is implanted into a subcutaneous pocket, and the catheter is inserted into the IT space and connected to the pump in the pump pocket. The pump location is determined by the patient's body composition and implanter preference. In cancer patients with terminal disease, the implanter should place the pump anteriorly for ease of access at end of life.

Constant-Flow Pumps   There is only one commercially available constant-flow pump in the United States, the Arrow 3000 (Codman). The IsoMed (Medtronic) has been removed from the market and had not been widely used for malignant pain in the United States. The AccuRx (St. Jude Medical) pump has not received U.S. Food and Drug Administration (FDA) approval but has been used in Europe. The Arrow 3000 has been used in Europe extensively but has not gained acceptance in the U.S. market for malignant pain. The Arrow 3000 is available in 16-, 30- and 50-mL sizes. Constant-flow pumps are powered by trichlorofluoromethane or N-butane gas. The daily dose desired is calculated into a fixed-rate formula that is translated into drug concentration. The pump flow rate is fixed; therefore if side effects develop or pain increases, the medication needs to be replaced. The Codman 3000 has an accessible reservoir and bolus port access that directly connects to the cerebrospinal fluid (CSF) through the IT catheter. Boluses may only be delivered when the pump has been accessed by a needle. Advantages to the constant-flow systems are lower cost and the longevity of the device as compared to programmable systems. Disadvantages include an inability to change the dose without a drug concentration change and an inability to deliver boluses without a needle inserted into the device.

Programmable Systems   Currently, the SynchroMed II (Medtronic) is the only commercially available programmable pump in the U.S. market. It is available in 20- and 40-mL reservoir sizes. The pump is powered by a lithium battery and dichlorotetrafluoroethane gas. The pump includes two access ports, one to the reservoir and one to the catheter. Programmable features include constant-flow, constant-flow with bolusing option, and complex programming features that allow the provider to program multiple dosing regimens in a 24-hour period. Other programming variations allow for weekday and weekend dosing interval fluctuations.

The pump is driven by a microprocessor situated inside the electronic module. The microprocessor controls the velocity of the rotors that push the drug through the pump tubing and catheter into the IT space. The inert gas provides a constant gas pressure into the reservoir that forces the medication into the pump tubing. As reservoir volume decreases, gas expands from a liquid to gaseous phase and maintains constant pressure in the pump chamber. This action forces the contents into the catheter. The drug is stored in the pump reservoir and is transported from the pump reservoir through the pump tubing, catheter port, and catheter tubing before reaching the CSF. The catheter access port is only accessible by a 24-gauge noncoring needle to prevent accidental injection. The reservoir should never be accessed with a needle smaller than the recommended 22-gauge noncoring needle for safety purposes. The life of the battery is identified on the telemetry strip as the elective replacement indicator after a programming session as "ERI x months." The pump has an absolute hard stop of 7 years after which time it will shut off. The pump is accurate within ±14.5%. Changes in atmospheric pressure, body temperature, and other environmental conditions affect this accuracy.

Pump-associated complications include malposition in the pocket, motor stall, battery depletion, electronic reconfiguration, and magnetic pole alteration (**Fig. 19-1**). Pumps become dislodged from their anchoring sutures and may flip in the pocket, temporarily or permanently kinking the catheter. Solubilities and varying pH of compounded medications may allow the medication to leak through the pump tubing into the device motor and result in a motor stall and failure of the device. Either direct or scatter radiation may deplete battery life or cause electronic failure. If the pump is exposed to an excessive magnet force (>2 Tesla), the pump will incur MRI-induced demagnetization of the internal pump motor magnet and render the pump inoperable. These complications may result in drug withdrawal or overdose syndromes.

Catheters   The catheter designed for both the Arrow 3000 and SynchroMed II pumps are composed of radiopaque silicone. The catheters are between 70 and 105 cm long and have multiport tips. There are a varying amount of catheter anchors designed to minimize the risk of dislodgement and kinking. All have removable stylets that improve ease of insertion.

Catheter complications affecting the performance of the catheter may include kinking, dislocation, leakage, breakage, displacement, and formation of an inflammatory mass. These complications may result in drug delivery into the pump pocket or subcutaneous tissue, drug withdrawal symptoms, loss of pain control, underinfusion of medication, or CSF leak (**Fig. 19-2**).

Complications such as nerve root trauma and catheter displacement do not occur frequently but may have serious consequences. Although occurring frequently with externalized catheter systems, the displacement of catheters implanted for long-term use in patients undergoing treatment for chronic or cancer pain is approximately 7%. Inflammatory mass formation at the catheter tip has a reported incidence of 0.5% but is likely higher secondary to underreporting by clinicians to manufacturers and the FDA. Inflammatory mass formation at the catheter tip is thought to be secondary to high concentrations of opioids (hydromorphone and

morphine), high compounded drug pH resulting in precipitation of medication at the catheter tip, and low-flow velocity of medication out of the catheter and of the surrounding CSF.

Implantation of External and Internal Intrathecal Systems

In patients for whom long-term IT therapy is warranted, the patient, caregiver, and clinician should engage in a detailed discussion regarding compliance, risks, appropriate expectations, and pump positioning. Before implantation, care should be taken to optimize a patient's physical condition whenever possible. This population is immunocompromised, hypercoagulable, and malnourished as a whole. Perioperative antibiotics should be used as recommended by epidemiology at the implanting hospital facility. If the patient has a history of infections, particularly with methicillin-resistant *Staphylococcus aureus*, preoperative preparation should include a chlorhexidine scrub, nasal mupirocin swabs for 3 days, and vancomycin preoperatively and postoperatively. Patients in active chemotherapy treatment regimens should have a white blood cell count of at least 2,000/mL and platelets of 20,000/mL at implantation. Colony-stimulating factors should be given to ensure that neutropenia does not occur for 7 days postoperatively. If the patient has a history of deep vein thrombosis, pulmonary embolus, or tumor growth into a major vessel, stopping anticoagulant therapy may be detrimental. Placement of an inferior vena cava filter may be indicated preoperatively. In others, maintaining the patient on low-molecular-weight heparin or using a heparin drip may be recommended by a hematologist preoperatively. Postoperative anticoagulation should be restarted within 12 hours of implantation depending on risk stratification.[5] Also, postoperative anticoagulation should be considered in bedbound patients to avoid propagation of clots after functional status improves.

The catheters are placed intrathecally, and the tip is floated to the desired vertebral level. Type of pain, location of pain generators, and solubility of medication selected determine the tip position. Many drugs used in IT therapy when infused at a constant rate diffuse more than a few dermatomes from the catheter tip. Recently, Flack and associates[6] demonstrated that drug distribution is extremely limited in chronic constant IT infusions. Limited drug distribution results in high drug concentrations and may influence inflammatory mass formation. Horizontal and vertical location of the catheter tip should be recorded to monitor for catheter-related complications.

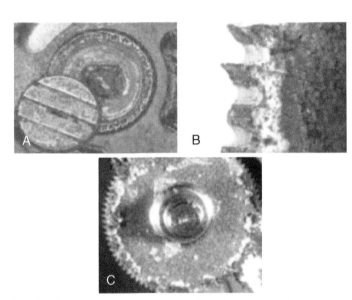

Fig. 19-1 Damage to the components of the pump motor assembly screws (**A**), gear teeth (**B**), and motor assembly gears (**C**) caused by corrosion. The pH conditions of certain medications may allow the medication to infiltrate the pump tubing, causing corrosion that can interfere with the pump's performance (e.g., motor stall).

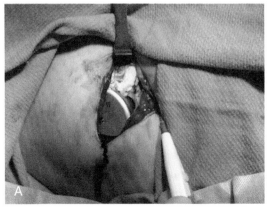
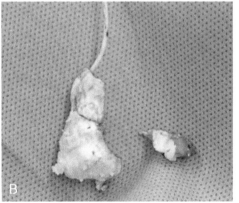

Fig. 19-2 A, Complications of the catheter. **B**, Dislodged catheter with drug precipitation.

In externalized systems, the catheter is tunneled laterally and connected to a port or externalized from the skin. For ease of care at end of life, it is recommended that catheters be tunneled to the anterior flank or abdominal wall where the site is easily accessed by nursing personnel. Anchoring externalized catheters to prevent dislodgements and fractures is essential. Patients with terminal delirium often pull at their catheters, resulting in breakage and loss of pain control at a critical time.

Internal pumps should likewise be placed as anterior as possible to simplify care at end of life. Dependent edema, anasarca, and other terminal physiologic syndromes make pump fills technically difficult.

Catheter

Implantation of the spinal end of an IT catheter is the same for both external and internal systems. The procedure may be performed under sedation or regional or general anesthesia. The patient is placed in either the prone or lateral decubitus position. The author prefers the lateral decubitus position for easy access to the abdominal wall for pump pocket formation or exteriorization of the IT catheter. A small (<1.5 inch) incision is placed in the lower lumbar area. Electrocautery is used for hemostasis, and the tissues are dissected to the supraspinal ligament. The spinal needle is placed below the L2 vertebral level to avoid spinal cord injury. Fluoroscopy is used to verify needle position. When free flow of spinal fluid is seen, the catheter is passed under fluoroscopic guidance to the desired level. If the catheter coils or becomes entangled laterally in the nerve roots, the needle is removed from the spine. The catheter is pulled back until it is free in the CSF and may be manipulated into position with careful guidance. The provider should not manipulate the catheter with the needle within the spine secondary to the risk of catheter shearing. Listening to the rhythm of the pulse oximetry helps the implanter to synchronize with the venous pulsations of the CSF and allow the catheter to float freely to the desired level. Catheters may be passed as high as C1 without difficulty from the lumbar region. Care should be taken to encourage radiology technicians to maintain catheter-tip visualization throughout catheter placement to help the implanter from passing the catheter into the ventricles of the brain. Many cancer patients have kyphosis, scoliosis, and underlying physiologic conditions, which inhibit ideal positioning on the table for fluoroscopy. It is recommended that the radiology technician perform a test run before placing the catheter to allow for smooth catheter flotation. When the catheter is in place, a purse-string suture may be placed to minimize leakage of CSF and catheter migration. The stylet is then removed, and the catheter is anchored to the supraspinous ligament or paraspinal fascia. The catheter is tunneled to the desired catheter exit site for external catheters or to the port or pump pocket.

In the externalized catheter system, the catheter is anchored in the abdominal fascia, to the abdominal skin, or both. The catheter connection device is likewise anchored to the skin. A purse-string suture around the catheter exit site helps to limit exudate leaking from the catheter exit site. In patients with anasarca, as much as 200 mL of fluid may weep from the wound daily.

A localized skin infection at the catheter exit site may track down the catheter to the IT space, resulting in meningitis if not attended to. Contamination of the system may occur during medication bag changes if sterile technique is not strictly followed. It is recommended that 100- or 250-mL infusion bags be used to minimize infection risk.

In the externalized catheter port-a-cath system, a small pocket is created anteriorly in the flank or abdomen. The catheter is tunneled to the pocket and connected to the port. The port is then anchored to the fascia using the anchoring suture loops on the device. The overlying skin is closed, and the port may be used immediately after surgery.

Pump Implantation

In patients for whom long-term IT therapy is warranted, the patient, caregiver, and clinician should engage in a detailed discussion regarding compliance, risks, appropriate expectations, and pump positioning. A 3-inch incision is made anteriorly in the flank or abdominal wall. The tissues are dissected to the fascia. Anchoring sutures are placed to secure the pump to the abdominal wall. A Silastic pouch may be used for anchoring if the implanter prefers this to the four suture loops on the pump. The current pump suture loops have welds that are sharp and tend to cut the anchoring sutures if they are not secured firmly or if the patient has violent abdominal wall contractions as with vomiting. To prevent suture breakage, double looping the sutures around the loops is recommended.

When documenting the procedure in the operative report, the catheter tip location, spine entry site, and side port orientation should be recorded. Recording these items will help troubleshoot pump and catheter problems in the future. Documentation of the orientation of the side port access site may help to prevent a pocket fill in morbidly obese patients and in patients with terminal anasarca.

In patients with cachexia, the implanter may choose to place the pump subfascially to prevent wound breakdown (**Fig. 19-3**). This adds a degree of difficulty to the procedure with additional surgical time that may place immunocompromised patients at increased infection risk. Skin breakdown because of excessive pressure remains rare even in patients with malignant pain and cachexia. Encouraging increasing perioperative

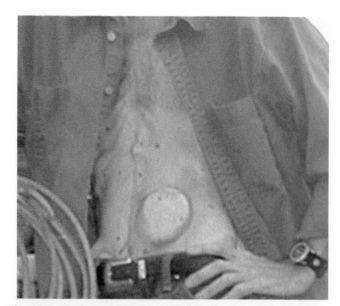

Fig. 19-3 Patient with cachexia and desmoids carcinoma. Even in the most cachexic patient, a 40-mL pump is usually tolerated. It may be placed subfascial if concern is present for pressure necrosis or pump extrusion.

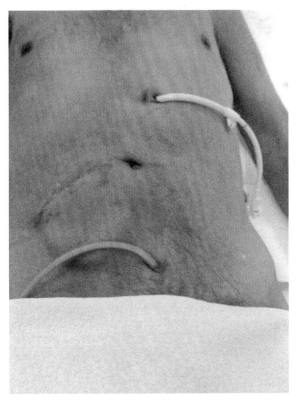

Fig. 19-4 Patient with suprapubic and gastrojejunal tubes.

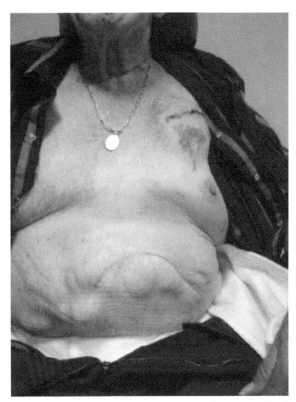

Fig. 19-5 Patient with pump implanted in the pectoral region.

nutritional intake, particularly protein intake, may improve wound healing in patients with cachexia. Also, when cleared by an oncologist, additional vitamin C supplements with zinc may improve healing, but specific supplementation in the patients with cachexia has not been defined and is controversial.[7,8] In protein-depleted patients, persistent pump pocket seromas may become problematic.

In patients with a large pannus or anasarca, the pump may be placed in the flank or over the ribs. This allows easy access for refills without patient or tissue manipulation. Likewise, patients with ostomies, fistulas, or abdominal wall tumors must be assessed for the best pump location before implantation. It is a good idea to discuss pump placement location with the patient and family before the procedure (**Fig. 19-4**). Some patients lack adequate fascia and muscular tissue secondary to multiple procedures or tumors and need to have the provider consider alternative locations. In the patient shown in **Fig. 19-5**, a large abdominal hernia caused excessive pressure on the pump, resulting in a femoral neuritis. When the pump was moved laterally over the ribs, the wound dehisced from external pressure while the patient was operating his wheelchair. The pectoralis site was discussed with the patient and his caregiver as the most rational choice for final pump placement. Here, it is easily accessed by providers, is comfortable for the patient, and does not limit motility or self-care.

Complications of Intrathecal Drug Delivery System Pump Implantation

Complications of pump system implantation can be divided into early and late complications.

Early Complications

Early complications include PDPH, infection, wound seroma formation, and bleeding at the spinal site or at the pump site. PDPHs occur in 10% of pump implantation surgeries. Conservative treatment with fluids, caffeine, antiemetics, and oral opioids usually allows the patient to recover without any intervention. With patients in whom severe nausea and vomiting occurs and conservative treatment has failed, an epidural blood patch may be indicated.[9]

Infections are related to breakage in sterile technique, predisposing clinical conditions of the patient, and poor wound healing. Patients with superficial infections typically respond to appropriate antibiotic therapy. In patients with pump pocket or spine incision infections, the device should be explanted and intravenous (IV) antibiotics given until culture and sensitivities have been obtained.

The diagnosis of aseptic or viral meningitis in the cancer patient with an IT catheter or pump should not cause alarm. Supportive care and neurological monitoring should be provided until symptoms resolve, but the pump and catheter do not need to be removed. In cases of bacterial meningitis, risk stratification, pain assessment, and life expectancy need to be considered. Removal of the pump and catheter is recommended[7] but may be undesirable because of potential uncontrolled pain. IV antibiotics should be initiated immediately, with more specific treatment prescribed after obtaining spinal bacterial cultures and susceptibilities. If the life expectancy of the patient is lengthy, the physician should proceed with pump and catheter removal after discussing it with the patient and family. After explantation, the patient should be monitored for signs of withdrawal and hospitalized until the danger of seizures has passed and pain is controlled. The system may be reimplanted after a course of antibiotics has been administered and the patient has been cleared for surgery by the infectious disease team. In terminal patients with vancomycin-sensitive *Staphylococcus* who refuse pump removal, IT vancomycin may be administered at 10 mg/day. Other published data demonstrate that IV vancomycin combined with epidural vancomycin (150 mg/day for 3 weeks) resolved infection.[4]

Seroma development in the pump pocket is a common early complication of implantation. Risk can be minimized with reduction in pump pocket size, strict adherence to abdominal binder placement, and improvement of nutritional status. Persistent seromas should be aspirated and sent for culture to rule out infection. If the fluid is clear and colorless, the system should be checked for leaks or catheter dislodgement. Clear, colorless fluid is usually CSF. Persistent noninfected seromas may be treated with tetracycline. One gram diluted into 30 mL of 0.5% bupivacaine is injected into the pump pocket after draining the seroma. Bupivacaine is used to minimize the burning from the caustic tetracycline. An abdominal binder is then placed over the pump, and the patient wears the binder for 72 hours. If the seroma reoccurs, the wounds should be explored for a leak or an infection.

Bleeding at the spine or pump site can be disastrous. Any acute change in neurological function in the immediate postoperative period needs to be assessed and examined radiographically with a computed tomography (CT) scan and coagulation studies. Patients with lumbar spine superficial bleeds typically respond to pressure dressings. Persistent bleeding into the pump pocket may be secondary to anticoagulation or perforating arteriole or venous vessels. If the patient does not respond to pressure dressings, the wound will need to be explored to evaluate the cause of bleeding.

Late Complications

Late complications of pump implantation include pump malposition, catheter malposition, pump pressure dehiscence as a complication of cachexia, and inflammatory mass formation.

Pump malposition occurs when the sutures anchoring the pump have been broken. This typically occurs after increased abdominal wall contractions such as with coughing or vomiting in the first few weeks after implantation. These pumps may not have anchored firmly to the fascia, and with added contracture of the abdominal muscles against the sharp welds of the catheter loops, the anchoring sutures break. Instructing patients to wear a tight abdominal binder or double looping suture through the suture loops may help to decrease the incidence of pumps from becoming dislodged. Some patients play with the pump in the pocket, which loosens the pump from the wall. This is also known as "pump fiddler's syndrome." If this is suspected, a Silastic sleeve may be placed on the pump and the pump anchored both inferiorly and superiorly.

Pump pressure dehiscence occurs as a complication of severe cachexia. After pump implantation, the patient continues to lose weight, and lack of postoperative healing with adequate pump capsule formation combined with fat necrosis of the anterior wall can lead to this problem. Care should be taken to place the pump in the area where the greatest percentage of adipose tissue lies under the skin. The pocket should be made small but not so tight as to place excessive pressure on the overlying skin in the first few postoperative weeks.

Development of an inflammatory mass at the catheter tip can occur at any time after pump implantation. The provider needs to be diligent during the physical examination and question any subtle findings. MRI or CT myelography can differentiate inflammatory mass formation from progression of disease. Either way, early detection is key. An inflammatory mass is thought to be the result of high concentrations of medication in a relative low-flow state. Added to this may be the high pH of compounded drugs. Drug concentrations should be kept as low as reasonably possible to help avoid these devastating complications. Late detection may result in permanent neurological injury and paralysis.

Intrathecal Drug Delivery Management Considerations

Pain secondary to malignancy may be neuropathic, somatic, sympathetic, or mixed pain. Patients with neuropathic pain only may respond to single-agent ziconotide, clonidine, or bupivacaine. Patients with somatic pain may be treated with opioids as a single agent. For patients with neuropathic or mixed pain pathologies, IT opioids alone may not be sufficient, and treatment may require a nonopioid medication (e.g., a local anesthetic, antispasmodic, or nonopioid pain medication) added to the spinally delivered opioid.

Because spinal drug infusion delivers drugs directly to the IT space, patients with nociceptive, neuropathic, or mixed pain syndromes and who have failed to respond to more conservative therapies may respond to IT therapy. Patients with postlaminectomy surgery syndrome, CRPS, intractable abdominal pain, diffuse cancer pain, or osteoporotic compression fractures have received benefit from this form of therapy.[2]

Only three agents have been approved by the FDA for IT use: morphine sulfate, ziconotide, and baclofen. Many other agents are routinely used intrathecally whose efficacy has been supported in the literature. A team of experts meets regularly to review and publish consensus guidelines for the use of both FDA-approved and off-label agents. A secondary subcommittee also makes recommendations for the use of agents to manage malignant pain. In 2007, the Polyanalgesic Consensus Conference (PACC) recommended the algorithm for IT medication shown in **Box 19-2**.

For patients with malignant pain, the Polyanalgesic Consensus Guidelines for Malignant Pain were established (**Box 19-3**). Its recommendations centered around survivorship of the patient. If the patient is expected to live longer than 1 year, the PACC 2007 guidelines were to be followed. Because end-of-life issues include escalating pain that may require more rapid dose escalation and more complex polyanalgesia as well as the need to maintain quality of life, the panel agreed that the revised management algorithm needed to allow more flexibility and more aggressive therapy for patients whom were not expected to live longer than 1 year. If in this group, a patient's functional status improves and response to chemotherapy is noted, the patient's medication regimen should be adjusted to the more conservative PACC 2007 guidelines.

Medication Titration

Titration of multiple medications in an IT infusion is usually based on one of the component drugs. For simplicity, this drug is usually the opioid or local anesthetic in the solution because these medications tend to have the greatest side effects when titrated too aggressively. Other component medications are compounded with dosage safety margins and target effect in mind. Individual responses to

First line: Morphine or hydromorphone or ziconotide
Second line: Fentanyl or morphine/hydromorphone + ziconotide or morphine/hydromorphone + bupivacaine/clonidine
Third line: Clonidine or morphine/hydromorphone/fentanyl + bupivacaine and/or clonidine + ziconotide
Fourth line: Sufentanil or sufentanil + bupivacaine and/or clonidine + ziconotide
Fifth line: Midazolam, meperidine, or ketorolac (little safety information; use as a last resort with informed consent)
Sixth line: Gabapentin, octreotide, conopeptides, neostigmine, XEN2174, AM336, CGX1160 (experimental only)

In addition, the panel recommended maximum concentrations as follows:

- Morphine 20 mg/mL
- Hydromorphone 10 mg/mL
- Fentanyl 2000 µg/mL
- Sufentanil 50 µg/mL
- Bupivacaine 40 mg/mL
- Clonidine 2000 µg/mL
- Ziconotide 100 µg/mL

First line: Morphine/hydromorphone monotherapy or morphine/hydromorphone + bupivacaine or bupivacaine monotherapy or ziconotide (After the FDA approval of ziconotide, it was added to the first-line recommendations for neuropathic pain when appropriate. The need for rapid titration and side effect profile should be assessed.)
Second line: Morphine/hydromorphone/fentanyl/sufentanil + bupivacaine + clonidine or morphine/hydromorphone/fentanyl/sufentanil + bupivacaine
Third line: Opiate + more than two adjuvants or opiate + bupivacaine + clonidine or baclofen for spasticity, myoclonus, neuropathic pain, or second opiate (hydrophilic/lipophilic) as adjuvant
Fourth line: Opiate + more than three adjuvants or opiate + second line adjuvants + droperidol or midazolam or ketamine (*neurotoxic*) (The addition of droperidol for intractable nausea and vomiting was recommended at any line. Ketamine should be used only in terminal care or as last resort because of neurotoxicity to the spinal cord.)

Later additions recommending opioid dosing as low as possible to avoid hyperalgesia.

each medication should be anticipated and often take precedence in titration tolerance. As in oral titration regimens, some patients need slow titration because tolerance develops to side effects. Infusion titration recommendations for implantable and external methods are described as follows. Titration should be guided according to a patient's pain level as determined by the Visual Analog Scale (VAS) and according to functional status.

If VAS scores are 2 to 4, the dose of an implanted device may be increased by 10% to 25% over 3 to 4 days. With externalized systems, dose rate may be increased 10% to 25% per hour per day until pain relief is satisfactory.

If VAS scores are 5 to 6, dose rates of implanted devices can be increased by 25% to 50% daily, and a therapeutic bolus dose should be considered. If local anesthetic is present in the solution, multiple small boluses should be used until pain relief is achieved to avoid motor blockade. With external systems, hourly rates should be adjusted 35% to 50% twice daily until pain relief is achieved.

Patients with VAS scores of 7 to 10 may require inpatient hospitalization, hospice, or equivalent care for treatment of pain crises. The panel recognizes that many patients desire to remain in the home environment. These patients may require a 50% to 100% rate increase in the external or implanted system. Therapeutic boluses should be administered until pain relief is achieved, with subsequent daily medication adjustments until pain relief is sustained. These significant rate increases may result in problematic drug toxicities in the initial 12 hours after the adjustment, and clinicians should be available to manage acute effects.

In patients whose pain is stable, IT medication combinations are limited to first- and second-line therapies. As the complexity of pain progresses, movement through the algorithm results in more complex combinations to achieve pain relief. Rotation between opiates alone may improve pain or the combination of a lipophilic opioid (fentanyl) to a hydrophilic opioid (morphine or hydromorphone [Dilaudid]) may be necessary to control some painful syndromes. Adjuvant medications are added according to minimal dosage guidelines to prevent toxicities and are titrated to effect. Baclofen and clonidine are typically started at a dosage of 25 µg/day. The initial dosage should be reduced to 10 µg/day in hemodynamically fragile patients. Concentrations of all medications in the polyanalgesic mix are altered to provide maximal time between pump refills, with safe pump rate increases for uncontrolled pain.

If a medication is not beneficial or causes adverse effects in a particular patient, it should be weaned appropriately or the caregiver and patient should be informed of likely withdrawal symptoms and arrange for outpatient interventions. Acute discontinuation of baclofen or clonidine may result in hemodynamic instability, seizures, or death. To avoid these complications, physicians should institute oral or transdermal replacement therapy on discontinuation of IT medications and provide an appropriate weaning schedule.

Cancer patients with complex pain may require several polyanalgesic combinations until satisfactory relief is achieved with minimal side effects. Medication regimens may need to be reformulated after two unsuccessful attempts to improve response with aggressive dosage adjustments. Medications should be selected to target specific receptor responses and pain syndromes. Local anesthetics are important in initial therapy until adjuvant medications reach therapeutic levels with minimal side effects, after which local anesthetic doses may be reduced to limit effects such as weakness, urinary retention, and hypotension.

Side Effect Management
Management of potential side effects of IT therapy is similar to that of oral therapies. Opioid-induced nausea is managed with traditional antiemetics, opioid rotation, or administration of droperidol intrathecally at 0.5 to 1.0 µg/kg/day. Constipation is typically managed with stimulant or bulk laxatives, stool softeners, and methylnaltrexone subcutaneously every other day. Urinary retention is treated with 10 to 50 mg of oral bethanechol four times daily. Medication doses may need to be modified in cases of persistent urinary retention not responsive to bethanechol. For cases in

which edema develops or escalates after initiation of IT therapy, opioids can be rotated or doses reduced and adjuvant medications adjusted to achieve pain control. Initiation of loop or potassium-sparing diuretics may be helpful. In most cases, edema secondary to opioid therapy resolves on its own with conservative treatment. Patients with lymphedema may benefit from fluid mobilization therapy.

Patients taking high-dose oral and IT opioids should be evaluated for effects of respiratory depression. In this patient population, a small change in the carbon dioxide curve may shift a patient into unconsciousness. When appropriate, patients should undergo formal sleep evaluations to determine the effect of treatment regimens on respiratory depression.

Patients with chronic disease have hormonal dysfunction as a consequence of the disease. High-dose long-term opioids worsen hormonal dysfunction. Hypogonadism in this population worsens negative nitrogen balance and weight loss, depression, osteoporosis, and weakness. These patients may become more prone to pathological fractures even in the face of bisphosphonates secondary to poor osteoblastic function.

Breakthrough Pain

Breakthrough pain may originate from a source different from that of background pain and requires immediate assessment. Oral immediate-release opioids should be provided for rescue; patients should also have a small amount of a benzodiazepine on hand for treatment of acute anxiety related to severe pain onset until an IT dose titration can be provided.

Personal Therapy Manager

The Personal Therapy Manager (PTM) is a handheld device used to deliver physician-programmed boluses with the SynchroMed II infusion system. It is helpful for controlling breakthrough pain without additional oral medications. This device is similar to the demand dose with patient-controlled analgesia. The clinician sets the parameters for the bolus amount, the lockout period, and the number of allowed boluses per day. This device allows patients to become more actively involved in their therapy, in which unpredictable increases in their pain can be treated with additional doses of medication through the pump. Opiate dosing is similar to oral rescue dosing at 10% to 25% of the daily dose. The rate of bolus delivery depends on the physician's desire to increase spread or control spread of the medication in the IT space. The bolus delivery rate also depends on the infusate and the catheter-tip position. Bolusing bupivacaine or clonidine too rapidly can have devastating effects. In the author's clinic, clonidine boluses are limited to 10 to 25 μg with a 5-minute lockout, and bupivacaine boluses are limited to a 0.5- to 1-mg bolus over a 5-minute period. The first therapeutic bolus is given in the office before instituting the PTM. The patient is monitored for 30 minutes after the bolus. The type of pain and patient dysfunction determine the frequency of boluses. End-stage cancer patients may be allowed to bolus every hour to limit need for frequent reprogramming at the end of life, and long-term survivors with malignant pain are typically limited to four boluses in a 24-hour period. Patients with ziconotide should not use the PTM because of neurological sequelae of bolus dosing with this medication unless the clinician has monitored the patient's response to boluses directly. The use of the PTM improves patient's satisfaction of therapy by allowing the freedom to control pain without the side effects of oral medications. The PTM is also beneficial because it allows the patient to ensure that the pump automatically resumed infusing medication after the temporary interruption of

pump rotor function because of the magnetic field. If the pump motor does not return to normal function, the screen of the PTM will display a symbol indicating that the patient should contact the provider.

Overall, when programming the PTM, thought should be given to short- and long-term side effects of all the medications in the admixture. Short-term sequelae to be considered are hypotension and paralysis. Long-term sequelae to be considered are weakness, sedation, respiratory depression, and mental status changes.

Troubleshooting Intrathecal Drug Delivery Systems

Patients with indwelling IDDS may present to the pain clinic with loss of pain relief, acute or worsening neurological deficits, withdrawal symptoms, or decreased mental status. The patient should be seen with a complete history and physical examination. Available family members should be consulted for accuracy of time course of events. Physical examination findings should be compared with those from previous visits.

Loss of Pain Control

Loss of pain control may occur secondary to disease progression, hyperalgesia secondary to opioid escalation, catheter migration, catheter kinking or dislodgement, or pump malfunction. If no signs of withdrawal are present, a simple anteroposterior (AP) spine radiograph may be used to determine if the catheter has migrated or become dislodged. If the patient has signs of withdrawal or progressive neurological decline, an urgent workup is warranted. An AP spine radiograph should be used to locate the catheter tip. Then an MRI with contrast should be performed if there no contraindications, looking both at the catheter tip and the area of neurological changes on physical examination. If the patient is unable to have an MRI, CT myelography should be performed. These tests will identify spinal cord–compressing lesions, an inflammatory mass at the catheter tip, or tumors that may be compressing the catheter (**Fig. 19-6**). When indicated, the patient should be brought to the operating room for device revision as soon as possible. If no problems are found with the system or the spinal canal and hyperalgesia of opioids is suspect, opioid rotation or aggressive opioid weaning should be performed. The patient's pain may be treated with both oral and IT adjuvant medications.

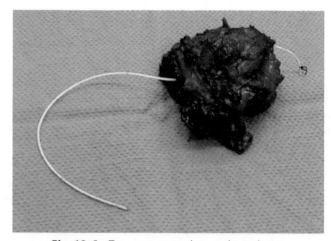

Fig. 19-6 Tumor compressing on the catheter.

Medication-Related Complications

Medication related complications involve programming errors, drug compounding errors, and technician errors.

Programming errors include medication concentration recording errors, dosage errors, and bridge bolusing errors. Vigilance must be taken to ensure that the correct medication is infused into the pump and entered into the programmer with the correct concentration. After reprogramming, it is recommended that a second individual review the telemetry against the prescription and drug invoice before the patient leaves the clinic. Failure to do so may result in patient overdose or death. Use of the current programmers and the SynchroMed II, bridge bolusing is calculated by the programmer software. When switching medication concentrations, the patient should be informed about when the new medication will arrive at the catheter tip. If the patient feels any different before that time, the clinician should be notified immediately.

The United States Pharmacopoeia and the American Society of Health System Pharmacists have issued statements on the preparation of sterile products that have clinical, legal, and practical significance. Physicians who use compounded products for IT therapy should only use pharmacies that follow these guidelines. The physician should have a strong working relationship with the compounding pharmacist because compounding errors could result in withdrawal symptoms, overdose, and death.

When the therapy seems to be producing adverse effects or lack of efficacy, the physician needs to have a systematic approach to problem solve the therapeutic options. If the patient no longer seems to be getting therapeutic benefit from a previously stable treatment dose of medication, evaluation needs to consider progression of disease, catheter problems, and pump malfunctions. CT scans, CT myelograms, and MRIs of the spine may help to diagnose changes in the patient's underlying condition. If these results are negative for changes in disease state or if they are positive and additional modalities such as pain blocks are ineffective, the clinician should progress to system evaluation. If the system checks out without problems, then drug should be aspirated from the reservoir and sent for analysis. Compounding errors and dilution or replacement of pump medication by the patient may be demonstrated with analysis.

Technician errors may occur with pump refills. The technician may mistake the scar tissue capsule for the port and inject the infusate into the pump pocket. Some pockets have a small chronic seroma that is slightly yellow in color similar to compounded drug on withdrawal from the pump reservoir. When the correct amount is withdrawn, the technician injects the infusate into the pump pocket. This mistake can result in vascular instability, respiratory depression, and death with complex pump formulas that include clonidine or in an opioid-naïve patient.

If a needle smaller than the recommended 22-gauge noncoring needle is used to access the port, the side port may be accidentally accessed. This results in direct CSF injection of the medication and will likely result in death if not recognized within seconds of the injection. If the side port is accessed to clear the drug from the catheter tubing, at least 1 mL of CSF should be withdrawn before pump bolusing under slow constant pressure. Accurate calculations are mandatory in pump tubing volume and catheter volume if the technician desires to clear the pump system of old drug. As many as three separate catheter aspirations and subsequent catheter bolusings may be needed to clear the pump tubing of old medication. Patients suspected in receiving a drug overdose from a programming error, pump pocket infusion, or side port injection should be admitted to a hospital and possibly an intensive care unit for observation for a minimum of 24 hours.

Pump Motor Stalls

Pump motor stalls occur infrequently but may result in loss of pain relief, withdrawal symptoms, or seizures. If the patient is experiencing therapy failure or increased pain, the pump should be interrogated and the event logs examined. If the logs do not point to an electronic or battery problem, a rotor study should be conducted. Under fluoroscopy, a small bolus is given to the patient. The pump is monitored for 45 seconds. The rotors should change configuration during the bolus. In the SynchroMed II, apertures will appear to open and close with the movement of the rotors. If the patient has normal pump rotor study results, then the pump reservoir should be drained to compare actual versus calculated volumes remaining. If pump volumes vary more than 20% of expected volume or if the event log has documented motor stalls, the device should be explanted and returned to the company for evaluation. If neither a discrepancy of volume nor motor stall on log examination are noted, the catheter should be examined for problems.

Conclusion

IT drug delivery is an attractive option for pain management in patients with refractory cancer pain as well as analgesic-related toxicities. Patients who are intolerant of oral opioids or concerned about dependence or addiction may be receptive to intraspinal therapy. Additionally, cancer patients receiving highly toxic chemotherapy regimens may benefit from IDDS because of the lower risk of additive adverse effects compared with conventional pain treatments. In patients with visceral tumors or autonomic dysfunction that results in gut dysmotility, anorexia, early satiety, and nausea, IDDS improves gut function through chemical sympatholysis.[2] In a study by Smith et al,[4] drug toxicity and fatigue were significantly reduced in the IDDS group, but the conventional medical management (CMM) group had a significantly higher rate of depressed level of consciousness versus the IDDS group. Perhaps most importantly, the Kaplan-Meier survival curves estimated a 53.9% survival rate at 6 months for the IDDS group compared with 37.2% for the CMM group. Although it is impossible to draw any definitive conclusions from the survival rate analysis, it does seem to correlate that more effective pain management with minimal side effects may lead to increased survival in patients and a sustained "will to live."

References

1. Fortner BV, et al: Description and predictors of direct and indirect costs of pain reported by cancer patients. *J Pain Symptom Manage* 25(1):9-18, 2003.
2. Smith TJ, Staats PS, Deer T, et al: Randomized clinical trial of an implantable drug delivery system compared with comprehensive medical management for refractory cancer pain: impact of pain, drug-related toxicity, and survival. *J Clin Oncol* 20(19):4040-4049, 2002.
3. The cost of dying: end of life care, *CBS 60 Minutes*, accessed February 17, 2001, from http://www.cbsnews.com/stories/2010/08/05/60minutes/main6747002.shtml.
4. Stearns L, Boortz-Marx R, Du Pen S, et al: Intrathecal drug delivery for the management of cancer pain: a multidisciplinary consensus of best clinical practices. *J Support Oncol* 3(6):399-408, 2005.

5. Follett KA, Boortz-Marx RL, Drake JM, et al: Prevention and management of intrathecal drug delivery and spinal cord stimulation infections. *Anesthesiology* 100:1582-1594, 2004.

6. Flack SH, Anderson CM, Bernards C: Morphine distribution in the spinal cord after chronic infusion in pigs. *Anesth Analg* 112:460-464, 2011.

7. Gray D, Cooper P: Nutrition and wound healing: what is the link? *J Wound Care* 10(3):86-89, 2001.

8. Jamshed N, Schneider E: Is the use of supplemental vitamin C and zinc for the prevention and treatment of pressure ulcers evidence-based? *Annals of Long-Term Care* 28-32, 2010.

9. Du Pen SL: Complications of neuraxial infusion in cancer patients. *Oncology* 13(suppl 2):45-51, 1999.

IV Intrathecal Drug Delivery Systems for Spasticity

Chapter 20 Intrathecal Baclofen Trialing

Chapter 21 Baclofen Pump Management

20 Intrathecal Baclofen Trialing

Michael Saulino

CHAPTER OVERVIEW

Chapter Synopsis: Although intrathecal drug delivery systems (IDDS) are most often used to treat chronic pain, they can also be used for spasticity. Rather than analgesic drugs, therapy for spinal spasticity requires intrathecal baclofen (ITB) therapy. Spasticity can take on many forms, with muscle hypertonia usually resulting from some form of central nervous system damage. Delivery of the γ-aminobutyric acid agonist directly to receptors in the spinal cord can reduce this aberrant muscle contraction. Patients that might have the malady (and thereby may benefit from ITB) include those with cerebral palsy, multiple sclerosis, spinal cord or brain injury, or neurodegenerative diseases. *Spasticity* or *muscle overactivity* may in fact refer to a collection of positive symptoms that may need special attention to detect and classify, each of which can be influenced by other factors. Not surprisingly, patient selection and education remain key factors in success of ITB, much like other IDDS procedures. Certain procedural details require special consideration in patients with spasticity as well.

Important Points:
- Spasticity has diverse clinical presentations.
- Each intervention for spasticity, including IT therapy, has specific advantages and disadvantages.
- Before committing a patient to chronic ITB therapy, a trial exposure of ITB should be undertaken.
- Trialing centers should create an environment in which neuromuscular and functional changes, as well as adverse effects, can be observed and managed.

Clinical Pearls:
- Review patient's experience with previous interventions for spasticity management.
- Educate patients, family, and caregivers on the advantages and disadvantages of intrathecal baclofen therapy.
- Consider a functional assessment before and during an intrathecal baclofen trial.
- Manage long-term expectations for intrathecal baclofen therapy.
- Prepare patients, family, and caregivers for implant and chronic maintenance therapy.

Clinical Pitfalls:
Failure to:
- Implement protocols to manage adverse events including prolonged effects of an intrathecal baclofen bolus.
- Consider effects that intrathecal baclofen might have on other neurologic co-morbidities such as neurogenic bladder, seizures, hydrocephalus, etc.
- Coordinate results of screening trial relative to planned starting dose of permanent infusion (i.e., clear communication between trialing clinician and implanting surgeon).
- Recognize the complex relationship between spasticity and pain.
- Acknowledge limitations of intrathecal baclofen therapy.

Introduction

Intrathecal baclofen (ITB) therapy is a powerful technique for management of spastic hypertonia, a condition that is frequently observed after injury to the central nervous system (CNS). Similar to intrathecal (IT) therapy for pain control, ITB infusion exerts its therapeutic effect by delivering baclofen directly into the cerebrospinal fluid (CSF), thus affording enhanced distribution of this agent to target neurons in the spinal cord. IT administration of baclofen is typically undertaken through use of an externally programmable or surgically implanted pump, delivering drug at precise flow rates via a catheter placed in the spinal canal. Patients with a wide variety of CNS pathology, including cerebral palsy, spinal cord injury, multiple sclerosis, and acquired brain injury in both adult and pediatric populations, have achieved therapeutic benefit from this treatment strategy.[1] This chapter reviews the nature of spasticity; techniques for spasticity management; patient selection for ITB; and procedural details, assessments, measures, and adverse event management of ITB trials.

Defining Muscle Overactivity

CNS pathology often creates a constellation of signs or symptoms that encompasses both positive and negative components. Weakness and loss of dexterity, the most commonly encountered negative phenomena, are relatively easy to define. The positive components are more complex with diverse pathophysiological mechanisms. Observable phenomena include increased resistance to passive stretch, muscle–tendon hyperreflexia, clonus, co-contraction of synergistic muscle groups, and spontaneous flexor and extensor spasms (**Box 20-1**). Spasticity is only one of these features, namely a velocity-dependent increase in resistance to passive range of motion (ROM). Collectively, all positive signs can be called "muscle overactivity" with the recognition that abnormal pathology extends beyond the muscle itself. Frequently, and perhaps unfortunately, the term *spasticity* is often applied to the entire collection of signs. Given this common practice, the terms *spasticity* and *muscle overactivity* will be used somewhat interchangeably in this and the subsequent chapter.[2,3]

The clinical presentation of muscle overactivity is quite diverse because of the various categories of CNS disease. One distinction is the number of muscle groups involved. Diffuse patterns of spasticity can involve all four limbs (quadriplegic), both lower extremities (paraplegic or diplegic), or the upper and lower extremities on the same side of the body (hemiplegic). Combinations of these patterns can also be seen (e.g., paraplegic and hemiplegic) in the same patient. The axial musculature can similarly be involved. Alternatively, a more localized appearance that involves only a few muscles or muscle groups can be detected. Mixtures of focal and diffuse patterns can also be recorded in the same patient. Flexion (the movement of a limb to decrease the angle of a joint), extension (the opposite movement) or combined flexion and extension synergies can be observed. Spasticity can also be graded on severity (mild, moderate, and severe) by both objective and subjective measures. Assessment measures are discussed shortly. Clinicians must exert some degree of caution when applying severity descriptors to muscle overactivity so as not to misrepresent their clinical impact on the patient. Relatively slight resistance to passive motion, which could be evaluated as mild to the physician, may have a quite significant functional impact to the patient, who could describe the same phenomena as severe.[3]

Spasticity can be both beneficial and deleterious. Advantageous effects of spasticity potentially include assistance with mobility, maintenance of posture, improvement of vascular circulation, preservation of muscle mass and bone mineral density, prevention of venous thrombosis, and assistance in reflexive bowel and bladder function. Conversely, spasticity can also interfere with positioning, mobility, comfort, and hygiene. Spasticity has also been linked to increased metabolic demands, which can be problematic in nutritionally compromised patients. Spontaneous spasms can interfere with sleep or duration of wheelchair use. Spasms can also lead to skin breakdown because of shearing effect or impaired healing of surgical wounds because of tension along suture lines.[4] The relationship of spasticity to pain is complex. Spasticity can limit the ROM about a joint and result in musculoskeletal pain. A reduction of spasticity may reduce the pain associated with biomechanical pain. However, CNS disease can also produce neuropathic pain. Modulation of spasticity may not be effective in reducing neuropathic pain.[5,6] Clinicians who care for patients with spasticity must consider all aspects of a patient's spasticity before embarking on a treatment plan. The goal may not be complete elimination of spasticity but rather titration to maximize the risk-to-benefit ratio.

Techniques for Spasticity Management

Given the diversity of spasticity presentations and the variety of diseases that create spasticity, it is not unexpected there are a multiplicity of treatment options. These modalities can be divided into nonpharmacological, oral medications, chemodenervation techniques, IT therapy, orthopedic surgical techniques, and neurosurgical interventions.[7-13] A detailed review of each of these modalities is beyond the scope of this chapter. **Table 20-1** summarizes the nature of each intervention with their associated advantages and disadvantages. How each of these techniques is applied to each patient population is an evolving art and science. Some practitioners have advocated a sequential approach to hypertonia (**Fig. 20-1**). In this algorithm, ITB is reserved until nonpharmacological, oral medications, and chemodenervation have been attempted and proved either unsuccessful or intolerable. Graham and colleagues[14] used a matrix configuration to describe the various characteristics of spasticity interventions, contrasting reversible versus irreversible options and focal versus global effects (**Fig. 20-2**). In this model, each modality is used in a rather individualistic fashion. In this paradigm, ITB is considered reversible (neural structures are not surgically altered, and rate of dose administration is adjustable) and global (CNS effects of ITB distribution are typically observed in all extremities and the trunk). An alternative model applies possible modalities in combination depending on individual patient characteristics (**Fig. 20-3**). The role of ITB therapy with this schema is to potentially combine this technique with other modalities for synergistic therapeutic effects.[9] Physical techniques such as stretching, strengthening, bracing, and gait retraining are essential for attaining maximal functional benefit that may follow tone reduction. Patients might continue to use oral spasticity agents for a variety of reasons, including ongoing ITB titration, "breakthrough" spasms, an irregular spasticity pattern, disease progression, or residual upper extremity tone. Combining ITB therapy and neurolytic procedures is appropriate for patients manifesting both focal dystonic features and global hypertonicity or residual upper extremity hypertonia.[15,16] The indications for combining neuro-orthopedic procedures and ITB therapy include correction of fixed deformities in the presence of ongoing spastic hypertonia.[10] Concomitant use of orthopedic surgery and ITB in children with cerebral palsy may reduce the need for subsequent orthopedic surgery.[17] In summary, the role of ITB within the armamentarium of spasticity modification continues to evolve and define itself.

Patient Selection for Intrathecal Baclofen Therapy

Patient selection and education are fundamental concepts to all aspects of medical practice. These principles are of enhanced importance with interventional procedures involving implantable technology. Appropriate candidates need to be counseled before proceeding with this form of therapy. Patients should be apprised of all aspects of the therapy, including trialing, implantation, postoperative rehabilitation, and chronic maintenance issues. The recognition by the patient that this treatment modality represents a long-term commitment cannot be understated. In general, patients can be considered candidates for ITB therapy when:

- Spasticity is poorly controlled despite maximal therapy with other modalities.
- Spasticity is poorly controlled because of limited patient tolerance of other modalities.
- Adjustable spasticity reduction afforded by a programmable variable flow pump would be advantageous.

The diagnoses approved by the U.S. Food and Drug Administration (FDA) for ITB therapy include spasticity of spinal (traumatic spinal cord injury and multiple sclerosis) and cerebral origin (acquired brain injury, cerebral palsy, and stroke). There is greater

Table 20-1: Spasticity Interventions

Category	Intervention	Description	Advantages	Disadvantages
Nonpharmacological	Removal or avoidance of noxious stimuli	Treatment of neurogenic bladder, neurogenic bowel, decubitus ulcers, and so on	• Returns patient to baseline hypertonia • May eliminate ongoing stimuli • Relatively low cost • Minimal adverse effects	• May not be easily reversible • Modulation may not be predictable
	Manual stretching	Physical movement of involved limbs by caregivers	• Low cost • Minimal risk	• Short duration of effect
	Passive stretching	Bracing, splinting, serial casting	• Low cost • Minimal risk	• Potential for skin breakdown • Restricts patient movement
Oral medications	GABAergic agents α_2-Adrenergic agents Serotonin antagonists Peripherally-acting agents GABA analogues	Benzodiazepines (e.g., diazepam, lorazepam) Baclofen Clonidine Tizanidine Cyproheptadine Dantrolene Pregabalin Gabapentin	• Non-invasive • Low cost • Allows patient control • Global effectiveness • Secondary indications (e.g., sleep aide, pain)	• Potential poor patient tolerability • Weakness • Sedation • Hepatotoxicity
Chemodenervation	Motor point or nerve blocks Botulinum toxins	Local anesthetics Alcohol Phenol Botox Myobloc Dysport	• Excellent effect for focal hypertonia	• Multiple injections needed for global tone • Technical skill for localization • Cost • Need to repeat injections
IT therapy	GABAergic agents	Baclofen	• Highly potent • Affords precise delivery control	• Surgical procedure • Risk of overdose and withdrawal • Need for constant maintenance
Orthopedic surgery	Tendon lengthening Tendon transfers	Alter length–tension relationship Reduces efferent signaling from muscle spindles	• Corrects underlying deformity • Long duration of effect	• Invasive • Destructive • May require extensive motor control analysis
Neurosurgical	Rhizotomy Myelotomy	Ablation of involved spinal nerve roots (rhizotomy) or spinal cord (myelotomy)	• Long duration of effect	• Invasive • Destructive • Neuropathic pain

GABA, γ-aminobutyric acid; IT, intrathecal.

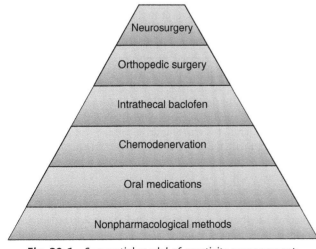

Fig. 20-1 Sequential model of spasticity management.

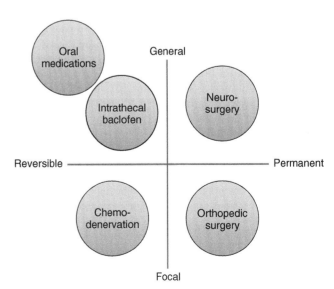

Fig. 20-2 Individualistic model of spasticity management.

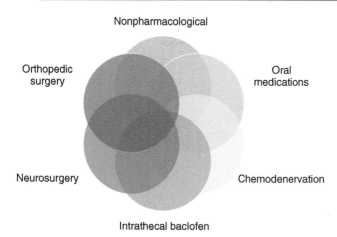

Fig. 20-3 Synergistic model of spasticity management.

experience with spasticity of spinal origin compared with cerebral origin because the former indications had earlier FDA approval. Other diseases, such as degenerative conditions of the brain and spinal cord (e.g., amyotrophic lateral sclerosis, hereditary spastic paraparesis) have also shown efficacy with ITB.[18-20]

Patients should be clinically stable, comprehend the advantages and disadvantages of ITB therapy, be able to return to clinic for titration and refills, and have demonstrated a positive response to a test dose of ITB. For individuals with cognitive impairment and in pediatric patients, caregivers must be involved in the medical decision making. Typically, a sufficient amount of time after a neurological insult should pass before considering IT therapy, allowing a reasonable amount of natural recovery to occur. For multiple sclerosis, in which the neurologic presentation may vary, patients should not be solely evaluated during an exacerbation. In severe cases, this therapy can be considered early in the post-injury recovery period (e.g., <12 months[21]). ITB therapy generally reduces lower limb hypertonia to a greater extent compared to the upper extremities. Perhaps more cephalad catheter tip placement can potentially improve upper limb effects,[22] although the upper limb response to this strategy is not uniform.[23] Other advantages of ITB therapy include higher potency with potentially less adverse effects compared with oral baclofen, the ability to have a global effect on all affected limbs, and the possibility of later adjustment with changing patient need or progressive disease. Disadvantages include surgical risks (bleeding, infection, damage of neural structures), the potential for serious adverse effects, including overdose and withdrawal, and the requirement for ongoing follow-up with health care professionals for dosing adjustments and pump refills. Ventricular shunting for hydrocephalus is not a contraindication to ITB therapy, but practitioners should be aware of potential interactions between the devices on CSF flow.[24] ITB can also be used in patients with seizures with the understanding that this therapy has been occasionally associated with a risk of increased seizures.[25-27] Similarly, prior abdominal or pelvic surgery (e.g., gastrostomy, suprapubic tube placement) that is relatively common in neurological patients does not represent a contraindication for IT pump placement but does require some consideration during surgical placement. Patients and caregivers should be fully apprised of these issues so they can make a sound decision in proceeding toward an IT trial.

Similar to IT therapy for chronic pain management, the purpose of performing an IT trial is to expose the patient to the potential agents that will be used on a more permanent basis. A trial allows the patient to temporarily experience the potential benefits (as well as deleterious effects) of the proposed IT agent and provides the clinician an opportunity to observe the effects and prepare potential management strategies for these effects. Although both subjective and objective measures of improvement can be measured for both pain and spasticity trials, it is of paramount importance to recognize that pain assessment is primarily subjective (i.e., rating of pain intensity), but spasticity evaluation can have a much more objective basis (e.g., changes in tone, ROM, strength). Clinicians must tailor their trialing protocols to represent this profound difference.

Procedural Details

The typical method for ITB trialing is to perform a lumbar puncture and inject a bolus of a baclofen solution into the CSF. The most commonly used initial screening dose of baclofen is 50 μg.[28,29] The onset of clinical effects from a screening bolus occurs within 1 to 3 hours after the injection, and peak effects are typically observed 4 to 6 hours after the injection. The effects of the screening bolus are always temporary with the effects routinely lasting 6 to 8 hours.[30,31] Prolonged effects of single-test bolus have been reported.[32] Screening boluses can be repeated if the initial injection is unsuccessful. It is a commonly accepted practice to wait at least 24 hours before repeating a trial to ensure that the patient's neuromuscular status has completely returned to baseline. "Positive" responses are reported in 80% to 90% of bolus trials.[28] Generally, antibiotic prophylaxis is not needed for a bolus trial.[33] For patients on antiplatelet or anticoagulant therapy, recommendations from the American Society of Regional Anesthesia are followed.[34] Fluoroscopic guidance can assist needle localization into the IT space because anatomical landmarks for lumbar puncture can be variable,[35] and low CSF flow is possible in this patient population.

An alternative method for conducting trials involves placement of a temporary IT catheter and monitoring patient response to a short-term continuous infusion of baclofen.[36] This technique is more commonly used for evaluating patients with chronic pain for IT therapy. The potential advantages of catheter ITB trials include (1) avoidance of sequential lumbar punctures, (2) presumably improved approximation of chronic post-implant IT infusion response compared with single bolus injections, (3) the ability to control catheter tip placement, and (4) the ability to adjust infusion rate while assessing favorable (and unfavorable) effects of ITB administration. The disadvantages of catheter trials include increased technical difficulty, increased need for observation, and increased risk of meningitis and structural damage. The technique for IT catheter placement is discussed in the next chapter. Fluoroscopic guidance is generally considered mandatory for catheter placement. Although antibiotic prophylaxis is usually not needed for bolus trials, it is unclear whether antibiotic prophylaxis is needed for short-duration IT catheter trials. Factors to consider include the duration of the trial, patient immunocompetency, and potential chronic bacterial colonization. Evidence suggests that trial duration is a key risk factor for development of infectious complications. Thus, the trial should last only as long as is required to indicate a potential benefit of chronic ITB therapy.[33,37] There is no consensus regarding the optimal method of anesthesia used for catheter placement. Local anesthesia potentially lowers the risk of inadvertent damage to neural structures. However, if excessive patient movement or severe anxiety is anticipated, deep sedation or general anesthesia may be warranted.[38] There is little evidence to suggest that catheter trials provide better long-term outcomes compared with bolus trials when used as predictors of post-implant response. Prospective data in the pain management literature suggest no difference in outcomes from either IT trial method.[39]

Definitions of "success" for screening trials vary. A liberal description of a successful trial might be any improvement in spasticity that suggests future benefit from chronic long-term infusion. The most commonly cited criterion for a successful ITB trial is a 2-point reduction on the Modified Ashworth Scale.[28] The nature of this scale is discussed below. Patients may also demonstrate improvement in joint ROM, both actively and passively. Sequential assessments every few hours are warranted to evaluate the onset, peak, and resolution of ITB effects. ITB trials can potentially differentiate ROM deficits attributable to severe spasticity, which are potentially reversible without surgery, from fixed contractures. Although these evaluation techniques are often useful for patients with hypertonia in resting positions, these assessments may be inadequate for prediction of ITB effect during active functional tasks. In these patients, excessive tone reduction may impede performance of activities such as transfers and walking. Observation of ambulation, transfers, posture, and wheelchair propulsion during the trial is thus warranted. Adjunctive objective evaluation techniques may be helpful and include neurophysiologic assessment[40] and instrumented gait analysis.[30] During a screening trial, some individuals may experience excessive spasticity reduction during the peak effect of the ITB bolus. This occurrence is not a contraindication for pump implantation because the chronic infusion system has the ability to modulate the dose and subsequent desired effect. If excessive or prolonged hypotonia is observed during a screening trial, a repeat trial at a lower dose or continuous trial may be warranted. Particular care should be paid to patients who demonstrate an improvement on "passive" measures of spasticity (thus qualifying for long-term infusion on the basis of trial "success") yet demonstrate functional worsening during the trial. Post-implant rehabilitation in this subset of patients is particularly important.

Some centers proceed directly to pump implantation without a screening trial. For stroke patients, two justifications have been proposed: (1) the increased risk of spinal hemorrhage while patients are on anticoagulation or antiplatelet therapy and (2) the risk of recurrent stroke if these agents are discontinued. This method reduces the ability to differentiate fixed contracture from spasticity before implantation. Although patients may still benefit,[41]

it should only be undertaken after a full discussion with the patient and caregiver regarding the risks and benefits of a "no trial" approach.

Assessment Measures

As acknowledged previously, hypertonia assessment can demonstrate a much more objective component compared with a chronic pain evaluation. This does not mean that tonal assessment is by any means straightforward. From a technical standpoint, spasticity levels can be affected by many factors, including temperature, emotional status, time of day, level of pain, body position, and the amount of prior stretching. Given this potential variability, interpretation of serial measurements can be problematic.

Hypertonia can be evaluated clinically using a number of well-established rating scales.[42] The most commonly used scales include the Ashworth,[43,44] Modified Ashworth,[45] and Tardieu Scales.[46,47] **Table 20-2** summarizes these scales. The inter- and intrarater reliability of these scales is generally considered fair to good with occasional reports of suboptimal consistency.[48,49] One potential criticism of the Ashworth and Modified Ashworth Scales is the inability to distinguish between the rheologic properties of the soft tissues and the neural contributions to hypertonia. The Tardieu Scale attempts to address the difficulty by measuring two angles, the angle (R1) at which resistance is first encountered with a quick muscle stretch, and the final angle (R2), which reflects the maximum range of movement with a slow muscle stretch. The difference between the two is claimed to represent the true amount of spasticity or spasticity angle. More sophisticated measures of hypertonia include neurophysiologic testing that attempts to quantify the muscle response to stretch (surface electromyographic activity, H-reflex response, the H-reflex standardized to the M-wave max, or the F-wave response) or instrumented measurements of stiffness and torque with accelerometers.[31,50] The Wartenberg pendulum score is calculated during the gravity-induced pendulum-like movement of the lower limb as the ratio of joint angles measured by goniometry or computerized video motion analysis.[51] Some subjective measures include patient assessment of spasm intensity or logs of spasm frequency. There is an inconsistent correlation between subjective report and objective measures of spasticity.[52]

	Table 20-2: Commonly Used Spasticity Rating Scales		
	Ashworth Scale	**Modified Ashworth Scale**	**Tardieu Scale**
0	No increase in muscle tone	No increase in muscle tone	No resistance to passive ROM
1	Slight increase in muscle tone manifested by a catch and release or by minimal resistance at the end of the ROM when the affected part is moved in flexion or extension	Slight increase in muscle tone manifested by a catch and release or by minimal resistance at the end of the ROM when the affected part is moved in flexion or extension	Slight resistance to passive ROM
1+		Slight increase in muscle tone manifested by a catch followed by minimal resistance throughout the remainder (less than half) of the ROM	
2	More marked increase in muscle tone through most of the ROM, but affected part(s) easily moved	More marked increase in muscle tone through most of the ROM, but affected part(s) easily moved	Catch followed by a release
3	Considerable increase in muscle tone; passive movement difficult	Considerable increase in muscle tone; passive movement difficult	Fatigable clonus (<10 sec)
4	Affected part(s) rigid in flexion or extension	Affected part(s) rigid in flexion or extension	Infatigable clonus (>10 sec)

ROM, range of motion.

Adverse Event Management

Adverse effects can occur during IT trialing. Spinal headache or post-lumbar puncture syndrome is a complication of an injection-related dural leak and is not a direct medication effect. Spinal headaches occur in up to 30% of patients undergoing lumbar punctures and vary in severity from mild to incapacitating. Headache typically worsens when the patient sits or stands up and decreases in the supine position. These headaches typically begin within 2 days but may be delayed for as long as 2 weeks. Spinal headaches can be accompanied by dizziness, neck or arm pain, cranial nerve palsies, tinnitus, nausea, and distorted vision. Spinal headaches are more common in younger women with a low body mass index and in people who have a headache history in general. The risk of spinal headaches increases with use of larger needles. The headache resolves spontaneously in the majority of patients. Supportive measures include bedrest, caffeine, and abdominal binders. Epidural blood patches are reserved for recalcitrant cases.[53] Other procedure-related complications include bacterial and aseptic meningitis. Adverse effects that are more likely related to a pharmacological effect include nausea and vomiting, urinary retention, hypotension, seizures, drowsiness and sedation, respiratory depression, and coma. Nausea and vomiting and drowsiness and sedation are the most common adverse effects observed during ITB trial with reported incidences of 2% to 3%.[28] Management of overdose events is discussed in Chapter 21.

Although the procedural component of the trial should take place in a setting where injection sterility is assured, a number of settings are suitable for monitoring the effects of the trial. Examples include outpatient clinics, ambulatory surgical centers, inpatient hospitals, and inpatient rehabilitation facilities. Furthermore, it is helpful to use practice protocols or pathways to facilitate consistent assessment of key trial response indicators and reduce the risk of complications. Sequential evaluations of tone, ROM, and strength are required. For patients who use spasticity to assist with functional mobility, similar sequential evaluations of posture, transfers, and gait should be undertaken. Protocols for management of adverse events, including spinal headache, bowel and bladder changes, seizures, and respiratory depression, should be in place. Because the effects of ITB trials are occasionally prolonged, the practice setting should have the capacity for extended observation. Many experienced practitioners of ITB therapy believe that inpatient rehabilitation facilities are an optimal site for trials because these locations offer the best ability to assess functional changes and potentially manage adverse effects.

References

1. Francisco GE, Saulino MF, Yablon SA, Turner M: Intrathecal baclofen therapy: an update. *PM R* (9):852-858, 2009.
2. Sheean G: The pathophysiology of spasticity. *Eur J Neurol* 9(suppl 1):3, 9, discussion 53-61, 2002.
3. Sheean G, McGuire JR: Spastic hypertonia and movement disorders: pathophysiology, clinical presentation, and quantification. *PM R* 1(9):827-833, 2009.
4. Satkunam LE: Rehabilitation medicine: 3. management of adult spasticity. *CMAJ* 169(11):1173-1179, 2003.
5. Ward AB, Kadies M: The management of pain in spasticity. *Disabil Rehabil* 24(8):443-453, 2002.
6. Slonimski M, Abram SE, Zuniga RE: Intrathecal baclofen in pain management. *Reg Anesth Pain Med* 29(3):269-276, 2004.
7. Elovic EP, Esquenazi A, Alter KE, et al: Chemodenervation and nerve blocks in the diagnosis and management of spasticity and muscle overactivity. *PM R* 1(9):842-851, 2009.
8. Watanabe TK: Role of oral medications in spasticity management. *PM R* 1(9):839-841, 2009.
9. Kunz KD, Ames SL, Saulino MF: Multimodality approach to spasticity management: how patients treated with intrathecal baclofen also utilize other spasticity interventions. *Am J Phys Med Rehabil* 88(suppl 3):S57, 2009.
10. Lynn AK, Turner M, Chambers HG: Surgical management of spasticity in persons with cerebral palsy. *PM R* 1(9):834-838, 2009.
11. Pasquier Y, Cahana A, Schnider A: Subdural catheter migration may lead to baclofen pump dysfunction. *Spinal Cord* 41(12):700-702, 2003.
12. Abbruzzese G: The medical management of spasticity. *Eur J Neurol* 9(suppl 1):30, 34, discussion 53-61, 2002.
13. Oppenheim WL: Selective posterior rhizotomy for spastic cerebral palsy. A review. *Clin Orthop Relat Res* (253):20-29, 1990.
14. Graham HK, Aoki KR, Autti-Ramo I, et al: Recommendations for the use of botulinum toxin type A in the management of cerebral palsy. *Gait Posture* 11(1):67-79, 2000.
15. Gill CE, Andrade EO, Blair CR, et al: Combined treatment with BTX-A and ITB for spasticity: case report. *Tenn Med* 100(10):41, 42, 44, 2007.
16. Santamato A, Panza F, Ranieri M, et al: Effect of intrathecal baclofen, botulinum toxin type A and a rehabilitation programme on locomotor function after spinal cord injury: a case report. *J Rehabil Med* 42(9):891-894, 2010.
17. Gerszten PC, Albright AL, Johnstone GF: Intrathecal baclofen infusion and subsequent orthopedic surgery in patients with spastic cerebral palsy. *J Neurosurg* 88(6):1009-1013, 1998.
18. Francisco GE, Yablon SA, Schiess MC, et al: Consensus panel guidelines for the use of intrathecal baclofen therapy in poststroke spastic hypertonia. *Top Stroke Rehabil* 13(4):74-85, 2006.
19. Sadiq SA, Wang GC: Long-term intrathecal baclofen therapy in ambulatory patients with spasticity. *J Neurol* 253(5):563-569, 2006.
20. Francisco GE: The role of intrathecal baclofen therapy in the upper motor neuron syndrome. *Eura Medicophys* 40(2):131-143, 2004.
21. Francisco GE, Hu MM, Boake C, Ivanhoe CB: Efficacy of early use of intrathecal baclofen therapy for treating spastic hypertonia due to acquired brain injury. *Brain Inj* 19(5):359-364, 2005.
22. Burns AS, Meythaler JM: Intrathecal baclofen in tetraplegia of spinal origin: efficacy for upper extremity hypertonia. *Spinal Cord* 39(8):413-419, 2001.
23. Sivakumar G, Yap Y, Tsegaye M, Vloeberghs M: Intrathecal baclofen therapy for spasticity of cerebral origin-does the position of the intrathecal catheter matter? *Childs Nerv Syst* 26(8):1097-1102, 2010.
24. Fulkerson DH, Boaz JC, Luerssen TG: Interaction of ventriculoperitoneal shunt and baclofen pump. *Childs Nerv Syst* 23(7):733-738, 2007.
25. Buonaguro V, Scelsa B, Curci D, et al: Epilepsy and intrathecal baclofen therapy in children with cerebral palsy. *Pediatr Neurol* 33(2):110-113, 2005.
26. Schuele SU, Kellinghaus C, Shook SJ, et al: Incidence of seizures in patients with multiple sclerosis treated with intrathecal baclofen. *Neurology* 64(6):1086-1087, 2005.
27. Solaro C: Incidence of seizures in patients with multiple sclerosis treated with intrathecal baclofen. *Neurology* 66(5):784, 785; author reply 784-785, 2006.
28. Stempien L, Tsai T: Intrathecal baclofen pump use for spasticity: a clinical survey. *Am J Phys Med Rehabil* 79(6):536-541, 2000.
29. Hoving MA, van Raak EP, Spincemaille GH, et al: Intrathecal baclofen in children with spastic cerebral palsy: A double-blind, randomized, placebo-controlled, dose-finding study. *Dev Med Child Neurol* 49(9):654-659, 2007.
30. Horn TS, Yablon SA, Stokic DS: Effect of intrathecal baclofen bolus injection on temporospatial gait characteristics in patients with acquired brain injury. *Arch Phys Med Rehabil* 86(6):1127-1133, 2005.
31. Stokic DS, Yablon SA, Hayes A: Comparison of clinical and neurophysiologic responses to intrathecal baclofen bolus administration in moderate-to-severe spasticity after acquired brain injury. *Arch Phys Med Rehabil* 86(9):1801-1806, 2005.
32. Baguley IJ, Bailey KM, Slewa-Younan S: Prolonged anti-spasticity effects of bolus intrathecal baclofen. *Brain Inj* 19(7):545-548, 2005.

33. Rathmell JP, Lake T, Ramundo MB: Infectious risks of chronic pain treatments: injection therapy, surgical implants, and intradiscal techniques. *Reg Anesth Pain Med* 31(4), 2006.

34. Horlocker TT, Wedel DJ, Benzon H, et al: Regional anesthesia in the anticoagulated patient: defining the risks (the second ASRA Consensus Conference on Neuraxial Anesthesia and Anticoagulation). *Reg Anesth Pain Med* 28(3), 2003.

35. Snider KT, Kribs JW, Snider EJ, et al: Reliability of Tuffier's line as an anatomic landmark. *Spine (Phila Pa 1976)* 33(6):E161-E165, 2008.

36. Bleyenheuft C, Filipetti P, Caldas C, Lejeune T: Experience with external pump trial prior to implantation for intrathecal baclofen in ambulatory patients with spastic cerebral palsy. *Neurophysiol Clin* 37(1):23-28, 2007.

37. Burgher AH, Barnett CF, Obray JB, Mauck WD: Introduction of infection control measures to reduce infection associated with implantable pain therapy devices. *Pain Pract* 7(3):279-284, 2007.

38. Staats PS: Complications of intrathecal therapy. *Pain Med* 9(suppl 1):S102-S107, 2008.

39. Deer T, Chapple I, Classen A, et al: Intrathecal drug delivery for treatment of chronic low back pain: report from the national outcomes registry for low back pain. *Pain Med* 5(1):6-13, 2004.

40. Yablon SA, Stokic DS: Neurophysiologic evaluation of spastic hypertonia: implications for management of the patient with the intrathecal baclofen pump. *Am J Phys Med Rehabil* 83(10 suppl):S10-S18, 2004.

41. Gwartz BL: Intrathecal baclofen for spasticity caused by thrombotic stroke. *Am J Phys Med Rehabil* 80(5):383-387, 2001.

42. Platz T, Eickhof C, Nuyens G, Vuadens P: Clinical scales for the assessment of spasticity, associated phenomena, and function: a systematic review of the literature. *Disabil Rehabil* 27(1-2):7-18, 2005.

43. Pierson SH: Outcome measures in spasticity management. *Muscle Nerve Suppl* 6(suppl):S36-S60, 1997.

44. Ashworth B: Preliminary trial of carisoprodol in multiple sclerosis. *Practitioner* 192:540-542, 1964.

45. Bohannon RW, Larkin PA, Smith MB, Horton MG: Relationship between static muscle strength deficits and spasticity in stroke patients with hemiparesis. *Phys Ther* 67(7):1068-1071, 1987.

46. Tardieu G, Shentoub S, Delarue R: Research on a technic for measurement of spasticity. *Rev Neurol (Paris)* 91(2):143-144, 1954.

47. Gracies JM, Marosszeky JE, Renton R, et al: Short-term effects of dynamic Lycra splints on upper limb in hemiplegic patients. *Arch Phys Med Rehabil* 81(12):1547-1555, 2000.

48. Mehrholz J, Wagner K, Meissner D, et al: Reliability of the modified Tardieu scale and the modified Ashworth scale in adult patients with severe brain injury: a comparison study. *Clin Rehabil* 19(7):751-759, 2005.

49. Ansari NN, Naghdi S, Arab TK, Jalaie S: The interrater and intrarater reliability of the modified Ashworth scale in the assessment of muscle spasticity: limb and muscle group effect. *NeuroRehabilitation* 23(3):231-237, 2008.

50. Dachy B, Dan B: Electrophysiological assessment of the effect of intrathecal baclofen in spastic children. *Clin Neurophysiol* 113(3):336-340, 2002.

51. Graham HK: Pendulum test in cerebral palsy. *Lancet* 355(9222):2184, 2000.

52. Lechner HE, Frotzler A, Eser P: Relationship between self- and clinically rated spasticity in spinal cord injury. *Arch Phys Med Rehabil* 87(1):15-19, 2006.

53. Ahmed SV, Jayawarna C, Jude E: Post lumbar puncture headache: diagnosis and management, *Postgrad Med J* 82(973):713-716, 2006.

21 Baclofen Pump Management

Michael Saulino

CHAPTER OVERVIEW

Chapter Synopsis: In addition to treating patients with chronic pain, intrathecal drug delivery systems can also be used to treat those with various forms of muscle spasticity or hypertonia. In this case, the drug delivered intrathecally is baclofen, a γ-aminobutyric acid receptor agonist that works like a brake on spinal motor neuron activity. This chapter considers the issues of pump implantation methods and management. The choice of implantation site may vary with the patient according to his or her body type and drug needs. Additionally, the patient and clinician must work together to set up and maintain this multifaceted therapy, particularly in ambulatory patients. Dose titrations carried out after implantation also vary for each patient and can take up to 9 months. As with any intrathecally delivered drug, one must consider the risks of baclofen overdose or withdrawal caused by improper delivery or device complications. Successful treatment with intrathecal baclofen (ITB) requires a team approach with attention to detail.

Important Points:
- Create post-implantation rehabilitation programs, especially for ambulatory patients.
- Maintain protocols for management of ITB withdrawal and overdose.
- Formulate troubleshooting algorithms based on physician familiarity and local resources.

Clinical Pearls:
- Review implant site and catheter tip placement based on the patient's characteristics.
- Monitor carefully the effects of intrathecal baclofen titration and weaning of oral agents.
- Consider post-implantation rehabilitation.
- Manage long-term expectations for intrathecal baclofen therapy.

Clinical Pitfalls:
Failure to:
- Implement protocols to manage adverse events including overdose and withdrawal.
- Institute mechanisms that reliably coordinate patient follow-up for dosing adjustments, refills, and battery replacements.
- Institute a troubleshooting algorithm based on clinical experience and local resources.

Introduction

Intrathecal baclofen (ITB) therapy has been used for more than two decades in the management of patients with spastic hypertonia associated with the upper motor neuron syndrome. Chapter 20 reviews the nature of the spastic condition, techniques for spasticity management, patient selection for ITB therapy, and procedures for executing ITB trials. This companion chapter describes the methods for intrathecal (IT) pump implantation, management of the implanted patient, the nature of chronic maintenance therapy, and the procedures for managing ITB overdose and withdrawal.

Implantation

After a positive trial response has been observed (i.e., a significant reduction in hypertonicity without unmanageable adverse effects), a patient may proceed to pump implantation. Some centers proceed immediately to implantation, but others have patients undergo more extensive pre-admission testing for permanent implantation compared with the initial trial. Although the implantation procedure might be considered a relatively minor surgery, the patient population served by ITB therapy can be somewhat fragile. Special attention should be paid to the cardiac, pulmonary, and nutritional status of preoperative subjects.[1] Patients should be clinically stable before surgery to minimize perioperative complications. Preoperative antibiotics are typically used with attention to potential bacterial colonization relative to neurogenic bladder or decubitus ulcers. Patients on chronic anticoagulation need to discontinue medications in the days preceding the procedure.[2] The risks of the permanent pump implantation and infusion are the same as the screening trial (e.g., excessive hypotonia, structural damage to neurologic structure, infection) with the additional risks of drug overdose, drug withdrawal, and device complications. These latter complications are described below.

Various options for pump and catheter placement should be considered before the procedure. The size of the implanted pump should be determined based on the patient's body habitus and anticipated IT dosing. Smaller and thinner individuals might prefer a smaller pump size, either for esthetic reasons or to prevent erosion of the pump through the skin and subcutaneous tissue. Similarly, the pump can be placed under abdominal fascia for similar reasons.[3,4] Patients who are anticipated to require high ITB doses or who reside a great distance from the follow-up clinic will benefit from larger pumps with larger drug reservoirs and longer refill intervals. The tip of the IT catheter is routinely placed in the mid-lower thoracic region, particularly if reduction of lower extremity spasticity is the primary concern. More rostral tip placement can be attempted to improve upper extremity hypertonicity.[5,6]

Pump implantation and continuous catheter are typically performed under sedation or, in some cases, under general anesthesia after careful considerations. The patient is placed either in a prone or lateral decubitus position. Spinal anatomy is confirmed fluoroscopically. The typical site of insertion into the spinal canal is posteriorly at the L2-L3 or L3-L4 interspace. A spinal needle is inserted through the skin several millimeters lateral to the midline and one or two spinal levels caudal to the proposed thecal sac penetration. Advancement of the needle should be monitored with fluoroscopic guidance, which ideally permits penetration into the thecal sac. Multiple dural punctures can potentially allow cerebrospinal fluid (CSF) leakage, which might result in inadvertent subdural or epidural catheter placement as well as increasing the possibility of postoperative spinal headache. After the needle tip is placed in the thecal sac, the inner cannula is removed, and freeflowing CSF should be observed. The IT catheter is then placed through the spinal needle and advanced cephalad.[7] The catheter tip is then positioned to the spinal level appropriate for the individual patient, usually T10-T12 for paraplegic patients and more rostrally for tetraplegic or hemiplegic patients.[5] Catheter tip placement into the upper thoracic spine, cervical–thoracic junction, and even the cervical spine has become increasingly commonplace for management of upper extremity hypertonia. The spinal needle is then removed. The catheter should be secured without undue tension to avoid kinking. The pump is generally implanted under the skin or abdominal fascia in the right or left lower quadrant. Subfascial placement may be particularly beneficial in thin patients. Alternative sites include the buttock (similar to placement of spinal cord stimulator systems) and the anterior chest wall (similar to placement of pacemakers). The catheter is then tunneled subcutaneously and connected to the pump. The use of abdominal binder has been used by some centers to reduce the incidence of incisional seroma and spinal headache. The management of spinal headache is described in Chapter 20.

Typically, liquid baclofen is placed in the reservoir intraoperatively with immediate commencement of IT infusion. The initial dosage of ITB is often determined by the patient's response to the test dose. A reasonable starting dose is 100% to 200% of the bolus dose divided over a 24-hour period. If a patient demonstrated prolonged or excessive hypotonia during the screening phase, it may be prudent to start at 50% of the bolus dose divided over a 24-hour period. It is imperative for the implanting physician to have a close relationship with the trialing physician to determine the appropriate starting dose. The concentration of the initial solution placed in the pump reservoir should be as low as possible to afford downward adjustments in case adverse effects are encountered. The patient should continue all oral antispasticity medications until a weaning schedule is prescribed. Typically, the acute hospitalization for pump implantation is 1 to 2 days.[8]

Titration Phase and Post-Implantation Management

Dose adjustments can commence immediately after pump implantation. In general, 24 hours is a reasonable time to wait between each dosing adjustment to allow for the full effects of the ITB to be observed. Dose modifications are performed by interrogating the pump with a handheld programmer, programming the needed adjustments, and then updating the pump's dosing schedule. The programmer communicates with the pump via radiotelemetry. Various modes of administration include simple continuous (dose delivered continuously throughout 24-hour cycle), complex continuous (variable dose delivered continuously during 24-hour cycle), and periodic bolus (regularly scheduled boluses of ITB within 24-hour cycle). These various modes of delivery are represented diagrammatically in **Fig. 21-1**. In this example, the total daily dosing for the three modes of delivery is the same, but the dose at any particular time is variable. The complex continuous dosing mode allows for differential effects throughout the course of the day. For example, a patient may find it beneficial to be on a lower dose during the day (to minimize weakness and maximize functional mobility) and a higher dose during the night (to minimize nocturnal spontaneous spasms). Periodic bolus dosing delivers several boluses rapidly over a few minutes with relatively low delivery between the boluses. This mode of delivery may allow for greater distribution of drug with enhanced access to more cephalad spinal levels. This mode of delivery may be particularly beneficial for addressing upper extremity hypertonia. The periodic bolus delivery mode potentially places a patient at a higher risk of overdose, although this has not been observed clinically. Both the complex continuous and periodic bolus modes of delivery are purported to be beneficial for the management of pharmacological tolerance. If a clinician is unsure if a dosing adjustment is warranted, a single bolus (at a given dose per day) can be programmed

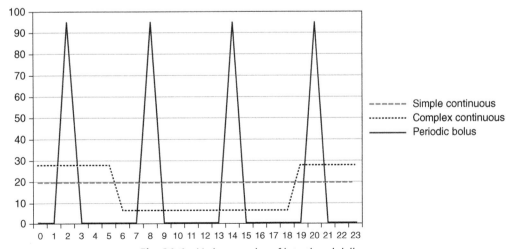

Fig. 21-1 Various modes of intrathecal delivery.

for several days followed by an automatic return to the baseline delivery. This mode of delivery is called single bolus with simple continuous delivery and allows the patient to be exposed to two different dosing levels automatically without the need for a physician visit. This mode of delivery can also be used for stepwise titration of IT delivery.

More recently, a handheld accessory for IT delivery has become available that allows for patient-controlled preprogrammed boluses of IT delivery. The amount, frequency, and lockout period for these boluses are set by the physician. At present, the only FDA-approved use for this device is management of breakthrough pain in a patient previously implanted with a permanent intrathecal delivery system. Although this device allows patients to vary their IT dosing to address for the variability of the spastic condition, it does have the theoretical risk of masking ongoing or progressive noxious stimuli that may be driving the increased tone. In patients with neurological conditions, increased spasticity may be the only sign of a potentially serious medical condition, such as urolithiasis or appendicitis. Thus, use of the handheld patient-activated device could potentially delay the patient's need to seek medical attention. The patient activation device could also be used as a tool for guiding IT titration. Further investigation is warranted into the safety and efficacy of using patient-controlled ITB delivery.[9] The combination of programming options allows for extraordinarily wide variety of options for IT delivery. This programmability, as well as the precise delivery of the IT delivery system, cannot be obtained with any other method of spasticity management.

During titration, some patients require ITB dose increases with a subsequent increase in refill frequency. Under these circumstances, a higher concentration of baclofen solution will extend the refill interval. When changing concentrations, it is imperative to program the pump correctly by incorporating a bridge bolus to compensate for the residual baclofen solution in the pump and catheter.[10] Failure to compensate for this residual solution may result in serious under- or overdosing. Traditionally, the therapeutic effect of ITB, as well as other agents delivered to the subarachnoid space, has been considered mostly closely linked to the dose administered. Until recently, relatively little attention has been paid to mode of delivery, concentration of the baclofen solution, and flow rate of IT delivery. These components of the therapy are beginning to demonstrate significant influence on the effectiveness of IT therapy, including baclofen. It is reasonable to postulate that lower drug concentrations and higher flow rates can potentially have larger areas of distribution within the spinal fluid compared with concentrated solutions with slower flow rates.[11] This hypothesis may be especially pertinent in this population because CSF flow can be dramatically altered in the presence of neurological disease. Practitioners are encouraged to consider this possibility in the management of patients who use this therapy.

During the titration phase of ITB therapy, patients are usually weaned from oral antispasticity medications. The amount of each IT adjustment varies depending on patient tolerability. Nonambulatory patients may tolerate dose adjustments of 20% of total daily dose, but others, especially ambulatory patients, require lower titration increments (5% to 10%). Adverse effects that may be seen during this phase of therapy include excessive hypotonia, changes in bowel[12,13] and bladder status,[14] and increased thromboembolic risk.[15,16] The frequency and size of dosing adjustments should be individualized based of the response to prior changes. Some patients tolerate rapid titration with daily dosing adjustments, but others may require longer periods of observation and accommodation before undertaking further adjustments. It is common for patient to demonstrate irregular spasticity patterns. Thus, some individuals may also benefit from some residual use of oral medications to address variable breakthrough spasms or to address upper extremity spasticity that is not addressed by ITB therapy.[17-19] The prevalence of irregular spasticity patterns is not completely known. There is no reliable conversion of oral to IT medications, so health care providers should use appropriate clinical judgment in simultaneously prescribing IT and oral agents. The titration phase of therapy could last 6 to 9 months after implantation.

If ITB is anticipated to affect the patient's active functional status, a rehabilitation program after implantation is appropriate. Post-implant rehabilitation may also be needed for caregiver training. The setting, scope, and complexity of this program vary depending on the patient's individual goals as well as the availability of these services in a given region. The timing of rehabilitation is also subject to some debate. Some centers defer therapies for few weeks after the implant because of concerns of catheter fracture or incisional dehiscence, but others favor immediate post-implant rehabilitation. Some implanters limit thoracolumbar flexion or twisting for a few weeks to minimize any potential issues. However, there have been no reports of incisional or catheter difficulties related to a specific activity. Potential disciplines involved in the rehabilitation process include physiatry or neurorehabilitation, physical therapy, occupational therapy, and rehabilitation nursing. Issues that potentially require attention include incisional care, medical management (spinal headache, pain assessment, medication adjustment, dosing changes), mobility, self-care ability, and bowel and bladder function. Patients, especially ambulatory individuals, should be thoroughly counseled on the need for post-implant rehabilitation to maximize the benefits of ITB therapy.

Because spasticity may provide some protection against venous thrombosis, rapid reduction of hypertonia may place patients with neurological disorders at higher risk of thromboembolic phenomena in the postoperative phase. Both lower extremity venous thrombosis and secondary pulmonary embolism have been reported in the postoperative phase of ITB therapy. Consideration of mechanical or chemical prophylaxis is warranted. This intervention must be balanced against the risk of spinal hemorrhage or incisional hematoma with anticoagulant use. There is no standard of care for the length or type of prevention measures, so each clinician must make decisions based on each individual patient's risk factor profile.

Long-Term Maintenance and Troubleshooting

After the titration phase of ITB therapy, the patient enters the chronic maintenance phase of therapy. Aspects of this treatment phase include refilling the pump reservoir with new medication, troubleshooting any infusion system malfunction, and replacing the pump for battery replenishment.

Reservoir refills are sterile, office-based procedures that occur every few weeks to few months for the duration of treatment. Standard baclofen solutions are stable in the pump reservoir for up to 6 months. The pump has a low residual reservoir volume, which is the lowest volume that supports stable flow through the catheter. The refill interval is the time required for the pump to dispense the volume of solution from a full reservoir to the low reservoir volume. The refill interval reflects the baclofen concentration and daily dose. Pump refills are scheduled to have sufficient residual reservoir volume before the alarm date to avoid "low reservoir syndrome" and associated symptoms of ITB withdrawal.[20] Patients should always be aware of their next clinic appointment and alarm date. Pump refills are typically accomplished by palpating the pump externally and using a template to guide a needle into the reservoir chamber. Fluoroscopy or ultrasonography can be used to assist in port localization and needle placement.[21] The remaining solution of the previous refill is aspirated and should correspond to the calculated volume by the pump programmer. The new baclofen solution is then instilled through the same needle. The needle tip must be reliably determined to be within the reservoir chamber. Inadvertent injection of an IT solution into the subcutaneous tissue can result in serious adverse events.[22]

Two concentrations of ITB (Lioresal Intrathecal) are FDA approved and commercially available for use in reservoir refills, 500 and 2000 µg/mL. Higher concentrations of liquid baclofen are available through specialized pharmacies. These nonstandard concentrations are considered "compounded," which is defined as providing pharmaceuticals in dosage forms or combinations that are not commercially available. The potential benefits of higher concentrations include lower cost and less frequent pump refills. Although the use of compounded solutions for IT pain delivery is relatively common, the role of compounded ITB solution is less well defined. One study of 27 samples of compounded baclofen obtained from seven compounding pharmacies demonstrated that more than 40% were more than 5% above or below their labeled concentration, and 22% deviated more than 10% from the labeled concentration.[23] Thus, compounded baclofen may lead to inaccurate or inconsistent dosing because of concentration variations, causing symptoms of under- or overdose. There is also anecdotal evidence that baclofen concentrations above 2000 µg/mL may contribute to catheter tip abnormalities, although this abnormality has also been reported in noncompounded solutions.[24] Additional risks that are potentially associated with compounded baclofen solutions include contamination or drug precipitation. The use of compounded ITB should only be used with a full realization of the potential risks and benefits associated with this strategy. Patients and caregivers should be involved in this decision-making process.

Other issues related to long-term ITB therapy include precautions for use and battery replacement. Current IT delivery systems are considered magnetic resonance imaging (MRI) compatible and have been formally tested in magnets up to 1.5 Tesla. IT delivery will automatically stop in the presence of the magnetic field and restart when removed from the magnetic field. An electronic check of the IT delivery can be done with the programmer to ensure restart of IT delivery. Normally, the duration of an MRI scan is of insufficient duration to result in clinically significant withdrawal.[25-27] Whole-body shock-wave lithotripsy is relatively contraindicated with IT delivery systems because of the potential for electronic damage by the sound waves. Hyperbaric oxygen therapy has been reported to result in a degree of underdosing, so clinicians should proceed with caution with this therapy in patients who have IT pumps.[28] There is also a case report of battery failure of an IT delivery system after exposure to high-dose radiation therapy.[29]

Battery replenishment, typically a same-day surgical procedure, is undertaken approximately every 5 to 6 years. There may be some benefit in planning a pump replacement before detecting alarm condition in an effort to avoid serious withdrawal symptoms.[30]

For patients with chronic, nonprogressive neurological conditions, ITB dosing should be relatively stable during the maintenance phase of therapy. Individuals with progressive diseases such as amyotrophic lateral sclerosis or multiple sclerosis may require increasing dosages over time. Patients with previously well-controlled hypertonia on a stable dosing regimen who present with increased spasticity should be examined carefully. Although pharmacological tolerance to ITB is a possible cause for increasing dosing,[31-33] this phenomena should not be assumed until a thorough clinical evaluation has been undertaken. Co-morbidities of

neurological disease (e.g., urinary tract infection, bladder distention, urolithiasis) can serve as noxious stimuli that act as "triggers" for increased spasticity.[14] If no cause for increased spasticity is discovered, an investigation for a system malfunction should be promptly undertaken. An approach to this exploration is discussed below.

Causes for Loss of Baclofen Effectiveness

Potential causes of loss of effectiveness of ITB therapy include programming errors and mechanical problems involving the pump or catheter (e.g., kinks, holes, occlusions).[34] Some of these problems are readily detectable, but others are more challenging to discover. In general, programming and refilling errors tend to be easily identified and corrected. Malfunctions involving the pump mechanism are rare but when present are also rather simply confirmed. Catheter problems are relatively frequent, however, and may vary in their presentations and ease of diagnostic identification. Fig. 21-2 illustrates potential sites of catheter disruption. Approaches to pump and catheter malfunction are presented next. It is important to note that no absolute consensus exists regarding an optimal diagnostic algorithm. Physicians should make decisions based on their individual resources and familiarity with each diagnostic technique.[13] Prompt identification of any delivery system problem is imperative given the potential serious effects of ITB overdose and withdrawal.

Two initial techniques for investigation of pump malfunction include pump interrogation and checking the pump residual reservoir volume. Interrogation of the pump's dosing parameters should match the prescribed dosing. The presence of an audible alarm (as well as electronic alarm during pump interrogation) or discovery of an unexpected "extra" residual volume in the reservoir suggest a pump-related malfunction. Alarm conditions generally occur either in a low battery or low reservoir situation. A low battery alarm will sound when the battery has reached significant discharge. A low reservoir alarm will indicate that the pump has delivered near all of the contents of the reservoir and that the patient needs an immediate refill. An increase in reservoir residual volume might indicate an abnormality of the pump rotor. Rotor failure is diagnosed by imaging of the pump rotors, programming a specific bolus that rotates the rotor axis either 60 or 90 degrees, and then repeating the imaging. Failure to rotate the expected amount is an indication of possible rotor failure. Rotor stall can also be seen with a severely kinked catheter. If there is any doubt as to the concentration of reservoir solution, then a new solution should be instilled. Similarly, if a low reservoir alarm is detected, then a timely refill should be undertaken. The presence of a permanent rotor stall or low battery condition should prompt urgent replacement of the pump.[35]

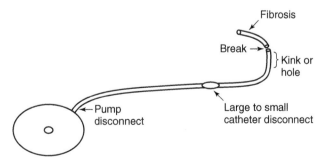

Fig. 21-2 Sites of potential catheter disruptions in intrathecal delivery systems.

After mechanical pump abnormalities and programming and solution difficulties have been eliminated from consideration, attention must then be turned to potential catheter problems. Most commonly, this undertaking will involve imaging techniques.[36] Plain radiography is a typical first step. An anteroposterior and lateral lumbar and thoracic spine radiography series should be obtained to visualize all tubing, connectors, and entrance of the catheter into the spinal canal. If the films are normal, a catheter access port (CAP) aspiration can be undertaken. This procedure involves accessing a port (i.e., the CAP) that is in direct continuity with the catheter. Because the distal end of the catheter lies within the subarachnoid space, CSF should be able to be readily withdrawn through the catheter. Aspiration of at least 2 to 3 mL is necessary for determination of a "normal" aspiration because the volume of the catheter is typically less than 0.25 mL. Failure to aspirate fluid can suggest catheter disruption or occlusion with the recognition that some patients with neurological disorders may produce minimal CSF in the region of the catheter tip. The presence of significant fluid on side port aspiration does not eliminate the possibility of a catheter problem but does confirm some degree of catheter continuity. After the catheter has been cleared of the drug solution and CSF obtained, contrast medium can be injected and visualized fluoroscopically or with computed tomography. Extravasation of dye out of the catheter can diagnose catheter breaks, catheter tip loculations, and migration of the catheter into the subdural or epidural spaces.[37] Contrast should not be injected if 2 to 3 mL of CSF cannot be easily aspirated because this can potentially expose the patient to ITB overdose from infusion of drug remaining in the catheter.[38]

Other imaging techniques for diagnosis of catheter malfunction include radionuclide scintigraphy and MRI. Indium I-111 DTPA (diethylenetriamine pentaacetic acid) can be injected into the pump reservoir and used as a tracer to determine the patency of the infusion system. After injection, serial sequential scanning occurs every 24 hours for 2 to 3 days. Normal study results should demonstrate an intact catheter and full ventriculogram. This technique can detect evidence of catheter occlusion, pump malfunctions, and large leaks. Disadvantages of this procedure include cost, the need for 2 to 3 days to confirm the abnormality, and limited anatomical resolution.[39] MRI of the thoracic spine can demonstrate spinal hemorrhage, an abscess, and other soft tissue abnormalities near the catheter tip. Rarely, granulomas can develop at the catheter tip, but these have only been pathologically confirmed with IT opiate therapy for chronic pain. Although rare, granulomas have the potential to cause serious neurological injury from spinal cord compression. MRI imaging of the catheter tip with gadolinium contrast is the diagnostic test of choice for granuloma detection.[40]

Abrupt reduction or cessation of ITB delivery may result in withdrawal syndrome, which can have serious, if not fatal, consequences. The severity of ITB withdrawal syndrome is not consistently related with dosing levels. Perhaps the most common symptomatic presentation is return of the patient's "baseline" degree of hypertonia. Additional characteristics of this syndrome may include pruritus, seizures, hallucinations, and autonomic dysreflexia. Some patients demonstrate a life-threatening syndrome exemplified by exaggerated or rebound spasticity (i.e., greater than baseline degree of hypertonia), fever, hemodynamic instability, and altered mental status. If not treated aggressively, this syndrome can progress over 24 to 72 hours to include rhabdomyolysis, elevated liver function test levels, hepatic and renal failure, disseminated intravascular coagulation, multiorgan system failure, and rarely death.[41] Typically, the withdrawal symptoms will abate in several

---

Box 21-1: Symptoms of and Interventions for Intrathecal Baclofen Withdrawal

Symptoms of Intrathecal Baclofen Withdrawal
Rebound hypertonia
Pruritus
Seizures
Behavioral abnormalities, altered mental status, hallucinations
Cardiovascular abnormalities, autonomic dysreflexia
Rhabdomyolysis
Hepatic and renal failure
Disseminated intravascular coagulation
Multiorgan system failure

Interventions for Intrathecal Baclofen Withdrawal
General cardiopulmonary support
Oral or intrathecal baclofen
Oral or intravenous benzodiazepines
Oral or intravenous dantrolene
Oral cyproheptadine

---

days, although there have been reports of prolonged ITB withdrawal syndrome.[42] After recognition of ITB withdrawal, initial treatment includes supportive care, careful observation, and replacement of baclofen via intervenous infusion or preferably through restoration of IT delivery. There is no consistent oral to IT conversion rate. Thus, oral baclofen administration may require frequent modification to attenuate the withdrawal syndrome. Adjunctive pharmacotherapy may also include administration of benzodiazepines (enteral or intravenous),[43] dantrolene,[25] or cyproheptadine.[44] Management of withdrawal should be executed in an urgent, if not emergent, fashion and should precede diagnostic investigation into the cause of the malfunction. After the withdrawal syndrome has been modulated, then identification and correction of the delivery system malfunction can be done. The symptoms of and intervention for ITB withdrawal are summarized in Box 21-1.

Pharmacological tolerance refers to adaptive changes that have taken place within systems affected by the drug so that clinical response to the drug is reduced.[31-33] Tolerance has been implicated as a cause of acquired loss of response to ITB despite escalating doses, often in the context of failure to demonstrate radiological evidence of an ITB system malfunction. Controversy exists, however, regarding whether response failure in such scenarios represents undiagnosed problems with drug administration through the pump and catheter system rather than actual pharmacologic tolerance in γ-aminobutyric acidergic target neurons of the spinal cord.[45] Accordingly, a thorough analysis of any potential system malfunction should be undertaken before attributing dose escalation to tolerance. Neurophysiological assessment may be particularly helpful in this scenario. Assuming that these steps have been unsuccessfully attempted, interventions for tolerance include decreasing the concentration of baclofen solution with a concomitant increase in flow rate, utilization of periodic bolus delivery, and substitution with IT morphine.[46]

In contrast to withdrawal, which can occur despite vigilant attention, ITB overdose is generally caused by human miscalculation during dosing adjustments or concentration changes. Mechanical difficulties leading to overdosing are exceeding rare. Subdural encapsulation of the IT catheter with subsequent rupture of the subdural pocket could lead to inadvertent excessive baclofen exposure.[47,48] There have been rare reports of inadvertent injection of a refill solution into the CAP, resulting in massive overdose.[48] Overdose can occur during catheter patency studies if the drug within the catheter is inadvertently injected into the subarachnoid space. Additionally, if a catheter disruption is detected and the patient is undergoing restoration of IT delivery, overdosing can occur if IT delivery is resumed at the same dosing level before disruption. In this clinical scenario, patients should be started on dosing levels similar to levels initiated at pump implantation.

Symptoms of baclofen overdose include profound hypotonia or flaccidity, hyporeflexia, respiratory depression, apnea, seizures, coma, autonomic instability, hallucinations, hypothermia, and cardiac rhythm abnormalities.[49,50] Plasma and CSF levels of baclofen can be obtained, but the results may be misleading because there is no direct correlation between the programmed IT dosing and CSF baclofen levels.[51] Initial management of overdose is supportive and includes maintenance of airway, respiration, and circulation. Intubation and ventilatory support may be necessary. Secondary measures include reduction or temporary interruption of IT delivery by pump reprogramming. Optional measures for ITB overdose include CSF drainage via CAP aspiration or lumbar puncture and administration of an "antidote." Although not true antidotes, both physostigmine and flumazenil have been reported to reduce central side effects, such as somnolence and respiratory depression. Physostigmine is the more commonly used agent but may produce adverse affects such as bradycardia, seizures, and increased respiratory secretions. Patients who are treated for baclofen overdose must be watched closely for rebound withdrawal after the pump is stopped and the drug load is decreased.[50]

Summary

The efficacy of ITB therapy has been demonstrated for over two decades. Initially, patients with upper motor neuron syndrome who demonstrated difficulties with passive function (e.g., positioning, hygiene) were the most common group referred for this therapy. More recently, patients with problematic active function (e.g., ambulation) have been referred and have successfully used this intervention. Both groups are best served by a dedicated medical, surgical, and rehabilitation team that is capable of managing all aspects of this therapy described in this chapter. As the sophistication of IT delivery systems increases and newer agents become available, the requirement for a team-based approach will become even more paramount. If clinicians are interested in using ITB therapy, they should develop a robust team environment to manage the routine, urgent, and emergent needs of their patient population.

References

1. Deer TR, Smith HS, Cousins M, Doleys DM, et al: Consensus guidelines for the selection and implantation of patients with noncancer pain for intrathecal drug delivery. *Pain Physician* 13(3):E175-E213, 2010.
2. Horlocker TT, Wedel DJ, Benzon H, et al: Regional anesthesia in the anticoagulated patient: defining the risks (the second ASRA consensus conference on neuraxial anesthesia and anticoagulation). *Reg Anesth Pain Med* 28(3), 2003.
3. Kopell BH, Sala D, Doyle WK, et al: Subfascial implantation of intrathecal baclofen pumps in children: technical note. *Neurosurgery* 49(3):753, 756, discussion 756-757, 2001.
4. Vanhauwaert DJ, Kalala JP, Baert E, et al: Migration of pump for intrathecal drug delivery into the peritoneal cavity: case report. *Surg Neurol* 71(5):610, 612, discussion 612, 2009.
5. Burns AS, Meythaler JM: Intrathecal baclofen in tetraplegia of spinal origin: efficacy for upper extremity hypertonia. *Spinal Cord* 39(8):413-419, 2001.
6. Motta F, Stignani C, Antonello CE: Upper limb function after intrathecal baclofen treatment in children with cerebral palsy. *J Pediatr Orthop* 28(1):91-96, 2008.
7. Albright AL, Turner M, Pattisapu JV: Best-practice surgical techniques for intrathecal baclofen therapy. *J Neurosurg* 104(4 suppl):233-239, 2006.
8. Penn RD: Intrathecal medication delivery. *Neurosurg Clin North Am* 14(3):381-387, 2003.
9. Ilias W, le Polain B, Buchser E, Demartini L, oPTiMa Study Group: Patient-controlled analgesia in chronic pain patients: experience with a new device designed to be used with implanted programmable pumps. *Pain Pract* 8(3):164-170, 2008.
10. Elovic E, Kirshblum SC: Managing spasticity in spinal cord injury: safe administration of bridge boluses during intrathecal baclofen pump refills. *J Spinal Cord Med* 26(1):2-4, 2003.
11. Flack SH, Bernards CM: Cerebrospinal fluid and spinal cord distribution of hyperbaric bupivacaine and baclofen during slow intrathecal infusion in pigs. *Anesthesiology* 112(1):165-173, 2010.
12. Kofler M, Matzak H, Saltuari L: The impact of intrathecal baclofen on gastrointestinal function. *Brain Inj* 16(9):825-836, 2002.
13. Morant A, Noe E, Boyer J, et al: Paralytic ileus: a complication after intrathecal baclofen therapy. *Brain Inj* 20(13-14):1451-1454, 2006.
14. Vaidyanathan S, Soni BM, Oo T, et al: Delayed complications of discontinuation of intrathecal baclofen therapy: resurgence of dyssynergic voiding, which triggered off autonomic dysreflexia and hydronephrosis. *Spinal Cord* 42(10):598-602, 2004.
15. Carda S, Cazzaniga M, Taiana C, Pozzi R: Intrathecal baclofen bolus complicated by deep vein thrombosis and pulmonary embolism. A case report. *Eur J Phys Rehabil Med* 44(1):87-88, 2008.
16. Murphy NA: Deep venous thrombosis as a result of hypotonia secondary to intrathecal baclofen therapy: a case report. *Arch Phys Med Rehabil* 83(9):1311-1312, 2002.
17. Krach LE, Kriel RL, Nugent AC: Complex dosing schedules for continuous intrathecal baclofen infusion. *Pediatr Neurol* 37(5):354-359, 2007.
18. Kunz KD, Ames SL, Saulino MF: Multimodality approach to spasticity management: how patients treated with intrathecal baclofen also utilize other spasticity interventions. *Am J Phys Med Rehabil* 88(3 suppl):S57, 2009.
19. Kofler M, Quirbach E, Schauer R, et al: Limitations of intrathecal baclofen for spastic hemiparesis following stroke. *Neurorehabil Neural Repair* 23(1):26-31, 2009.
20. Rigoli G, Terrini G, Cordioli Z: Intrathecal baclofen withdrawal syndrome caused by low residual volume in the pump reservoir: a report of 2 cases. *Arch Phys Med Rehabil* 85(12):2064-2066, 2004.
21. Hurdle MF, Locketz AJ, Smith J: A technique for ultrasound-guided intrathecal drug-delivery system refills. *Am J Phys Med Rehabil* 86(3):250-251, 2007.
22. Coyne PJ, Hansen LA, Laird J, et al: Massive hydromorphone dose delivered subcutaneously instead of intrathecally: guidelines for prevention and management of opioid, local anesthetic, and clonidine overdose. *J Pain Symptom Manage* 28(3):273-276, 2004.
23. Moberg-Wolff E: Potential clinical impact of compounded versus noncompounded intrathecal baclofen. *Arch Phys Med Rehabil* 90(11):1815-1820, 2009.
24. Deer TR, Raso LJ, Garten TG: Inflammatory mass of an intrathecal catheter in patients receiving baclofen as a sole agent: a report of two cases and a review of the identification and treatment of the complication. *Pain Med* 8(3):259-262, 2007.
25. Khorasani A, Peruzzi WT: Dantrolene treatment for abrupt intrathecal baclofen withdrawal. *Anesth Analg* 80(5):1054-1056, 1995.
26. Sawyer-Glover AM, Shellock FG: Pre-MRI procedure screening: recommendations and safety considerations for biomedical implants and devices. *J Magn Reson Imaging* 12(1):92-106, 2000.
27. von Roemeling R, Lanning RM, Eames FA: MR imaging of patients with implanted drug infusion pumps. *J Magn Reson Imaging* 1(1):77-81, 1991.
28. Akman MN, Loubser PG, Fife CE, Donovan WH: Hyperbaric oxygen therapy: implications for spinal cord injury patients with intrathecal

baclofen infusion pumps: case report. *Paraplegia* 32(4):281-284, 1994.

29. Wu H, Wang D: Radiation-induced alarm and failure of an implanted programmable intrathecal pump. *Clin J Pain* 23(9):826-828, 2007.

30. Leong MS, Carpentier BW: Pump battery assessment: cold, old, or dead! *Neuromodulation* 4(3):117-119, 2001.

31. Hefferan MP, Fuchigami T, Marsala M: Development of baclofen tolerance in a rat model of chronic spasticity and rigidity. *Neurosci Lett* 403(1-2):195-200, 2006.

32. Heetla HW, Staal MJ, Kliphuis C, van Laar T: The incidence and management of tolerance in intrathecal baclofen therapy. *Spinal Cord* 47(10):751-756, 2009.

33. Heetla HW, Staal MJ, van Laar T: Tolerance to continuous intrathecal baclofen infusion can be reversed by pulsatile bolus infusion. *Spinal Cord* 48(6):483-486, 2010.

34. Follett KA, Naumann CP: A prospective study of catheter-related complications of intrathecal drug delivery systems. *J Pain Symptom Manage* 19(3):209-215, 2000.

35. Sgouros S, Charalambides C, Matsota P, et al: Malfunction of SynchroMed II baclofen pump delivers a near-lethal baclofen overdose. *Pediatr Neurosurg* 46(1):62-65, 2010.

36. Dvorak EM, McGuire JR, Nelson ME: Incidence and identification of intrathecal baclofen catheter malfunction. *PM R* 2(8):751-756, 2010.

37. Turner MS: Assessing syndromes of catheter malfunction with SynchroMed infusion systems: the value of spiral computed tomography with contrast injection. *PM R* 2(8):757-766, 2010.

38. Lew SM, Psaty EL, Abbott R: An unusual cause of overdose after baclofen pump implantation: case report. *Neurosurgery* 56(3):E624, discussion E624, 2005.

39. Stinchon JF, Shah NP, Ordia J, Oates E: Scintigraphic evaluation of intrathecal infusion systems: selection of patients for surgical or medical management. *Clin Nucl Med* 31(1):1-4, 2006.

40. Deer T, Krames ES, Hassenbusch S, et al: Management of intrathecal catheter-tip inflammatory masses: an updated 2007 consensus statement from an expert panel. *Neuromodulation* 11(2):77-91, 2008.

41. Coffey RJ, Edgar TS, Francisco GE, et al: Abrupt withdrawal from intrathecal baclofen: Recognition and management of a potentially life-threatening syndrome. *Arch Phys Med Rehabil* 83(6):735-741, 2002.

42. Hansen CR, Gooch JL, Such-Neibar T: Prolonged, severe intrathecal baclofen withdrawal syndrome: a case report. *Arch Phys Med Rehabil* 88(11):1468-1471, 2007.

43. Cruikshank M, Eunson P: Intravenous diazepam infusion in the management of planned intrathecal baclofen withdrawal. *Dev Med Child Neurol* 49(8):626-628, 2007.

44. Meythaler JM, Roper JF, Brunner RC: Cyproheptadine for intrathecal baclofen withdrawal. *Arch Phys Med Rehabil* 84(5):638-642, 2003.

45. Francisco GE, Yablon SA, Schiess MC, et al: Consensus panel guidelines for the use of intrathecal baclofen therapy in poststroke spastic hypertonia. *Top Stroke Rehabil* 13(4):74-85, 2006.

46. Vidal J, Gregori P, Guevara D, et al: Efficacy of intrathecal morphine in the treatment of baclofen tolerance in a patient on intrathecal baclofen therapy (ITB). *Spinal Cord* 42(1):50-51, 2004.

47. Pasquier Y, Cahana A, Schnider A: Subdural catheter migration may lead to baclofen pump dysfunction. *Spinal Cord* 41(12):700-702, 2003.

48. Sorokin A, Annabi E, Yang WC, Kaplan R: Subdural intrathecal catheter placement: experience with two cases. *Pain Physician* 11(5):677-680, 2008.

49. Yeh RN, Nypaver MM, Deegan TJ, Ayyangar R: Baclofen toxicity in an 8-year-old with an intrathecal baclofen pump. *J Emerg Med* 26(2):163-167, 2004.

50. Shirley KW, Kothare S, Piatt JH Jr, Adirim TA: Intrathecal baclofen overdose and withdrawal. *Pediatr Emerg Care* 22(4):258-261, 2006.

51. Albright AL, Thompson K, Carlos S, Minnigh MB: Cerebrospinal fluid baclofen concentrations in patients undergoing continuous intrathecal baclofen therapy. *Dev Med Child Neurol* 49(6):423-425, 2007.

Chapter 22 Future of Intrathecal Drug Delivery Systems (Including New Devices)

Chapter 23: Trialing for Ziconotide Intrathecal Analgesic Therapy

Chapter 24: Perioperative Management of Patients with Intrathecal Drug Delivery Systems

22 Future of Intrathecal Drug Delivery Systems (Including New Devices)

Erin R. Lawson and Mark S. Wallace

CHAPTER OVERVIEW

Chapter Synopsis: Intrathecal (IT) drug delivery of analgesic or antispastic agents has provided some significant improvements over systemic drug delivery in certain patients, including the need for lower doses of drug. Delivery devices have undergone improvements that allow for more complex delivery schedules and allow patients to reap the benefits for many years after implantation. These improvements have allowed for better analgesia and fewer adverse side effects, but the procedure has room for further improvement, particularly in the areas of battery lifetime and device size and durability. More sophisticated devices require more space and power and therefore more frequent battery and drug refills. A better understanding of drug combinatorial effects may open the therapy to expanded patient populations in the future. This chapter also considers some of the pitfalls seen with the procedure's 20-year history, which should be avoided in future development.

Important Points:
- Technological advances in spinal drug delivery have been slow over the past two decades.
- The most significant advance is the addition of the ability of patients to self-administer boluses through an implanted IT pump. The clinical benefits of this addition have not been determined.
- The precision of spinal drug delivery is adequate; however, there is a need for better catheter technology that resists shearing and breaks. New technology is in clinical trials, but the clinical benefits have not been determined.
- Catheter-tip granuloma formation continues to be a concern, and future efforts need to focus on the prevention of this complication.

Clinical Pearls:
- Recommendations for detection of catheter tip granulomas include vigilant monitoring for a decreasing analgesic effect of drug, new and progressive neurological symptoms, or both.
- Recommendations for preventing granuloma formation include using the lowest possible drug doses and placing the catheter tip in the lumbar thecal sac when possible.
- Using thick-walled catheters is recommended for avoiding catheter fracture or disconnect. Presently, most of the catheters in use are thick walled. It is yet to be determined if improvements in catheter technology actually decrease catheter-related complications.
- Extreme caution should be taken when programming and refilling the pump to avoid accidental drug overdose.

Clinical Pitfalls:
- Catheter-tip granulomas are a potentially catastrophic adverse outcome with IT drug delivery. Prevention and early detection are keys to successful outcome.
- The catheter is the most vulnerable component of the system and the one most prone to problems, including disconnection from the pump or port, large to small catheter disconnect, kinks or holes in the catheter, catheter breaks, and catheter dislodgements.
- Postoperative catheter migration caused by pulling of the catheter by pump movement with patient ambulation and bending is another common yet frustrating occurrence that requires surgical revision.
- Incorrect programming, pump malfunction or fracture, and complications with pump refill all pose risks of drug overdose and possibly death.
- Abrupt withdrawal or otherwise improper dose titration is also a potential adverse outcome of improper system management.

Introduction

Since the late 1980s, intrathecal (IT) analgesic therapy has increasingly become an accepted alternative to standard medical management for the treatment of patients with persistent pain.[1] Because drug doses are much lower when applied directly to the IT space compared with oral or parenteral application, side effects and drug toxicities are often much less. With the development of implantable IT drug delivery devices, patients may benefit from continuous IT administration of analgesics or antispasmodics for years without fear of infection or dislodgment. Newer sophisticated implanted IT drug delivery systems (IDDS) and drug development allow clinicians to further improve analgesia and limit adverse effects through combination therapy and precise control over delivery.[2] Clinicians may take advantage of the wide variety of available agents and devices to tailor treatment regimens to individual patients.

Future Technology

The ideal IDDS would provide physicians and patients with a safe, comfortable, discrete, sturdy, durable, and effective method of drug delivery requiring infrequent drug refills, battery changes, or other intervention. There is currently no perfect system, and new technology continues to aim for improvement. Technology that can effectively and safely treat breakthrough pain as well as address intra-and interpatient variability are continued goals. Unfortunately, programming technology advances such as bolus options and individual programming features increase power expenditure, necessitating more frequent surgical battery change. Also, increases in technology of the system have made implantable pumps more bulky and decreased the space for infusate storage. Pumps that require less energy and rechargeable systems are a relatively new approach to this problem. A piezoelectric membrane pump has been developed that reduces both bulk and energy requirement.[3] Technology behind rechargeable spinal cord stimulators may be eventually applied to IT pumps.[4] However, risks associated with battery failure and withdrawal syndrome may limit this technology use in IT drug therapy. In addition, the power requirements for an IT pump are much lower than spinal cord stimulator requirements, making it difficult to justify the benefits compared with the risks. Finally, less fragile pump materials may have a future in reducing drug delivery system damage, breakdown, and failure.[4] IT drug delivery devices are becoming increasingly compatible with agents and admixtures. By broadening the available options of drug delivery, innovations in IT therapy may reach new subsets of patients.

The Prometra Programmable Pump System is a fully implantable device awaiting approval by the U.S. Food and Drug Administration (FDA) that is designed to improve precision in drug delivery. The system ensures dosing accuracy through a positive-pressure design in which drug is administered through a gate-controlled system into a 20-mL fixed-volume control chamber.[5] The system is 71 mm wide by 20 mm thick, weighs 150 g, and allows a flow rate of up to 28 mL/day. The pump is composed of highly durable, mostly immobile parts to promote usage for longer than 10 years.[5] A clinical trial of the Prometra pump conducted in individuals with intractable chronic cancer pain or chronic non-malignant pain demonstrated an overall 97.5% dose accuracy rate.[6-8] Patients had statistically significant improvements in visual analog scale score, numeric rating scale score, and Oswestry disability index assessments from baseline to 1 year.[9]

The MedStream Programmable Infusion System is another implantable device currently under investigation. This implantable drug delivery system offers improved catheter technology and pump durability. Its SureStream intraspinal catheter has been designed to resist kinking and tearing. The MedStream ceramic drive system maintains the infusion rate without motors, gears, or rotating parts.[10] The pump has either a 20- or 40-mL reservoir, measures 76 mm by 21.6 mm (20 mL) or 28.2 mm (40 mL).[10] The MedStream is currently pending FDA approval, although it is already available for sale in several European countries.[10]

The Medallion is an implantable drug delivery system awaiting FDA approval for study in humans. The Medallion system focuses on safety improvements with the creation of a negative pressure reservoir. If a break in the system occurs, medication would not leak out of the reservoir into the patient. The negative pressure draws medication from the syringe during pump refills rather than requiring syringe plunger manipulation, further reducing the risk of inadvertent injection into the patient rather than the pump.[11] A pressure sensor is present to detect flow resistance. The Medallion, with either a 20- or a 40-mL pump, measures 2.6 inches in diameter and is 0.72 inches thick across the flat portion of the can.[11] Both sizes include a sutureless connector and a radiopaque IT catheter and are compatible with an 8-year battery at 0.5 mL/day.[11] The Medallion clinical trials will assess the system's pressure sensor in addition to the overall safety and efficacy of the device.[11]

The Personal Therapy Manager (PTM) is a compatible hand-held device to be used with an existing IDDS. This technology is designed to address breakthrough pain by allowing patients to self-administer a bolus dose of infusate. The PTM was approved by the FDA in 2005 for concomitant use with the SynchroMed II pump.[12] Maximum bolus dosing is specified to avoid administrative over-dose. The device also records usage, pre- and postbolus pain scores and technical events and calculates predicted refill requirements based on background infusion and bolus doses.[4,13,14] Patients using the device have reportedly experienced a 29% reduction in pain, improved quality of life, and reduced need for supplemental analgesics, and there have been no reported major adverse events associated with its use.[13] The PTM is only compatible with the newer SynchroMed pumps and is not covered by many managed care organizations or Medicare. The out-of-pocket cost for patients is estimated at $500. It is unclear at this time if this device will significantly shorten the pump battery life.

Concerns and Pitfalls

As recently described by Coffey et al,[15] IT opioid drug infusion is not a completely harmless technique. Coffey et al found higher than expected mortality among noncancer pain patients treated with IT opioid infusion attributable to inadvertent drug overdose.[15] Incorrect programming, pump malfunction or fracture, and complications with pump refill all pose risk of drug overdose. Likewise, abrupt withdrawal or otherwise improper dose titration is a potential adverse outcome of improper system management.

Catheter-tip granulomas are another potential source of adverse outcome with IT drug delivery. IT inflammatory masses are relatively common. A recent online survey of health care professionals in the United States who commonly use IDDS in their patients revealed that 63% of responding physicians had experience with granulomas in their patients. Of those practitioners, 63 reported having a patient who experienced permanent or temporary neurological injury because of a granuloma.[16] Most agents used in implantable infusion systems, including baclofen, have been associated with granuloma formation.[2] Only fentanyl and sufentanil as single infusions have not been reported in the literature in association with granuloma formation.[2] IT granulomas are predominantly innocuous, but they do have the potential to cause irreversible neurological injury, including complete and permanent paralysis.[17] Granulomas typically shrink or resolve completely after cessation of drug administration over 2 to 5 months.[18] Small granulomas that do not cause neurological compromise may be managed by drug discontinuation and observation. However, larger masses or those that cause neurological dysfunction require surgical removal.[18] Granuloma formation typically presents with decreasing analgesic effect of drug and new and progressive neurological symptoms.[18] Therefore, current recommendations for detection include vigilant monitoring for these signs. Routine imaging without signs or symptoms of granuloma is not recommended. Granuloma formation is thought to be related to properties of the drug, cerebrospinal fluid (CSF) flow dynamics, and possibly catheter tip location.[19] The risk of granuloma formation appears to increase with dose escalation and increases in drug concentration, especially in areas of relatively low CSF flow. Therefore, recommendations for prevention are to use the lowest possible drug doses and placement of catheter tip in the lumbar thecal sac when possible.[18] There is no current technology aimed at reducing risk of catheter-tip granuloma. Initially, granuloma formation was partially attributed to single-orifice catheters, and catheters were redesigned with multiple orifices for drug infusion to lower this risk.[19] However, granulomas have continued to form on these multiorifice catheters.[19] The theory that high drug concentrations at the catheter tip increase the risk of granuloma formation suggest that the use of the PTM may reduce this risk by administering bolus dosing with resultant drug dispersion from the tip. Additional research is needed on CSF kinetics to determine the best location for the catheter tip to prevent granuloma formation. One would assume that catheter-tip locations with a high CSF circulation would be less prone to granuloma formation because of drug dispersion.

Catheter and pump-related problems persist as an opportunity for improvement. A recent systematic review of programmable IT opioid delivery systems for chronic noncancer pain found on average 27% of patients require equipment-revision surgery.[20] The catheter is the most vulnerable component of the system and the one most prone to problems. The frequency of catheter-related complications has been reported to be more than 30%.[21] A previous study of IT delivery systems by Penn et al[22] found catheter malfunction occurring at rates varying from 10% to 40%. Catheter malfunction can be divided into the following categories: (1) disconnection from the pump or port, (2) large to small catheter disconnect (if present), (3) kinks or holes in the catheter, (4) catheter breaks, and (5) catheter dislodgements. The implantable infusion pumps have two locations where the catheter may become disconnected—from the pump or port or from the large to small catheter disconnect. Over time, the catheters may develop a kink or hole and may also break anywhere along the catheter. Penn et al[22] performed a prospective study of thin- and thick-walled IT catheter reliability in 102 patients. Sixty percent of the patients had no catheter complications; the remaining patients had one to five complications. Most of the complications occurred in the thin-walled Silastic catheter, and the authors concluded that the thin-walled Silastic catheter does not perform well and that larger, thick-walled catheters should be used.[22] Presently, most of the catheters in use are thick walled. Since this article was published, there have been improvements in catheter technology; however, it is unclear if improvements have actually decreased catheter-related complications. Further improvements are needed.

Surgical technique to reduce the risk of complications is primarily practitioner dependent. Postoperative catheter migration caused by pulling of the catheter by pump movement with patient ambulation and bending is a common yet frustrating occurrence that requires surgical revision. Therefore, surgical anchors and anchoring technique to limit catheter migration is a common focus. Right-angled anchors used in concert with straight anchors have been supported by some to limit migration.[23]

Failures and Recalls

On August 27, 2009, the FDA notified health care professionals of a Class 1 recall of Medtronic Sutureless Connector Catheters and Revision Kit Models 8709SC, 8731SC, 8578, and 8596SC when paired with Medtronic IsoMed pumps. Medtronic Neuromodulation recalled the use of INDURA 1P Intrathecal Catheter and Sutureless pump Connector Revision Kit with IsoMed infusion pumps. A design incompatibility prohibits the sutureless connector catheter from connecting properly to the IsoMed pump, resulting in catheter disconnection or blockage. As of August 2009, Medtronic Neuromodulation had received 10 reports worldwide

of improper connection of the Sutureless Connector Catheter to the IsoMed pump requiring medical interventions to correct the problem.[24] Currently, the Sutureless Connector may be used for connection of the IT catheter to the implanted Medtronic SyncroMed II and SynchroMed EL infusion pumps only.

Finally, surgical complications such as infection and bleeding pose risk of complications. There have been no controlled trials on surgical implantation technique.[4] Future investigation into optimal perioperative care, percutaneous approach, and surgical technique to improve outcome and reduce complications is warranted.

References

1. Smith HS, Deer TR, Staats PS, et al: Intrathecal drug delivery. *Pain Physician* 11(suppl):S89-S104, 2008.
2. Deer TR, Krames ES, Hassenbusch SJ, et al: Polyanalgesic Consensus Conference 2007: recommendations for the management of pain by intrathecal (intraspinal) drug delivery: report of an interdisciplinary expert panel. *Neuromodulation* 10:300-328, 2007.
3. Kan J, Yang Z, Tang K, et al: [Pumping performance of a new piezoelectric pump for drug delivery]. *Sheng Wu Yi Xue Gong Cheng Xue Za Zhi* 21:297-301, 2004.
4. Ilias WT: Optimizing pain control through the use of implantable pumps. *Med Dev* 1:41-47, 2008.
5. InSet Technologies Inc: Information on file with the company. 500 International Drive, Suite 141 Mt. Olive, NJ 07828.
6. Rosen SD, Rauck R, Barsa J, et al: Multi-center evaluation of drug delivery accuracy with the Prometra intrathecal infusion pump. *Pain Med* 10:124, 2009.
7. Trials C: *Prometra implantable programmable pump (PUMP)*, accessed from http://clinicaltrials.gov/ct2/show/NCT00817596; 2009.
8. Trials C: *Prometra's utilization in mitigating pain II (PUMP2)*, accessed from http://clinicaltrials.gov/ct2/show/NCT00866164; 2009.
9. Berg AB, Deer T, Dunbar E, et al: *Efficacy of morphine sulfate infusion via the Prometra® intrathecal infusion pump. A prospective multicenter evaluation*. New York, 2009, Presented at the 5th World Congress Institute of Pain.
10. Codman & Shurtleff Inc.: MedStream. Information on file with the company. 325 Paramount Drive Raynham, MA 02767.
11. Alfred Mann Foundation: Medallion pump. Information on file with the company. 25134 Rye Canyon Loop, Suite 200 Santa Clarita, CA 91355.
12. U.S. Food and Drug Administration: *PMA-premarket approval*, 2009, accessed from http://www.accessdata.fda.gov/scripts/cdrh/cfdocs/cfPMA/PMA.cfm?ID=4499.
13. Ilias W, Buchser E, Demartini L: Patient-controlled analgesia in chronic pain patients: experience with a new device designed to be used with implanted programmable pumps. *Pain Pract* 8:164-170, 2008.
14. Rainov N: Making a case for programmable pumps over fixed rate pumps for the management of fluctuations in chronic pain and spasticity: a literature review. *Neuromodulation* 5:88-99, 2002.
15. Coffey RJ, Owens ML, Broste SK, et al: Mortality associated with implantation and management of intrathecal opioid drug infusion systems to treat noncancer pain. *Anesthesia* 111:881-892, 2009.
16. Deer TR, Krames E, Levy RM, et al: Practice choices and challenges in the current intrathecal therapy environment: an online survey. *Pain Med* 10:304-309, 2009.
17. Ghafoor VL, Epshteyn M, Carlson GH, et al: Intrathecal drug therapy for long-term pain management. *Am J Health Syst Pharm* 64:2447-2461, 2007.
18. Hassenbusch S, Burchiel K, Coffey RJ, et al: Management of intrathecal catheter-tip inflammatory masses: a consensus statement. *Pain Med* 3:313-323, 2002.
19. Murphy P, Skouvaklis, D, Amadeo, R, et al: Intrathecal catheter granuloma associated with isolated baclofen infusion. *Anesth Analg* 102:848-852, 2006.

20. Turner J, Sears, J, Loeser J: Programmable intrathecal opioid delivery systems for chronic noncancer pain: a systematic review of effectiveness and complications. *Clin J Pain* 23:185-190, 2007.

21. Albright AL, Gilmartin R, Swift D, et al: Long-term intrathecal baclofen therapy for severe spasticity of cerebral origin. *J Neurosurg* 98:291-295, 2003.

22. Penn RD, York MM, Paice JA: Catheter systems for intrathecal drug delivery. *J Neurosurg* 83:215-217, 1995.

23. Li TC, Chen MH, Huang JS, et al: Catheter migration after implantation of an intrathecal baclofen infusion pump for severe spasticity: a case report. *Kaohsiung J Med Sci* 24:492-497, 2008.

24. U.S. Food and Drug Administration: *Medtronic neuromodulation, INDURA 1P intrathecal catheter, intrathecal catheter, sutureless pump connector revision kit, and intrathecal catheter pump segment revision kit*. Class 1 recall, August 27, 2009. Online at http://www.fda.gov/MedicalDevices/Safety/RecallsCorrectionsRemovals/ListofRecalls/ucm183735.htm.

23 Trialing for Ziconotide Intrathecal Analgesic Therapy

Allen W. Burton

CHAPTER OVERVIEW

Chapter Synopsis: In the realm of intrathecal drug delivery systems (IDDS) for chronic intractable pain, ziconotide presents a new therapeutic avenue. This nonopioid drug acts as an antagonist at voltage-dependent calcium channels in the spinal cord. Accordingly, the side effect and dosage profiles differ substantially from the more familiar opioid effects. Although ziconotide carries its own risks, clinicians should educate themselves to the specific benefits and considerations associated with this relatively new tool in their arsenal. Patients and their families should also receive substantial education about the drug and its possible effects in starting IDDS. The drug's cost contributes additional reason for serious patient commitment to the drug trial procedure. Patients either with or without an existing pump may be candidates for ziconotide therapy. Patients with pain refractory to opioids or with untenable side effects represent another population that potentially could benefit from ziconotide.

Important Points:
- Ziconotide is a novel intrathecal (IT) calcium channel blocking, potent analgesic agent that should be considered in patients with refractory pain syndromes.
- Clinicians need not be intimidated or fear the ziconotide side effect profile because the side effects are dose dependent and reversible unlike many of the lethal side effects that can be seen with conventional IT therapies.
- With careful, methodical attention to low starting doses, clinicians can add another potent weapon to their pain treatment armamentarium.

Clinical Pearls:
- Ziconotide is a nonopioid with subtle central nervous system side effects at low doses; it must be approached cautiously but not overly so.
- Ziconotide is potent at microgram doses; as such, clinicians need to pay careful attention to precise dosing and adjustments during the trial.
- If a patient experiences side effects during the trial, it is acceptable to back down the dose slightly and continue the trial.

Clinical Pitfalls:
- Ziconotide is expensive (compared with other IT agents), and patients need to understand their commitment to the trial procedure.
- The patient and family should understand the side effect profile when embarking on the trial because the drug has unique side effects.

Introduction

Ziconotide is a nonopioid intrathecal (IT) analgesic approved in the management of severe chronic pain patients for whom IT therapy is indicated. Many refractory chronic pain patients may be candidates for this therapy. Because of the narrow therapeutic window of ziconotide, many clinicians remain uncertain as to how to trial the medication. Many experts disagree on the best trial methodology, including the duration, dose, and measured parameters. In this chapter, two basic scenarios are addressed: the existing pump patient and the pump candidate.

Establishing Diagnosis

Diagnoses that are amenable to ziconotide therapies are diverse with the common thread being refractory, difficult-to-manage pain. Ziconotide has been studied extensively in pain populations, including the chronic pain population, mostly with failed back surgery syndrome (FBSS), as well as a cancer pain and HIV/AIDS-related pain syndromes.[1-3] Many of the patients in these studies had neuropathic pain, but nociceptive and visceral pain were also noted to respond. Many potential candidates for ziconotide may already have an IT pump in place and are failing to respond to their analgesic regimen, but others may not have a pump or catheter in place.

Guidelines

Exact guidelines and timing for considering ziconotide therapy exist in the form of the spinal Polyanalgesic Consensus Conference.[4] Patients who have existing IT therapy in place with unsatisfactory analgesia or overwhelming side effects may be ziconotide candidates. Existing pump patients who appear to be developing tolerance to opioids or intolerable side effects, whether cognitive, edema, endocrine related, or others, should be considered.

Patients refractory to medical management, specifically opioid medications—whether oral, transdermal, or parenteral—may be good candidates for a ziconotide trial as a first IT therapy. The Polyanalgesic Consensus Conference guidelines support consideration of ziconotide as a first-line IT medication as opposed to only considering the failed pump patients.

Patient Management and Evaluation

Patients being considered for ziconotide therapy should have a careful review to ensure that all more conservative therapies have failed to provide adequate relief or caused side effects. Next, the patients should be educated about ziconotide because of the unique neurocognitive side effect profile of this agent. The family or caregivers should be included in the education session so they may provide an independent corroboration or assessment of trial efficacy or monitor for side effects. Lastly, any contraindications to a spinal catheter or ziconotide should be elucidated. Catheter contraindications include coagulopathy, active infection, thecal sac compromise by tumor, uncooperative patient, and others. Ziconotide contraindications include preexisting delirium, hypersensitivity to ziconotide, and psychosis per the drug label.[5]

Outcomes Evidence

Ziconotide trials have been done using several methodologies, including continuous infusion, short-term infusion, and bolus injection trials. Recently, a review of the available data comparing these trial methods was done; this is reviewed in this section.[6]

Continuous Infusion Trials: Open-Label Investigation with External Pumps

Three published reports that describe continuous infusion trialing studies were identified (**Table 23-1**). One was an open-label study, one was a retrospective chart review, and one was a case report.[7-9]

In this multicenter study[7], ziconotide was initiated at a dose of 2.4 µg/day and titrated upward over the course of 1 to 4 weeks; doses were increased in increments of 2.4 µg/day or less (up to 3 times per week) until meaningful analgesia or the maximum dose (21.6 µg/day; this dose was higher than the maximum recommended dose in the ziconotide prescribing information [19.2 µg/day])[7] was achieved or until intolerable adverse events (AEs) occurred. Effectiveness was assessed by Visual Analog Scale of Pain Intensity (VASPI) scores, the Categorical Pain Relief Scale (CPRS), and the Clinical Global Impression (CGI) scale (2 scales on which satisfaction with therapy and overall pain control were assessed).

A total of 71 patients with severe chronic malignant ($n = 2$) or nonmalignant ($n = 69$) pain were enrolled (39 men, 32 women; mean age, 52.8 years). Common pain types were neuropathic (70.4%), mixed (54.9%), nociceptive (40.8%), and degenerative (36.6%; patients could have been included in more than one pain classification). Mean ziconotide doses were 2.3 µg/day at initiation, 3.4 µg/day at week 1, and 4.0 to 4.1 µg/day for the remainder of the study. From baseline (before ziconotide exposure) to weeks 1, 2, 3, and 4, VASPI scores significantly ($P \leq 0.005$) improved by a median of 11.0% ($n = 69$), 32.6% ($n = 59$), 31.0% ($n = 48$), and 23.5% ($n = 23$), respectively. At the termination visit, 52.2% of patients reported moderate to complete pain relief on the CPRS, 53.6% of patients reported good to excellent pain control on the CGI scale, and 62.3% of patients reported they were at least somewhat satisfied with ziconotide therapy on the CGI scale. During the trial, the most common (experienced by >5% of patients) ziconotide-related AEs were dizziness, nausea, asthenia, vertigo, and headache. Although serious AEs were reported by 19 patients (26.8%), only one of these AEs (asthenia or leg weakness) was considered to be related to ziconotide. Five patients (7.0%) developed meningitis during the trial; however, none of the cases were considered to be related to ziconotide therapy. Four of the five cases resolved within 10 days, and none of the cases were ongoing at

---

Table 23-1: Ziconotide Continuous Infusion Trialing: Summary of Data

Reference	Type of Study	Patients (n)	Ziconotide Doses	Efficacy Results	Safety Results
Ver Donck et al[7a]	Open label	71	Mean initial dose, 2.3 µg/day; mean doses ranged from 3.4 to 4.1 µg/day for the remainder of the study	Median improvement from baseline in VASPI score ranged from 11.0% to 32.6% during the study	• Common AEs[b] were dizziness, nausea, asthenia, vertigo, and headache • SAEs occurred in 26.8% of patients; only one SAE was considered ziconotide related (asthenia or leg weakness)
Ting et al[8c]	Retrospective chart review	7	Initial dose, 1.2 or 2.4 µg/day; mean maximum dose,[d] 2.5 or 5.6 µg/day	Adequate analgesia[e] was achieved by 71.4% of patients	• The AEs of postdural puncture headache ($n = 3$), catheter dislodgment ($n = 2$), and deep vein thrombosis ($n = 1$) were reported
Wermeling & Berger[10f]	Case report	1	0.3 to 100.0 ng/kg/hr	Substantial analgesia: VASPI score <20 mm, achieved on day 5	• The AEs of confusion, double vision, memory impairment, sedation, and slurred speech were reported; all AEs resolved after temporary (24-hour) discontinuation of ziconotide

[a]The study was sponsored by Elan Pharmaceuticals, Inc.
[b]AEs that occurred in >5.0% of patients.
[c]This investigator-initiated study was supported by Elan Pharmaceuticals, Inc., by an educational grant to MD Anderson Cancer Center.
[d]Mean final doses for the groups receiving initial ziconotide doses of 1.2 or 2.4 µg/day, respectively.
[e]Adequate analgesia was defined as a decrease in Visual Analog Scale score of ≥3 points or a >50% self-reported improvement in pain relief.
[f]The authors of the study have conducted clinical research that was sponsored by Elan Pharmaceuticals, Inc.
AE, adverse event; SAE, serious adverse event; VASPI, Visual Analog Scale of Pain Intensity.

study completion. In all instances, meningitis occurred after more than 2 weeks of treatment with an external pump.[7]

In this retrospective chart review[8], patient response to therapy was evaluated on the basis of achieving adequate analgesia, defined as a decrease from baseline Visual Analog Scale (VAS) pain score (an 11-point scale, with higher scores indicating worse pain) of 3 or more points or a greater than 50% improvement in self-reported pain relief. Seven patients with chronic severe pain were included in the study. Patients were divided into two groups on the basis of their starting ziconotide dosage (1.2 or 2.4 µg/day). The first group consisted of four patients who started ziconotide at a dosage of 1.2 µg/day. Two patients had postlaminectomy syndrome, one had postthoracotomy pain, and one had central thalamic stroke pain. Among these patients, the mean trial duration was 14.5 days, and the mean maximum ziconotide dosage was 2.5 µg/day. All four patients achieved adequate analgesia. Patients reported the complications (AEs) of postdural puncture headache (n = 2), catheter dislodgment (n = 1), and deep vein thrombosis (n = 1). Both postdural puncture headaches resolved with an epidural blood patch; the patient who experienced catheter dislodgment reported adequate analgesia at the time of dislodgment, and the catheter was not replaced. None of the AEs were considered to be related to ziconotide. The second group consisted of three patients who started ziconotide at a dosage of 2.4 µg/day. One patient had breast cancer and postmastectomy pain, one had pudendal neuralgia, and one had central thalamic stroke pain. The mean trial duration was 18.3 days, and the mean maximum ziconotide dosage was 5.6 µg/day. Adequate analgesia was achieved by one patient. The complications (AEs) of postdural puncture headache (n = 1) and catheter dislodgment (n = 1) were reported. The postdural puncture headache resolved with an epidural blood patch, and the dislodged catheter was replaced; neither AE was considered to be ziconotide related. Five of the seven patients achieved adequate analgesia.[8]

Lastly, a case report of an external pump with an infusion trial follows.[9] The patient was a 54-year-old man with refractory peripheral neuropathy secondary to AIDS. He was implanted with an IT catheter and fitted with an external pump. Before starting ziconotide therapy, his VASPI score was 67 mm. For the first 24 hours of the trial, the patient was administered ziconotide at a dose of 0.3 ng/kg/hr (approximately 0.5 µg/day for a 70-kg patient). The ziconotide dosage was titrated upward rapidly from 1.7 to 168.0 µg/day over 6 days. On day 5, the patient reported a substantial improvement in analgesia (VASPI score, <20 mm). On day 6, the patient reported confusion, double vision, memory impairment, sedation, and slurred speech. To manage these AEs, the ziconotide dose was decreased to 33.6 µg/day. He had good pain relief for approximately 6 months until he was diagnosed with meningitis, and ziconotide therapy was discontinued; the meningitis was not believed to have been associated with ziconotide therapy.[9]

Limited-Duration Infusion Trials: Open-Label Study

In this study,[10] patients with chronic nonmalignant pain and average VASPI scores of 50 mm or greater during the 3 days before study entry were assigned to receive 1-, 5-, 7.5-, or 10-µg IT infusions of ziconotide via an external pump over the course of 1 hour (Table 23-2); patients had the option to receive an additional trial of ziconotide after at least 1 week had elapsed. Before the trial, patients were weaned from all spinal drugs. Effectiveness was evaluated via VASPI scores and the CPRS, which were assessed before initiating ziconotide treatment and periodically during the 48 hours after the start of the trial. A total of 22 patients with chronic neuropathic pain participated in the study. Two patients received two doses of ziconotide, for a total of 24 trials; five patients received the 1-µg dose, eight patients received the 5-µg dose, six patients received the 7.5-µg dose, and five patients received the 10-µg dose.[10]

The means of the maximum improvement from baseline in VASPI scores during the first 4 hours after the start of the infusion were 8.4, 14.0, 28.8, and 16.2 mm for the 1-, 5-, 7.5-, and 10-µg dose groups, respectively. The means of the maximum

Table 23-2: Ziconotide Limited-Duration Infusion Trialing: Summary of Data[a]

Reference	Type of Study	Patients (n)	Ziconotide Doses	Efficacy Results	Safety Results
Wermeling et al[9b]	Open label	22	1, 5, 7.5, and 10 µg	• Dose-related analgesia; • CSF levels of ziconotide were significantly positively correlated (P <0.05) with several indices of effectiveness	• AEs were reported by 40% of patients after the 1-µg infusion and by 100% of patients in the remaining dose groups • Three severe AEs were reported among patients who received 10-µg doses (myasthenia, dizziness, and headache) • Dose and CSF levels of ziconotide were significantly positively correlated (P <0.05) with the incidence of AEs
Wermeling and Berger[10c]	Case reports	2	5- or 10-µg epidural infusion	• Substantial analgesia for ≥7 hours; first patient, VASPI score of 0 mm (during hours 1 to 3 and 5 to 20); second patient, VASPI score <20 mm (during first 7 hours)	• Both patients reported the AEs of headache and somnolence • The AEs of light-headedness, pruritus, nausea, and hypotension were reported by one or the other patient • All AEs resolved within several hours

[a]Ziconotide was administered intrathecally unless otherwise noted.
[b]The study was sponsored by Elan Pharmaceuticals, Inc.
[c]The authors of the study have conducted clinical research that was sponsored by Elan Pharmaceuticals, Inc.
AE, adverse event; CSF, cerebrospinal fluid; VASPI, Visual Analog Scale of Pain Intensity.

improvement from baseline in the CPRS during the first 4 hours after the start of the infusion were 2.2, 1.8, 2.7, and 2.0 for the 1-, 5-, 7.5-, and 10-µg dose groups, respectively. On the basis of these and other effectiveness results, the authors concluded that analgesia was dose related. In addition, in this study, cerebrospinal fluid (CSF) ziconotide levels were drawn, and the area under the concentration-time curve for CSF ziconotide levels was significantly positively correlated (P <0.05) with the results of several effectiveness parameters.

Two of the patients (40.0%) in the 1-µg ziconotide dose group and all of the patients in the remaining groups experienced at least one AE during the study; however, most AEs were considered mild to moderate in severity. Although four patients experienced hypotension, there was no relationship between hypotension and plasma levels of ziconotide. Three severe AEs (myasthenia, dizziness, and headache) were reported, all of which occurred in the 10-µg ziconotide dose group. Both ziconotide dose and area under the concentration-time curve for CSF ziconotide levels were significantly positively correlated (P <0.05) with an increased incidence of AEs in general.[9,10]

Epidural Infusion Trial

The safety and effectiveness of limited-duration ziconotide *epidural* trials were reported in two case reports.[11] The first patient was a 47-year-old woman with right sacroiliac joint dysfunction and complex regional pain syndrome. Over the course of 1 hour, 10 µg of ziconotide was delivered via an *epidural* catheter. Results from VASPI scores and the CPRS indicated that ziconotide provided dramatic analgesia that lasted more than 20 hours; at some time points during the trial, her VASPI score was 0 mm (hours 1 to 3 and 5 to 20; baseline VASPI score, 68 mm), and her CPRS was 5 (hours 1 to 3 and 5 to 12). The patient experienced mild side effects of light-headedness.[10]

The second case was a 47-year-old woman with lumbar degenerative disc disease, facet syndrome, lumbar radiculitis, sciatica, and myofascial pain syndrome. Systemic analgesics provided limited pain relief (VASPI score, 85 mm), and the patient was administered 5 µg of ziconotide via an *epidural* catheter over the course of 1 hour. She experienced substantial analgesia during the trial with VASPI scores less than 20 mm. The patient reported the mild AEs of somnolence, pruritus, nausea, and headache; these AEs resolved within 10 hours.

Bolus Trials: Double-Blind, Placebo-Controlled Trial

One of each of the following types of ziconotide bolus injection investigations was identified: a small double-blind, placebo-controlled trial, an open-label study, a single-center trial, and a retrospective chart review (**Table 23-3**).[12-15] The value of ziconotide bolus injections in predicting patient response to long-term therapy was assessed in the last three bolus injection studies.[13-15]

Each patient with severe chronic pain in this study was administered up to 4 IT ziconotide injections (placebo [0 µg], 2, 4, and 8 µg in a randomized sequence) over a 1-month period. VASPI scores were assessed before each injection (baseline) and each hour after the injection for 6 hours.

Data were obtained from six patients, who received a total of 20 injections (four injections of placebo and of 4-µg ziconotide, six injections of 2-µg ziconotide and of 8-µg ziconotide). Pain (types) diagnoses were (postlumbar) lumbar postlaminectomy syndrome ($n = 4$), erythromelalgia ($n = 1$), and spinal cord injury ($n = 1$). The proportion of patients who reported a greater than 50% reduction from baseline in VASPI score was 0% after the placebo injection, 17% after the 2-µg ziconotide injection, 25% after the 4-µg ziconotide injection, and 50% after the 8-µg ziconotide injection. The proportion of patients that reported a greater than 30% reduction from baseline in VASPI score was 25% after the placebo injection, 17% after the 2-µg ziconotide injection, 50% after the 4-µg ziconotide injection, and 67% after the 8-µg ziconotide injection; these proportions included those patients who achieved greater than 50% reduction in VASPI score. The proportion of patients who reported 30% or less reduction from baseline in VASPI score

Table 23-3: Ziconotide Bolus Trialing: Summary of Data

Reference	Type of Study	Patients (n)	Ziconotide Doses	Efficacy Results	Safety Results
Rosenblum[12a]	Randomized, double blind, placebo controlled	6	Placebo (0 µg), 2, 4, and 8 µg	Dose-related analgesia	• Mild nausea or dizziness was reported after 38% of ziconotide injections and after 25% of placebo injections • 33% of patients reported nausea and vomiting and ataxia after the 8-µg injection
Grigsby and McGlothlen[13a]	Ongoing, single center, open label	42	1 µg with the possibility of up to two additional doses (3 and 5 µg)	18.5% ($n = 27$) of patients achieved effectiveness[b] after the 1-µg injection	• Three of 27 patients (11.1%) experienced AEs (nausea with or without vomiting); all AEs resolved spontaneously
Okano et al[14]	Single center	11	1.2, 2.4, and 5 µg	72.7% of patients reported a >50% improvement in pain relief	• Three patients (27.3%) experienced SAEs (urinary retention, hallucination, and motor weakness, respectively)
Baumgartl[15a]	Retrospective chart review	4	5, 40, and 50 µg	75% of patients reported pain score reductions of 2 to 5 points (on a 10-point scale)	• One patient reported dysphoria; one patient reported nausea and dizziness

[a]An investigator-initiated trial that was sponsored by Elan Pharmaceuticals, Inc.
[b]A ≥50% improvement over baseline in pain score.
AE, adverse event; SAE, serious adverse event.

was 75% after the placebo injection, 83% after the 2-μg ziconotide injection, 50% after the 4-μg ziconotide injection, and 33% after the 8-μg ziconotide injection. Two patients (33%) reported nausea and vomiting and ataxia after the 8-μg ziconotide injection. Patients reported mild nausea or dizziness after six of the 16 (38%) ziconotide injections and after one of the four (25%) placebo injections.[12]

Bolus Trials: Open-Label Study

The predictive value of IT bolus trialing for the effectiveness of long-term ziconotide therapy was assessed in this ongoing study (Table 23-3). Patients in this study had chronic nonmalignant pain that was refractory to systemic and/or IT opioid therapy. A 1-μg IT injection of ziconotide was administered to each patient; pain was rated on a VAS before, 1 hour after, and 24 hours after the injection. In addition, 1 and 24 hours after injection, patients were administered the Patient Satisfaction Questionnaire (PSQ), on which patients indicated whether they strongly disagree, disagree, neither agree nor disagree, agree, or strongly agree that they were satisfied with the trial of ziconotide. If effectiveness (a ≥50% improvement in pain score from baseline) was not achieved and no serious AEs were reported, patients had the option to receive up to two additional ziconotide injections (3 and 5 μg). Patients who experienced effectiveness at any time within 24 hours or who were satisfied with their trial were administered continuous IT ziconotide therapy (added to their existing IT regimen, if applicable). Pain was assessed on a VAS at 2 weeks and at 1, 3, 6, and 12 months of continuous infusion.[13]

At the last assessment, 42 patients had enrolled in the study. Common pain (types) diagnoses were FBSS (45.2%), degenerative disc disease (31.0%), and low back pain (16.7%). Twenty-seven patients received a 1-μg ziconotide injection; five of these patients (18.5%) experienced effectiveness, and the majority of patients either agreed or strongly agreed on the PSQ that ziconotide provided satisfactory pain relief at both 1 hour (55.6%; $n = 27$) and 24 hours (58.3%; $n = 24$) after the injection. One additional patient experienced partial effectiveness (relief of her back pain but not her hip pain) and proceeded to the 3-μg trial. Eight patients received a 3-μg ziconotide injection; three patients (37.5%) experienced effectiveness, and many patients either agreed or strongly agreed that ziconotide provided satisfactory pain relief at both 1 hour (42.9%; $n = 7$) and 24 hours (42.9%; $n = 7$) after the injection. The two patients who received a 5-μg injection did not experience effectiveness. Nausea or vomiting was reported by two patients during the 1-μg trial and by one patient during the 3-μg trial; these AEs resolved spontaneously in all patients.[13]

Sixteen patients received continuous ziconotide therapy (mean dose at last assessment, 1.19 μg/day; range, 0.60 to 5.00 μg/day), and two patients were scheduled to begin continuous ziconotide infusion in this ongoing trial. Improvements in pain scores from baseline (range, 12.5% to 100%) were experienced by four of 15 patients (26.7%) after 2 weeks of continuous ziconotide infusion, five of 12 patients (41.7%) after 1 month, five of seven patients (71.4%) after 3 months, and two of five patients (40.0%) after 6 months. On the PSQ, the number of patients who agreed or strongly agreed that ziconotide provided satisfactory pain relief during continuous infusion were eight of 15 patients (53.3%) after 2 weeks, six of 12 patients (50.0%) after 1 month, seven of seven patients (100%) after 3 months, and four of five patients (80.0%) after 6 months. Pain scores were either unchanged or had worsened for the remaining patients at each time point. Continuous infusion was discontinued in two patients; one patient discontinued because

of cognitive changes, and the other patient discontinued for personal reasons. These preliminary data indicates that a single-shot ziconotide trial may predict long-term response.[13]

Bolus Trials: Single-Center Study

The value of ziconotide bolus trialing in predicting long-term patient response to ziconotide was also investigated in this study[14] (Table 23-3). Eleven patients with existing IT pumps received a 1.2-μg ($n = 4$), 2.4-μg ($n = 5$), or 5.0-μg ($n = 2$) ziconotide bolus injection. Patients were evaluated 2 weeks after the injections. Serious AEs were reported by three of 11 patients (27.3%; urinary retention, hallucination, and motor weakness, respectively); both patients who received a 5-μg injection reported serious AEs (urinary retention and motor weakness, respectively). Eight of 11 patients (72.7%) experienced greater than 50% improvement in pain relief after the ziconotide injection; these patients had ziconotide added to their existing IT regimens. Seven of the eight patients (87.5%) who received continuous ziconotide infusion reported improved analgesia after 6 months of ziconotide treatment.[14]

Bolus Trials: Retrospective Chart Review

The predictive value of high-dose IT ziconotide bolus trialing was evaluated in this chart review (Table 23-3). Four patients who received IT bolus administration of ziconotide were identified (patients may have received more than one injection); two patients received a 5-μg injection, two patients received a 40-μg injection, and two patients received a 50-μg injection. After trialing, three patients (75%) reported a pain reduction of 2 to 5 points (on a 10-point scale); pain relief first occurred between the third and fourth hours after injection and lasted for approximately 3 to 6 hours. One patient reported the AE of short-term dysphoria after receiving a 5-μg injection, and one patient reported the AEs of nausea and dizziness after receiving a 50-μg injection. After trialing, three patients were administered continuous IT ziconotide via an external pump. During continuous infusion, one patient who had experienced analgesia during trialing experienced similar analgesia during infusion, one patient who had experienced no analgesia during trialing experienced no analgesia during infusion, and one patient who had experienced analgesia during trialing experienced no analgesia during infusion.[15]

Expert Opinion

A group of physicians familiar with ziconotide treatment published one potential protocol for trialing ziconotide.[16] Continuous IT ziconotide infusion was the recommended means of trialing, and the suggested dosing schedule was 1.2 μg/day at initiation with dose increases of 1.2 μg/day every 12 to 24 hours over the course of 3 days. The authors stated that the trial may be ended early if adequate analgesia is achieved before the end of 3 days and that the trial may be extended if adequate analgesia is not achieved after 3 days and AEs are absent or tolerable. If intolerable AEs occur, it was recommended that the trial be terminated immediately. Although the guidelines indicated that trialing may be performed on an inpatient or outpatient basis, it was suggested that patients be hospitalized for at least 24 hours and closely monitored thereafter.

The rate of upward titration recommended for ziconotide trialing in these guidelines is greater than the rate of upward titration recommended for beginning long-term ziconotide therapy;[17]

therefore the severity and frequency of AEs is likely to be higher during trialing than during long-term therapy. The guidelines stressed that administration of long-term ziconotide therapy should not start at the final dose achieved during the trial; long-term therapy should be reinitiated at a low dose (0.5 to 2.4 µg/day), and dose increases should occur one time or less per week.

Conclusion

Most of the studies reviewed were not randomized clinical trials. Although reviewing small nonrandomized trials (some of which are not published) is unconventional, the paucity of data in this area makes reviewing all available case reports relevant. Physician preferences for trialing spinal analgesia appear to have changed over the past decade. One report from 1996 indicated that only 6.4% of patients were trialed with continuous IT infusion[18]; however, 45% of respondents to a 2005 physician survey preferred trialing by continuous IT infusion.[19] Although most pain clinicians are aware of the value of IT analgesic trials, controlled studies to compare the safety and effectiveness of different trialing methods have not yet been performed. Instead, clinicians must rely on empiric or consensus-driven algorithms when determining trialing protocols. In one published algorithm, IT bolus injections are the suggested means of trialing in patients with refractory cancer pain with life expectancies longer than 3 months; however, continuous IT infusion trials are recommended for patients who experience inadequate analgesia with a bolus injection trial, patients who have a severe incidental pain syndrome, and patients with neuropathic pain.[11] Although long-term IT therapy is more closely simulated by continuous IT infusion trialing than by bolus trialing, bolus trialing is simpler to perform and is less expensive than is continuous IT infusion trialing.[20] Unlike continuous infusion trials, a bolus injection trial may provide an inadequate time frame to assess potential side effects; however, the likelihood of infectious complications is greater with continuous infusion trials than with bolus trials. Trialing ziconotide via continuous IT infusion is the method recommended in one expert opinion piece.[16]

The dose of ziconotide administered during a trial may be related to the effectiveness of that trial. Results from a limited-duration infusion study and a bolus injection study reveal that patients who received higher doses of ziconotide often experienced greater pain relief than patients who received lower doses of ziconotide.[9,12] Results from the limited-duration infusion study also indicated that several effectiveness parameters were significantly positively correlated (P <0.05) with the area under the concentration-time curve for CSF ziconotide levels. However, results from a small ($n = 7$) retrospective study of continuous ziconotide infusion trials indicate that effectiveness is not dose related.[8]

In addition to potentially being related to effectiveness, the dose of ziconotide administered to a patient during trialing may also be related to the incidence of AEs. Results from the largest ($n = 22$) ziconotide trialing study that compared the effects of different ziconotide doses revealed that both higher doses of ziconotide and higher CSF levels of ziconotide were significantly positively correlated (P <0.05) with an increased incidence of AEs.[9] In that study, serious AEs (myasthenia, dizziness, headache) were reported by only those patients who received the highest dose of ziconotide (10 µg). However, results from a retrospective study of continuous ziconotide infusion trials suggest that safety is not dose related.[8] In the remaining trialing studies, the relationship between ziconotide dose and the incidence of AEs was either not reported or difficult to ascertain because of the small sample sizes. In general, the AEs

reported in ziconotide trialing studies were similar to those reported in ziconotide clinical trials.[21-23]

Meningitis is a potential risk of continuous IT infusion trialing via an external pump. For example, 37 of the 40 (92.5%) cases of meningitis that occurred in ziconotide-treated patients during clinical trials were in patients with external drug pumps.[24] In the open-label continuous infusion trialing study of ziconotide, meningitis occurred in 7.0% of patients.[7] In that study, all cases of meningitis occurred after more than 2 weeks of IT infusion, suggesting that limiting the length of a continuous infusion trial may likely reduce the risk of meningitis. In an expert opinion piece on ziconotide trialing, the recommended length of a continuous IT ziconotide infusion trial was 3 days.[16] Clinicians may choose to trial patients with known risk factors for the development of meningitis (e.g., diabetes, severe rheumatological diseases, malignancies, or potentially altered immune states)[25-27] with bolus injections instead of continuous infusion or to use continuous infusion but limit the duration of each trial to a few days. A recent meta-analysis on externalized IT catheters for cancer pain revealed a rate of serious infectious complications to be very low (<1%).[28]

To date, the superiority of one particular trialing method over another in predicting long-term patient response to spinal analgesia has not been demonstrated. In a prospective, randomized investigation of morphine trialing, it was discovered that bolus injections were no more predictive of long-term patient response than were continuous epidural infusion trials.[29] The predictive value of ziconotide trialing was investigated in three studies; bolus injections of ziconotide were used in all of these investigations.[13-15] In two studies, patients who experienced analgesia or were satisfied with their trial also often reported pain relief during continuous infusion.[13,14] Results from the other study were mixed; however, it had a very small sample size ($n = 4$).[15] In all three studies, generally only those patients who experienced analgesia during trialing went on to receive continuous ziconotide infusion, indicating a selection bias. Controlled studies are necessary to determine which method of ziconotide trialing is most predictive of patient response to long-term ziconotide therapy.

Trialing ziconotide via the epidural route was associated with analgesia in two published case reports.[9,10] However, ziconotide is a large, hydrophilic molecule, and transport from the epidural to the IT space is likely inhibited[16]; the molecular weight of ziconotide (2639 Daltons [Da]) is greater than that of small-molecule drugs that may be delivered epidurally (e.g., morphine [285 Da], clonidine [230 Da]).[5,30,31] Furthermore, ziconotide is approved for IT administration only.[5]

A 2009 survey of health care professionals who use IT therapy in their practices revealed that the majority of practitioners (64.0%) indicated that between 26% and 50% of their pain management patients are insured by a government payer such as Medicare.[32] Numerous third-party payers, including Medicare, mandate a successful neuraxial analgesic trial (e.g., improved analgesia, tolerable AEs) before an implantable infusion pump will be reimbursed. The Medicare guidelines require that for a patient who requires spinally infused opioids for the treatment of chronic pain, an initial trial "must be undertaken with a temporary IT or epidural catheter to substantiate adequately acceptable pain relief and degree of side effects (including effects on the activities of daily living) and patient acceptance."[33] Notably, clinical experience with IT opioids was limited when this requirement was written; revision of the requirement on the basis of currently available data may be warranted. Although the method of trialing is not specified by Medicare, it is possible that regional carriers have distinct trialing requirements.

Therefore, the need exists for examples of different trialing procedures to be detailed in the published literature.

Although literature on this topic is scant and mainly consists of small nonrandomized trials, after careful review of the available data and their own clinical experience, the authors recommend continuous IT infusion trials of ziconotide be used when feasible. However, the authors also recognize the need for controlled studies to further investigate other trialing procedures.

Preliminary reports suggest that continuous ziconotide trialing, in addition to being the method recommended by an expert group, generally produced analgesia.[7,8,10] However, analgesia is also associated with limited-duration infusion trialing[9,10] and bolus trialing.[12-15] Thus, all three methods may be viable means of trialing ziconotide. Given the small samples sizes and lack of controlled studies, it is currently not possible to determine the relative safety and effectiveness of these trialing methods nor is it possible to determine if trialing predicts patient response to long-term ziconotide therapy. Controlled studies that compare different ziconotide trialing procedures may be warranted.

One acceptable approach that my group is presently using applies a continuous catheter trial of approximately 1 week's duration with daily dose adjustments in patients without existing IT systems. In our patients with IT systems, we use a single injection trial to determine whether to add or replace current IT therapy with ziconotide.

Acknowledgements

The author gratefully notes contributions made to this chapter by Drs. Tim Deer, Mark Wallace, Richard Rauck, and Eric Grigsby.

Disclosure

The author has received research grants and speaker's honorarium from Elan, Inc., and a research grant from Medtronic, Inc.

References

1. Rauck RL, Wallace MS, Leong MS, et al: A randomized, double-blind, placebo-controlled study of intrathecal ziconotide in adults with severe chronic pain. *J Pain Symptom Manage* 31:393-406, 2006.
2. Staats PS, Yearwood T, Charapata SG, et al: Intrathecal ziconotide in the treatment of refractory pain in patients with cancer or AIDS: a randomized controlled trial. *JAMA* 291:63-70, 2004.
3. Wallace MS, Charapata SG, Fisher R, et al: Intrathecal ziconotide in the treatment of chronic nonmalignant pain: a randomized, double-blind, placebo-controlled clinical trial. *Neuromodulation* 9:75-86, 2006.
4. Deer T, Krames ES, Hassenbusch SJ, et al: Polyanalgesic Consensus Conference 2007: recommendations for the management of pain by intraspinal (intrathecal) drug delivery: report of an expert interdisciplinary panel. *Neuromodulation* 10(4):300-328, 2007.
5. Elan Pharmaceuticals, Inc: *PRIALT® [package insert]*, South San Francisco, CA, 2008, Elan Pharmaceuticals, Inc.
6. Burton AW, Deer T, Wallace MS, et al: Considerations and methodology for trialing ziconotide: a review. *Pain Physician* 13:23-33, 2010.
7. Ver Donck A, Collins R, Rauck RL, Nitescu P: An open-label, multicenter study of the safety and efficacy of intrathecal ziconotide for severe chronic pain when delivered via an external pump. *Neuromodulation* 11:103-111, 2008.
8. Ting JC, Phan PC, Phan MV, et al: *External trialing of intrathecal ziconotide via tunneled catheter is safe and effective.* Poster presented at the 12th World Congress of Pain, Glasgow, Scotland, August 17-22, 2008.
9. Wermeling D, Drass M, Ellis D, et al: Pharmacokinetics and pharmacodynamics of intrathecal ziconotide in chronic pain patients. *J Clin Pharmacol* 43:624-636, 2003.
10. Wermeling DP, Berger JR: Ziconotide infusion for severe chronic pain: case series of patients with neuropathic pain. *Pharmacotherapy* 26:395-402, 2006.
11. Burton AW, Rajagopal A, Shah HN, et al: Epidural and intrathecal analgesia is effective in treating refractory cancer pain. *Pain Med* 5:239-247, 2004.
12. Rosenblum SM: *Intrathecal bolus injection of ziconotide for severe chronic pain: evaluation of analgesic response.* Poster presented at the American Society of Anesthesiologists Annual Meeting, Orlando, FL, October 18-22, 2008.
13. Grigsby E, McGlothlen G: *Value of single-shot trialing in predicting the effectiveness of long-term ziconotide therapy.* Poster presented at the 12th Annual Meeting of the North American Neuromodulation Society, Las Vegas, December 7, 2008.
14. Okano D, Akbik H, Zollet R, et al: Single-shot intrathecal ziconotide to predict its pump infusion effect [APPM meeting abstract 162]. *Pain Med* 9:116, 2008.
15. Baumgartl WH: *Pilot study results on the safety of high dose intrathecal bolusing of ziconotide.* Poster presented at the 10th Annual Meeting of the North American Neuromodulation Society, Las Vegas, December 7-10, 2006.
16. Caraway D, Saulino M, Fisher R, Rosenblum S: Intrathecal therapy trials with ziconotide: a trialing protocol before initiation of long-term ziconotide intrathecal therapy is presented. *Practical Pain Manage* 8:53-56, 2008.
17. Fisher R, Hassenbusch S, Krames E, et al: A consensus statement regarding the present suggested titration for Prialt (ziconotide). *Neuromodulation* 8:153-154, 2005.
18. Paice JA, Penn RD, Shott S: Intraspinal morphine for chronic pain: a retrospective, multicenter study. *J Pain Symptom Manage* 11:71-80, 1996.
19. Ahmed SU, Martin NM, Chang Y: Patient selection and trial methods for intraspinal drug delivery for chronic pain: a national survey. *Neuromodulation* 8:112-120, 2005.
20. Prager JP: Neuraxial medication delivery: the development and maturity of a concept for treating chronic pain of spinal origin. *Spine* 27:2593-2605, 2002.
21. Rauck RL, Wallace MS, Leong MS, et al: A randomized, double-blind, placebo-controlled study of intrathecal ziconotide in adults with severe chronic pain. *J Pain Symptom Manage* 31:393-406, 2006.
22. Staats PS, Yearwood T, Charapata SG, et al: Intrathecal ziconotide in the treatment of refractory pain in patients with cancer or AIDS: a randomized controlled trial. *JAMA* 291:63-70, 2004.
23. Wallace MS, Charapata SG, Fisher R, et al: Intrathecal ziconotide in the treatment of chronic nonmalignant pain: a randomized, double-blind, placebo-controlled clinical trial. *Neuromodulation* 9:75-86, 2006.
24. Ver Donck A, Collins R, Rauck RL, Nitescu P: An open-label, multicenter study of the safety and efficacy of intrathecal ziconotide for severe chronic pain when delivered via an external pump. *Neuromodulation* 11:103-111, 2008.
25. Durand ML, Calderwood SB, Weber DJ, et al: Acute bacterial meningitis in adults. A review of 493 episodes. *N Engl J Med* 328:21-28, 1993.
26. Meyer CN, Samuelsson IS, Galle M, Bangsborg JM: Adult bacterial meningitis: aetiology, penicillin susceptibility, risk factors, prognostic factors and guidelines for empirical antibiotic treatment. *Clin Microbiol Infect* 10:709-717, 2004.
27. Pappas PG, Perfect JR, Cloud GA, et al: Cryptococcosis in human immunodeficiency virus-negative patients in the era of effective azole therapy. *Clin Infect Dis* 33:690-699, 2001.
28. Aprili D, Bandschapp O, Rochlitz C, et al: Serious complications associated with external intrathecal catheters used in cancer pain patients. *Anesthesiology* 111:1346-1355, 2009.
29. Anderson VC, Burchiel KJ, Cooke B: A prospective, randomized trial of intrathecal injection vs. epidural infusion in the selection of patients

for continuous intrathecal opioid therapy. *Neuromodulation* 6:142-152, 2003.

30. PubChem Compound Database: Clonidine: compound summary (CID 2803), accessed March 17, 2009, from http://pubchem.ncbi.nlm.nih.gov/summary/summary.cgi?cid=2803.

31. PubChem Compound Database: Morphine: compound summary (CID 5288826), accessed March 17, 2009, from http://pubchem.ncbi.nlm.nih.gov/summary/summary.cgi?cid=5288826&loc=ec_rcs.

32. Deer TR, Krames E, Levy RM, et al: Practice choices and challenges in the current intrathecal therapy environment: an online survey. *Pain Med* 10:304-309, 2009.

33. Centers for Medicare & Medicaid Services, Medicare Coverage Database: NCD *for Infusion Pumps (280.14)* (publication number 100-3), accessed January 7, 2009, from http://www.cms.hhs.gov/mcd/viewncd.asp?ncd_id=280.14&ncd_version=2&basket=ncd%3A280%2E14%3A2%3AInfusion+Pumps.

24 Perioperative Management of Patients with Intrathecal Drug Delivery Systems

Thuong D. Vo, Ignacio Badiola, and F. Michael Ferrante

CHAPTER OVERVIEW

Chapter Synopsis: This chapter provides an overview of the procedure of intrathecal (IT) drug delivery on the whole. The treatment can provide a significant reduction in chronic pain (or spasticity) and a concurrent improvement in quality of life. Importantly, patient expectation and education appear to be critical factors in successful therapy. Careful consideration of patient selection, including a complete psychological assessment, also contributes to good outcomes. Patients receiving IT drug delivery generally have refractory pain or untenable side effects to opioid medications but should demonstrate drug sensitivity in a pre-implantation trial. Similar to any surgical procedure, pump implantation requires special precautions to avoid adverse reactions or outcomes, particularly in certain vulnerable populations. IT drug delivery can be used for both cancer and noncancer pain and has been used to treat neuropathic as well as visceral and nociceptive pain.

Important Points:
- The use of IT agents should be considered when other more conservative options fail or are not acceptable.
- New agents bring excitement to the field. The use of new agents should be based on an algorithmic thought process that involves animal safety studies, human safety, and clinical efficacy.

Clinical Pearl:
- IT opioids are the most commonly used drugs for IT therapy. Other options are considered when opioids are not effective or give unacceptable side effects.

Clinical Pitfalls:
- IT therapies have been available for many years and have had widespread use. Despite this, the U.S. Food and Drug Administration has approved only three drugs for labeled use. When using other agents, the decision should be based on scientific merit and clinical necessity.
- Recommendations have been made regarding drug doses and concentrations based on patient safety and adverse outcomes. These guides should be followed when possible, although the physician should use clinical judgment based on a risk-to-benefit analysis when treating individual patients.

The Evolution of Intrathecal Therapies

The concept of intrathecal (IT) therapies began in 1898 when August Bier performed "cocainization of the spinal cord." The use of IT phenol for cancer pain was described in the 1960s.[1] Work in the early 1980s on IT morphine in cancer patients paved the path for approval of IT delivery of morphine. Many investigators in the 1980s and 1990s expanded the roles of IT therapies to include noncancer patients. A multicenter retrospective study[2] showed that IT therapies were equally efficacious in noncancer patients. The same study also found that patients with somatic pain responded better than those with neuropathic pathology.[2] Over the years, monotherapy with morphine expanded to include various combinations of opioids with local anesthetics and α_2-agonists. The indications for IT therapy also expanded from the initial treatment of cancer pain and postlaminectomy (failed back

surgery syndrome) to encompass complex regional pain syndrome, postherpetic neuralgia, and painful peripheral neuropathy. At present, the list of indications for IT therapy continues to expand.

The potential advantages of IT therapy over other modes of drug delivery were quickly recognized. As the indications and the number of pharmacological agents for IT therapy rapidly evolved, so did the technology for IT delivery systems. An externally programmable and battery-powered IT delivery system, Medtronic SynchroMed (Minneapolis, MN) became available in 1991.[3] With this system, the flow rate (i.e., the dose of medication) could be externally programmed. A programmable IT delivery system for the treatment of patients with chronic pain is practical and allows numerous dosing alternatives. Today, the majority of IT delivery systems for treatment of cancer and noncancer pain are implantable programmable pumps.

Establishing Diagnosis

There are many factors to consider when considering permanent IT pump placement in a specific patient. **Box 24-1** shows selection criteria based on whether pain is malignant or nonmalignant in origin.

Basic Science of Spinal Analgesia

Conceptually, administration of an analgesic at a specific IT or epidural spinal level should avoid the dose-limiting side effects that would be produced with systemic opioids, as dosage would be dramatically reduced. The problem with this concept is that there have been multiple human studies demonstrating that the more lipophilic opioids produce analgesia via spinal and systemic mechanisms.[4] An intraspinally administered agent has many different tissues it must traverse on its journey to the receptor. Systemic uptake still occurs. These factors ultimately decrease the amount of opioid that reaches the site of action, the opioid receptors in the dorsal horn.

In the spinal cord, the gray matter can be divided into lamina, known as Rexed's laminae. The first six laminae are part of the dorsal horn and receive all afferent information from the periphery. Pain is modulated within the dorsal horn by descending pathways from higher rostral centers. The second lamina is known as the substantia gelatinosa. Opioid receptors are located in the substantia gelatinosa and are thought to assist in pain modulation.[5] The most important opioid receptors involved in pain modulation include the μ, δ, and κ receptors. These receptors bind endogenous or exogenous opioids and are coupled to G-proteins. These G-proteins lead to inhibition of adenylyl cyclase. This leads to activation of potassium currents, ultimately leading to membrane hyperpolarization. Other mechanisms may be involved including kinases and the phospholipase C cascade.[6] Adaptation in any of these pathways because of chronic opioid exposure may lead to tolerance.

Guidelines

At the dawn of IT therapy, preservative-free morphine sulfate was the first agent approved by the U.S. Food and Drug Administration (FDA) for IT use. Baclofen and ziconotide followed later. Off-label use of other narcotic and non-narcotic agents is common. These agents are used either individually or in combination and commonly include hydromorphone, fentanyl, clonidine, and bupivacaine.

Opioids

IT morphine reduces pain by more than 50% with the greatest efficacy in patients with somatic or mixed pain. There are reports of leg edema during morphine infusion. Besides catheter-tip granuloma, patients on IT morphine can develop hypogonadotropic hypogonadism, central hypocortisolism, growth hormone deficiency, and/or decreased libido.[7] In most patients, sexual function improves with gonadal steroid supplementation. Similar to other opioids, tolerance can develop with chronic therapy. Over time, escalating doses of morphine or morphine equivalents are needed to maintain pain relief. Some tolerant patients eventually require morphine in combination with other adjuvant medications or a different opioid because of inadequate pain control.

Hydromorphone is the alternative for patients who do not tolerate the side effects of IT morphine. Mean pain scores improve, and the side effects of drowsiness and nausea lessen. However, leg edema also occurs with protracted hydromorphone exposure. Catheter-tip granulomas also develop with hydromorphone but with less frequency. The oral equianalgesic ratio of hydromorphone:morphine is approximately 1:4 to 1:8.[8] Accordingly, the equivalent IT dose of hydromorphone is hypothesized to be 20% that of morphine in order to provide the same level of pain relief. Because the dose requirement of hydromorphone is relatively small, the side effects should also be less.

Other opioids have also been studied for IT administration. In a retrospective analysis, patients on fentanyl (10.5 to 115 μg/day) reported a 68% reduction in pain on average and an overall satisfaction rate of more than 75%.[9] Long-term exposure to sufentanil has not been studied. IT methadone has been studied in cancer and noncancer patients.

Local Anesthetics

The combination of bupivacaine with an intraspinal opioid results in a decrease in the dose of opioid to achieve the same level of analgesia (dose-sparing effect). Although rarely disabling, side effects of local anesthetics include numbness, urinary retention, and orthostatic hypotension. Because of its low cardiotoxicity profile, ropivacaine was compared with bupivacaine in a small double-blind, randomized, cross-over trial.[10] A higher dose of ropivacaine was required to achieve the same analgesic effect, although side effects were equivalent.

Adrenergic Agonists

IT clonidine used as monotherapy results in inadequate pain control and intolerable side effects. The combination of clonidine and opioid yields mixed results in somatic pain, but the same combination provides excellent pain relief in patients with neuropathic pain. Frequent side effects associated with clonidine are hypotension, fatigue, dry mouth, and sedation.

N-Methyl-D-Aspartic Acid Agonists

In rodent models, IT ketamine in combination with morphine provides analgesia. Possible mechanisms are synergistic interaction between ketamine and morphine, and/or attenuation of morphine-induced tolerance, or both.[11] Unfortunately, IT infusion of ketamine led to severe histologic and gross spinal cord toxicity.

Baclofen

Baclofen is a synthetic pre- and postsynaptic γ-aminobutyric acid type B receptor (GABA-B) agonist. Lamina II and III of the dorsal horn of the spinal cord contain a high concentration of baclofen receptors. Baclofen's mechanism of action is mediated by G-proteins. Presynaptic binding inhibits calcium influx, and postsynaptic binding augments potassium conductance, resulting in hyperpolarization. The net effect is decreased release of nociceptive neurotransmitters such as aspartate, glutamate, and substance P.

Although it is a poor antiepileptic agent, baclofen is effective in reducing tonicity in patients with spasticity. Candidates suitable for IT baclofen have failed oral management or did not tolerate the side effects of high-dose oral baclofen. Similar to other patients being considered for IT therapy, these patients need to undergo initial multidisciplinary assessment. The degree of spasticity must be quantitated before and after the therapy is initiated. Realistic goals are discussed with patients during these initial visits, and they include increased functionality, decreased contractures, care facilitation, overall comfort, and the need for continued refills. Poor compliance and unrealistic expectations are considered relative contraindications to IT baclofen therapy.

Approximately 10% to 75% of patients experience side effects with IT baclofen. The most common side effect is lethargy. Less frequent side effects include bradycardia and respiratory depression. These side effects can be minimized by slow drug titration. Patients with head trauma are at risk for new-onset seizures after institution of IT baclofen. There are case reports of IT baclofen exacerbating scoliosis. The exact mechanism is not known but could be related to the change in muscle tonicity of the paraspinous and truncal muscles.[12]

IT baclofen administration cannot be stopped abruptly because of a potentially life-threatening withdrawal syndrome. The withdrawal symptoms include fever, altered mental status, and profound muscular rigidity.

Gabapentin

IT gabapentin has been studied in rodent models. IT gabapentin reduces mechanical allodynia and thermal hyperalgesia. Compared with the subcutaneous and intraperitoneal routes, the increased potency of IT gabapentin is 10-fold greater. It also has minimal effect on heart rate and blood pressure. IT gabapentin and clonidine act synergistically.

Ziconotide

Ziconotide was approved by the FDA in 2004 for IT administration in patients with chronic pain refractory to other IT medications. The drug is a synthetic derivative of a toxin produced by the *Conus magus* sea snail. The toxin is a potent inhibitor of N-type voltage-sensitive calcium channels in the central and peripheral nervous systems.[13] Although approved for monotherapy, it is sometimes used in combination with other IT agents in clinical practice. A small observational study suggested that ziconotide in combination with an opioid is potentially safe and effective for patients with refractory chronic pain.[14] Side effects include abnormal gait, nausea, vomiting, urinary retention, dizziness, nystagmus, blurred vision, diplopia, memory impairment, and orthostatic hypotension. Side effects are associated with rapid titration and are usually improved with dose reduction.

Neostigmine, Adenosine, and Ketorolac

Much of the clinical experiences with neostigmine is derived from its use as a spinal anesthetic. Compared with bupivacaine, it has a quicker onset of sensory block and a longer duration of motor and sensory block. Side effects include nausea and vomiting. IT adenosine reduces the area of allodynia and hyperesthesia. Adverse effects include back pain. Prostaglandins are hypothesized to play a key role in central sensitization. However, IT ketorolac does not reduce pain.

Polyanalgesic Therapy

Polyanalgesic drug use to improve outcomes and safety has become an important issue when considering long-term care of patients receiving IT agents. In 2007, the Polyanalgesic Consensus Conference was convened, and recommendations were made to elevate ziconotide to first-line status along with morphine and hydromorphone. The consensus also recommended fentanyl as a second-line option as a solo agent largely because of its established safety, reduced risk of inflammatory mass, and efficacy when targeting pain generators near the catheter tip. The authors also recommended changes in concentration and maximum daily dosing. These recommendations were believed to represent ideal situations for the implanting and managing physician and the exception was made in the paper for complex patients requiring physician risk-to-benefit assessment. These dosing recommendations were also discussed in the accompanying consensus on IT inflammatory mass prevention and management. These represented changes to the previous consensus conference that was convened in 2003 based on a review of updated literature and clinical safety analysis. In 2003, recommendations were made by the Polyanalgesic Consensus Conference (**Fig. 24-1**), which concluded that morphine or hydromorphone are reasonable starting drugs in step 1.[15] If intolerable side effects or inadequate analgesia occur at the maximum recommended dose of morphine, then change to hydromorphone is warranted, and vice versa. An alternative is to go to step 2, especially in patients with neuropathic pain. In step 2, morphine or hydromorphone is either combined with bupivacaine or clonidine. Some clinicians favor bupivacaine because of clonidine's hypotensive effects. On the other hand, some are more comfortable with clonidine because its safety profile for intraspinal use has been well characterized. Step 3 is a combination of bupivacaine and clonidine with either morphine or hydromorphone. If the step 2 combination of drugs provides inadequate analgesia or intolerable side effects, then step 3 is reasonable. Before progressing to step 4, all of the combinations of drugs in step 3 should have been tried. Step 4 includes fentanyl, sufentanil, midazolam, and baclofen. A reasonable strategy is to replace morphine or hydromorphone in steps 1 to 3 with fentanyl or sufentanil. Growing evidence supports the use of IT baclofen in patients with pain primarily caused by spasticity, rigidity, or muscle cramping. The experience with IT midazolam is limited to cancer pain. A preservative-free formulation is available in Europe but not in the United States. Steps 5 and 6 approach the realm of the unknown. Step 5 includes neostigmine, adenosine, and ketorolac. Step 6 includes ropivacaine, meperidine, gabapentin, buprenorphine, octreotide, and others. The Consensus recommends using step 5 or 6 only when all other modalities have failed.

The guides and recommendations for granuloma were updated in 2007 and published in *Neuromodulation*.[15a] The concentrations of the drugs were also changed in the 2007 Consensus paper. To

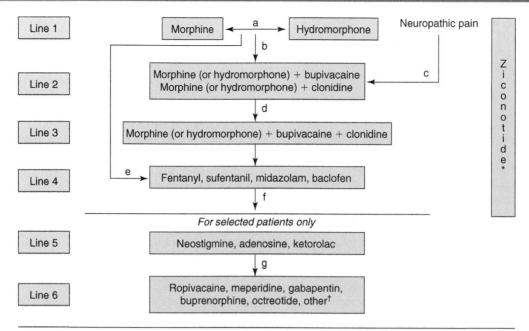

Fig. 24-1 Update of clinical guidelines for the use of intraspinal drug infusion in pain management. FDA, Food and Drug Administration; NMDA, *N*-methyl-D-aspartic acid. (Adapted from Hassenbusch JS, Portenoy KR, Cousins M, et al: Polyanalgesic Consensus Conference 2003: an update on the management of pain by intraspinal drug delivery—report of an expert panel, *J Pain Symptom Manage* 27:540-563, 2004.)

Table 24-1: Recommended Maximum Intrathecal Dosages and Concentrations

Drug	Dosage (mg/day)	Concentration (mg/mL)
Morphine	15	30
Hydromorphone	10	30
Bupivacaine	30	38
Clonidine	1.0	2.0

From Hassenbusch JS, Portenoy KR, Cousins M, et al: Polyanalgesic Consensus Conference 2003: an update on the management of pain by intraspinal drug delivery—report of an expert panel, *J Pain Symptom Manage* 27:540-563, 2004.

minimize complications of IT therapy, the Consensus also makes recommendations pertaining to the maximum dosages and concentrations of the four common agents (Table 24-1).[15] Morphine can be infused at a maximum concentration and rate of 30 mg/mL and 15 mg/day, respectively. The risk of catheter-tip granuloma parallels the increase in concentration and daily dose. At the recommended concentration and infusion rate, the risk of morphine-induced hyperalgesia is reduced. Hydromorphone can be maximally infused at a concentration of 30 mg/mL and at a rate of 10 mg/day. The maximum recommended concentration of bupivacaine is 38 mg/mL, and the rate is 30 mg/day. The total daily dose should attempt to preserve lower extremity motor function and bladder function. The concentration and dose should be kept

as low as possible. For most patients, the maximum recommended concentration and rate of clonidine is 2000 μg/mL and 1000 μg/day, respectively. Treatment should be initiated at 100 μg/day or lower in older and medically frail patients, hoping to reduce the risk of hypotension, sedation, peripheral edema, and cardiac arrhythmias. Before discontinuation, clonidine needs to be tapered to avoid withdrawal symptoms and rebound hypertension. Oral clonidine should be prescribed to patients if the infusion is abruptly discontinued. Interestingly, the dosages at which hypotension occur are in the range of 200 to 600 μg/day but rarely below or above this range. Please note the new recommendations on each of these drugs.

Indications and Contraindications

Proper patient selection, correct assessment of procedure benefit, and avoidance of iatrogenic exacerbation of the patient's existing medical condition are crucial for a successful IT therapy. One of the indications for IT therapy is failed oral analgesic therapy. If correctly identified, fewer than 10% of patients with chronic pain are suitable for IT therapy because more than 90% of patients will have adequate pain control on a combination of short- and long-acting analgesics. Besides patients taking high-dose analgesics, those with intolerable side effects are also appropriate for IT therapy. Contraindications to IT therapy include patient refusal or noncompliance, concurrent infection at time of implantation, patient failure to comprehend his or her responsibility after implantation, life expectancy, and unrealistic expectation of the level of pain relief. Some patients may fail the initial psychological evaluation, but their candidacy can be reinstated after the psychosocial issues are addressed.

Equipment

Tunneled Percutaneous Catheter

These are the same catheters used for acute pain management or continuous epidural anesthesia. The only difference is that the catheter itself is internalized or tunneled with the presumption that this will reduce catheter dislodgement from its intended location.[16] Thus, the duration of percutaneous catheter use can be prolonged with tunneling.

Implanted Catheter with Subcutaneous Injection Site

These catheters require surgical placement using fluoroscopy and sterile conditions. Catheters can be placed into the IT or epidural space. However, the two catheters that are most commonly used (the DuPen Silicone Rubber Epidural Catheter and the Port-a-Cath system) were only approved for epidural use. Final catheter tip location is several levels higher than point of entry into the epidural space to avoid migration out of the epidural space.

The DuPen catheter is essentially an exteriorized epidural catheter. The DuPen catheter was discontinued in April 2009. The Port-a-Cath system is totally internalized with a catheter in the epidural space and tunneled from the back to the reservoir site. The area selected for reservoir implant usually has a bone backstop (e.g., rib) to support the port during needle insertion. During placement, the port reservoir is secured to the fascia to prevent the port from inverting. The port is accessed using a noncoring needle (i.e., Huber needle) to prevent damage to the port septum from multiple needle insertions. The Huber needle can be connected to an external infusion device for a continuous infusion.

Totally Implanted Catheter with Implanted Infusion Pump

The first available infusion pump in the United States was the Infusaid Model 400. This pump was suitable only for continuous infusion. Because the rate of infusion could not be changed (the rate was set at the factory), the only way to change the amount of drug given to the patient was to change the concentration. It is easy to imagine how challenging this would be in patients who need frequent dose changes (i.e., cancer patients). Filling the pump was difficult, and inserting the needle incorrectly could lead to an overdose.

The Codman 3000 implantable constant flow infusion drug delivery system provides continuous infusion therapy for treatment of chronic pain, cancer, and spasticity. It is a battery-free system with no on-board electronic system. The system has an inner and outer chamber divided by an accordion style bellows. The outer chamber contains a propellant that is warmed by the patient's own body temperature. This leads to production of a constant pressure on the bellows, which causes the drug to flow out of the inner chamber through a filter and flow restrictor and then slowly out of the catheter.[17] Three reservoir sizes are available (16, 30, and 50 mL) with four preset flow rates available. Because it is a constant-flow pump, the only way to change the patient's dosage is to adjust the drug concentration during a pump refill. The flow rates are designated as high flow, medium flow, low flow, and ultra low flow. The actual flow rate for each depends on the size of the

reservoir with flow rates ranging from 0.3 mL/day to 3.4 mL/day. Bolus injections can be given through a closed tip needle with a needle shaft aperture that directs fluid away from the drug reservoir chamber and directly into the catheter. The needle has to be a special noncoring needle. Thus, the Codman system depends on proper needle type for refill or bolus in order to minimize the risk of overdose.

The new infusion systems, specifically the SynchroMed EL and now the SynchroMed II (Medtronic Inc, Minneapolis, MN), use the technology of pacemakers to allow programmability. The pump consists of a lithium battery, reservoir system, microprocessor, and antenna. An external programmer is used to communicate with the pump to change settings.

Technique

Pump Trials

The purpose of the trial is to determine which drug, if any, will benefit the patient. Trials can be performed by single-shot injection, continuous infusion, or intermittent bolus. In a study by Deer et al,[18] IT trials were successful in 93% of patients. In the implanted patients, numeric pain scores dropped by more than 47% for back pain and 31% for leg pain at 12 months of follow-up. At 12 months, 87% of patients were satisfied with the implant.

Patient Positioning

The trial procedure can be performed with the patient in a prone position on a fluoroscopic table that allows easy movement of a C-arm. A pillow under the abdomen help minimizes the normal lumbar lordosis. This greatly facilitates needle entrance into the IT space. It is recommended that the entire back from the lower scapular border to buttock be scrubbed and draped to minimize infectious risks.[19]

Trial Procedure

The technique of the trial procedure can use a continuous catheter with repeated boluses, infusion, or a single-bolus injection. At our institution, a pediatric Touhy needle is inserted at a level below the termination of the spinal cord. After the IT space is entered, as evidenced by cerebrospinal fluid (CSF) free flow, a radiopaque dye is injected to further confirm placement. After this is confirmed, either a single-bolus injection of the chosen opioid is administered or a catheter is placed through the needle and into the IT space. The catheter tip should be placed at the same spinal level where the permanent catheter tip will be placed. The location of the catheter tip depends on the condition being treated and the choice of opioid. Placement of the catheter tip near the spinal level mediating pain may be more important when using analgesic agents that are lipophilic, which penetrate further and faster into biological tissue than do hydrophilic agents (morphine and hydromorphone).[20]

The results of the trial are very important not only in their ability to guide which drug to use but also which patients would benefit from permanent implantation. The selection of who to permanently implant has to be carefully decided. Poor patient selection cannot be overcome by good technique or by using algorithms to salvage a poor response to trial.[21] A study performed by Deer and associates[21] showed no association between most factors and the success of the trial. Factors not associated with success included age and gender, previous pain treatments, use of psychological evaluations, duration of trial, and medical insurance. The only category shown to be associated with trial success was the type of pain upon presentation. Patients with neuropathic pain who underwent trial with opioid monotherapy had a success rate of 89% versus a 100% success rate with mechanical or mixed pain. The methodology of the trial (single bolus vs. continuous infusion) did not show a difference in outcome. During the trial, success can be evaluated by changes in numerical pain scores. Changes of greater than 50% are deemed to present efficacy. Presence of opioid side effects should be evaluated during the trial.

Implantation

The technique to place a permanent pump and catheter is usually performed in an operating room under sterile conditions. Permanent placement can be performed under local, spinal, or general anesthesia, but general anesthesia is usually chosen to ensure a more pleasant experience for the patient.

The patient is placed in the lateral decubitus position and is sterilely prepped to include the flank and abdomen. Intravenous antibiotics should be administered and should cover skin flora. Fluoroscopy can be used to identify the L2-L3, L3-L4, or L4-L5 levels. A level below the terminal portion of the spinal cord must be chosen. At this point, either the IT space can be entered percutaneously or a posterior midline incision that extends through the level of the needle placement can be made. The incision can be carried down to the supraspinous fascia followed by insertion of the Touhy needle into the IT space. Ideally, a shallow angled approach is used to avoid the need to make an acute bend as the catheter exits the needle and enters into the IT space, thereby facilitating insertion. After the catheter has been placed into the IT space, a purse-string suture with 2-0 silk is tied around the needle and subsequently tied down around the catheter as the needle is removed. This is done to minimize CSF leak around the catheter. The catheter is then anchored to the supraspinous fascia using an anchor that is provided by the manufacturer. The catheter fits through the anchor, and therefore puncture of the catheter is possible when suturing down the anchor. Free-flow CSF should be checked frequently. However, the proximal tip of the catheter should be clamped in between checks to prevent continuous CSF leakage.[22]

The pump is implanted in the lower abdominal quadrants below the belt line. Because of tissue movement when the patient is in the lateral decubitus position compared with when the patient is standing or sitting, it may be best to mark the incisions preoperatively with the patient in standing and sitting positions. The anterior ribs and the anterior superior iliac spine should be noted because a pump that is placed too high or too lateral may lead to patient discomfort. It is also important to not place the pump too deep because it may lead to problems in interrogation and refilling of the pump. The pump pocket incision should be made to approximate the size of the pump. The incision can be carried down to the rectus fascia in thin patients. This is followed by tunneling through the subcutaneous tissues from the pump pocket to the posterior incision. This must be done carefully to prevent accidental puncture of the peritoneum and possibly pleura. The catheter is then pulled through the tunnel to the pump pocket. The catheter can then be trimmed. It is important to again check for free flow of CSF before connecting the catheter to the pump. After it is connected, the pump can be placed back in the pocket and excess catheter placed behind the pump. The pump can be secured by suturing it to the underlying fascia, or the pump can be placed in a Dacron pouch, which can then be sutured to the underlying fascia. The Dacron pouch will ultimately endothelialize, assisting in forming a fibrous capsule around the pump. This will secure the pump but may make it difficult to remove in the future. After

adequate hemostasis is achieved, both the posterior and abdominal wounds should be irrigated and closed.

Patient Management and Evaluation

After a patient is identified as a candidate for IT therapy, he or she must undergo a multidisciplinary assessment to further evaluate his or her candidacy. The assessment includes psychological history and determination of support systems (or lack thereof), the pathophysiology of the pain, secondary gain issues, and life expectancy (especially for patients with cancer). IT therapy is cost-effective for cancer patients with life expectancies longer than 3 to 6 months and life expectancies longer than 11 to 22 months for noncancer patients.

When the patient satisfactorily completes the initial assessment, a trial is conducted to determine if the patient will benefit from IT opioid. Some pain specialists require patients to undergo detoxification before the trial. On the day of the trial, the patient should continue taking previous doses of oral analgesics to avoid symptoms of narcotic withdrawal, which may adversely confound the trial outcome. Immediately after the trial, the patient is placed in a monitored setting where periodic reassessment can be performed. The evaluation should, at a minimum, include pain relief and observation of side effects such as nausea or vomiting, urinary retention, and pruritus. At our institution, an IT catheter is left in place, and the patient is monitored overnight. The patient is evaluated periodically, and opioid is administered via the catheter as needed.

Because the IT dose of opioid is much less than via systemic routes of administration, the side effects should also be reduced. Nevertheless, they still exist. Common side effects are constipation, urinary retention, and pruritus. Myoclonus may develop after months of IT therapy and may be alleviated by dose reduction. Hydromorphone is a better choice for patients who experience pruritus and myoclonus with other opioids. Urinary retention is reversible and can be relieved by decreasing the dose.[23] Patients taking chronic opioids also have sex hormone deficiency requiring supplementation. Dependent edema has been associated with IT therapy.

Outcomes Evidence

There is a paucity of prospective, randomized, controlled trials examining the efficacy of IT therapy. Of the existing studies, it is difficult to make useful comparisons or to draw meaningful conclusions because of variations among study designs. There is moderate evidence to suggest the effectiveness of IT therapy in acute pain but limited or no evidence of efficacy for chronic pain. In other studies, there is moderate evidence to support IT therapy for long-term management of chronic noncancer pain. In a recent meta-analysis, patients with IT drug delivery systems (IDDS) have better pain control.[24] Based on a pain scale from 0 to 100, pain intensity decreased from a mean of 82 to 45 at 6 months and 44 at 12 months after permanent implantation of an IT pump. Another systematic review of IT therapy for long-term management of chronic noncancer pain demonstrated level II-3 or level III (limited) evidence.[25] More research is needed to determine the long-term benefits and risks of IDDS and therapy.

Mortality can be associated with IT therapy in patients with noncancer pain shortly after implant. The exact mechanism of death remains obscure. However, respiratory depression secondary to IT drug overdose or mixed IT and systemic drug interactions are plausible causes. Further analysis suggested the mortality rate to be 0.088% at 3 days, 0.39% at 1 month, and 3.89% at 1 year after implantation.[26] The mortality rates are higher than after spinal cord stimulator implant or lumbar discectomy.

Risk and Complication Avoidance

Techniques

IT access for catheter implantation places the patient at risk for postdural puncture headache (PDPH). Although many PDPHs resolve with conservative therapy consisting of hydration, caffeine, and analgesics, severe cases occasionally require an epidural blood patch. Epidural blood patches should be used judiciously (and avoided if possible) given the increased risk of infection when a non-sterile substance (blood) is placed in the region of a foreign body (catheter). It is advisable to perform the epidural blood patch under fluoroscopy to avoid inadvertent damage to the implanted catheter.

Light serosanguineous drainage from the wounds is to be expected, but continuous drainage should raise suspicion of CSF leakage, especially in the setting of headache. CSF leakage through the lumbar wound is an indication for surgical exploration.

In addition to the expected incisional pain, any pain out of proportion to the surgery may suggest damage to the nerve roots, spinal cord, or both.

Extensive dissection or cauterization may lead to pump pocket seroma. This complication is usually treated conservatively with a binder and should resolve in a couple of weeks. Part of the differential diagnosis of postoperative fluid collection is catheter leak or disconnect. Catheter leak or disconnect must be ruled out with a catheter dye study. Sometimes the source of CSF leakage is a persistent CSF fistula around the catheter, and the treatment is to place the catheter at a different level.

Pumps and Catheters

Despite our best attempt to maintain sterile barriers throughout the implantation process, infection still exists. Infection rates vary between 0.7% and 10.3% annually.[27] The majority of infections occur within 60 days after implantation. *Staphylococcus epidermidis* is the most commonly identified pathogen.[28] Measures to reduce surgical wound infection include preoperative antibiotics before incision, strict adherence to sterile techniques, minimization of traffic in the operating room, and use of postoperative antibiotics. Infection of the pump pocket or catheter track usually requires removal of the entire system. However, there have been case reports of nonsurgical treatment of infected pumps and catheters. One case report advocates systemic antibiotics and irrigation of the pocket site with antiseptic and antibiotic solutions for mild clinical signs and symptoms of infection.[29]

Suspected superficial would infection should be treated aggressively. The usual regimen involves oral antibiotics for 7 to 14 days and close observation. Most patients respond to this treatment, but the risk of developing a deep pocket infection or meningitis is always present. The system is explanted if the superficial infection progresses, if there is no resolution after a course of antibiotics, or if the infection recurs after cessation of antibiotics.

Mechanical complications (e.g., catheter displacement, disconnect, or breakage) can occur in any IDDS after implantation. Suspicion for a mechanical complication is high if the patient experiences a brief period of pain relief after implant or the expected pain relief is absent. A blockage to flow is suggested if aspiration of the pump reservoir reveals a larger quantity of drug than expected. Plain radiographs can demonstrate catheter displacement, disconnect, or breakage. A catheter dye study can assess the presence of catheter malfunction. A catheter is patent if CSF can be smoothly aspirated from the catheter access port. If contrast injected through the access port (after aspiration only) is seen in the IT space, it suggests the catheter is intact from the tip to the catheter access port. Surgical exploration is indicated if clinical suspicion of mechanical complication remains high despite normal diagnostic studies. Failure to take appropriate measures to investigate a possible mechanical complication can lead to detrimental consequences, especially for patients on IT baclofen therapy. On average, 27% of patients undergo equipment revision surgery, and 5% require permanent pump removal.[24]

The pump can sometimes rotate or "flip" within the pocket after implantation. This complication is related to the creation of an oversized subfascial pocket.[30] This complication can be minimized by creating a pump pocket of appropriate proportions. The pump can also be anchored to the tissue using different techniques. First, a Dacron pouch is tightly fitted over the pump before placement into the pocket. The pouch promotes scar formation over time and facilitates anchoring of the pump. Second, hooks on the deep surface of the pump can be anchored to the fascia using nonabsorbable sutures.

Abdominal pocket fluid collection can occur after implantation. It is usually noticeable after 2 weeks. The risk is reduced with an abdominal binder in the postoperative period. If the clinical signs and symptoms of local or systemic infection are absent, initial therapy can be observation and a pressure dressing simply consisting of gauze and tape. If the fluid pocket persists or increases in size, abdominal radiographs are performed to rule out mechanical complication. If at any time infection is suspected, the fluid is aspirated with a small-gauge needle, keeping in mind that the catheter or pump nozzle can be damaged by the procedure. If infection is not suspected, fluid collections should not be aspirated. Catheters can be damaged, and commensal skin flora can be introduced into the pocket as pathogens. Aspiration should be performed under direct vision using fluoroscopy.

Catheter-tip granuloma is the dreaded complication of IT therapy. IT catheter-related granulomas are underreported in the literature.[31] Granulomas are inflammatory masses at the tip of the IT catheter and can cause pain or lead to neurologic injury from spinal cord compression. Histologically, granulomas are characterized by activated macrophages with an epithelioid appearance. IT morphine-related granulomas often have necrotic tissue surrounded by macrophages, plasma cells, eosinophils, or lymphocytes. Catheter-tip granuloma is associated with the infusion of highly concentrated drugs or high daily dosage of opioids. Other possible causes that have been postulated include inadvertent addition of preservative, an indolent organism causing a chronic infectious process, or local pH or environmental changes.[32]

A sudden escalation of dosage required to alleviate pain in a patient whose pain was previously well controlled is a classic presentation of a granuloma. Positioning the catheter tip below the conus medullaris is not a proven method to eliminate the risk of developing a granuloma.[31] Anatomically, it makes sense that there is less chance of injury to the spinal cord if the catheter tip is below the conus medullaris. However, a granuloma may become adherent to the conus medullaris and present as cauda equina syndrome.[33] Vigilance and attention to symptoms and neurological signs are the best methods of early detection. Motor deficits typically occur late in the development of catheter-tip granuloma.[33] Magnetic resonance imaging is warranted for patients with an IT catheter who experience acute new-onset radicular pain with or without sensory or motor deficits. In the absence of significant or worsening neurological compromise, the patient can be observed. The granuloma may resolve spontaneously if the IT therapy is discontinued. If significant signs and symptoms of spinal cord compression exist, surgical exploration is indicated.

Medications

In a recent review, approximately one-quarter to one-third of patients undergoing IT therapy experience nausea or vomiting, urinary retention, and pruritus. A previous review of cancer and noncancer pain and different types of IT therapy found nausea or vomiting at 25%, urinary retention at 19%, myoclonic activity at 18%, sedation at 17%, and pruritus at 17%.

Medication overdose is an ever-present danger of IT therapy. Sources of overdose include injection into subcutaneous tissue next to the pump during attempted refill, injection in the side port during attempted refill, and misprogramming. Management of an opioid overdose requires cessation of drug administration via the pump, administration of naloxone, and initiation of supportive care. Similar measures are undertaken for baclofen overdose in addition to administration of physostigmine. Supportive care may include airway protection and intubation. A lumbar puncture to drain the drug-laden CSF is an option for rapid drug removal. An uncommon cause of overdose can be from an inadvertent infusion of drug into the subdural space followed by drug diffusion into the subarachnoid space. Management is expectant and depends on the presenting signs and symptoms.

Conclusion

IT drug therapy has traditionally been the last option in the chronic pain treatment paradigm. Recently, the pendulum has shifted, and IT therapy can be considered at an earlier time in the natural history of treatment. Given the correct patients and indications, IT drug therapy is a powerful tool in the armamentarium of treatment for patients with cancer pain and chronic noncancer pain.

References

1. Belverud S, Mogilner A, Schulder M: Intrathecal pumps. *NeuroTherapeutics* 5:114-122, 2008.
2. Paice JA, Penn RD, Shott S: Intraspinal morphine for chronic pain: a retrospective, multicenter study. *J Pain Symptom Manage* 11:71-80, 1996.
3. Wallace M, Yaksh TL: Long-term spinal analgesic delivery: a review of the preclinical and clinical literature. *Reg Anesth Pain Med* 25:117-157, 2000.
4. Bernards Christopher M: Recent Insights into the pharmacokinetics of spinal opioids and the relevance to opioid selection. *Curr Opin Anesthesiol* 17:441-447, 2004.
5. Morgan GE, Mikhail MS, Murray MJ: Pain management. In *Clinical anesthesiology*, ed 4, New York, 2006, McGraw-Hill, pp 359-411
6. Gutstein HB, Akil H: Opioid analgesics. In *Goodman and Gilman's the pharmacological basis of therapeutics*, ed 11, New York, 2006, McGraw-Hill.
7. Abs R, Verhelst J, Maeyaert J, et al: Endocrine consequences of long-term intrathecal administration of opioids. *J Clin Endocrinol Metab* 85:2215-2222, 2000.
8. Anderson VC, Cooke B, Burchiel KJ: Intrathecal hydromorphone for chronic nonmalignant pain: a retrospective study. *Pain Med* 2:287-297, 2001.
9. Willis KD, Doleys DM: The effects of long-term intraspinal infusion therapy with noncancer pain patients: evaluation of patient, significant-other, and clinic staff appraisals. *Neuromodulation* 2:241-253, 1999.
10. Dahm P, Lundborg C, Janson M, et al: Comparison of 0.5% intrathecal bupivacaine with 0.5% intraspinal ropivacaine in the treatment of refractory cancer and noncancer pain conditions: results from a prospective, crossover, double-blind, randomized study. *Reg Anesth Pain Med* 25:480-487, 2000.
11. Miyamoto H, Saito Y, Kirihara Y: Spinal coadministration of ketamine reduces the development of tolerance to visceral as well as somatic antinociception during spinal morphine infusion. *Anesth Analg* 90:136-141, 2000.
12. Sansone JM, Mann D, Noonan K, et al: Rapid progression of scoliosis following insertion of intrathecal baclofen pump. *J Pediatr Orthop* 26:125-128, 2006.
13. Wermeling D, Berger JR: Ziconotide infusion for severe chronic pain: case series of patients with neuropathic pain. *Pharmacotherapy* 26:395-402, 2006.
14. Deer T, Kim C, Bowman R, et al: Intrathecal ziconotide and opioid combination therapy for noncancer pain: an observational study. *Pain Physician* 12:E291-E296, 2009.
15. Hassenbusch SJ, Portenoy RK, Cousins M, et al: Polyanalgesic Consensus Conference 2003: an update on the management of pain by intraspinal drug delivery-report of an expert panel. *J Pain Symptom Manage* 27:540-563, 2004.
15a. Deer T, Krames ES, Hassenbusch S, et al: Management of intrathecal catheter-tip inflammatory masses: an updated 2007 consensus statement from an expert panel. *Neuromodulation* 11(2):77-91, 2008.
16. Ferrante, FM: Neuraxial infusion in the management of cancer pain. *Oncology* 13:30-36, 1999.
17. Codman & Shurtleff, Inc.: *Codman pumps*, accessed April 1, 2010, from http://www.codmanpumps.com.
18. Deer T, Chapple I, Classen A, et al: Intrathecal drug delivery for treatment of chronic low back pain: report from the National Outcomes Registry for Low Back Pain. *Pain Med* 5(1):6-13, 2004.
19. Kreis P, Fishman S: *Spinal cord stimulation percutaneous implantation techniques*, New York, 2009, Oxford University Press.
20. McCall T, MacDonald J: Cervical catheter tip placement for intrathecal baclofen administration. *Neurosurgery* 59:634-640, 2006.
21. Deer T: *Intrathecal drug delivery: overview of the proper use of infusion agents. In Raj's practical management of pain*, ed 4, Philadelphia, 2008, Mosby Elsevier, pp 945-954.
22. Knight HK, Brand MF, Mchaourab SA, et al: Implantable intrathecal pumps for chronic pain: highlights and updates. *Croat Med J* 48:22-34, 2007.
23. Uppal GS, Haider TT, Dwyer A: Reversible urinary retention secondary to excessive morphine delivered by an intrathecal morphine pump. *Spine* 19:719-720, 1994.
24. Turner JA, Sears JM, Loeser JD: Programmable intrathecal opioid delivery systems for chronic noncancer pain: a systematic review of effectiveness and complications. *Clin J Pain* 23:180-195, 2007.
25. Patel VB, Manchikanti L, Singh V: Systemic review of intrathecal infusion systems for long-term management of chronic non-cancer pain. *Pain Physician* 12:345-360, 2009.
26. Coffey RJ, Owens ML, Broste SK: Mortality associated with implantation and management of intrathecal opioid drug infusion systems to treat noncancer pain. *Anesthesiology* 111:881-891, 2009.
27. Fluckiger B, Knecht H, Grossman S, et al: Device-related complications of long-term intrathecal drug therapy via implanted pumps. *Spinal Cord* 46:639-643, 2008.
28. Follett KA, Boortz-Marx R, Drake JM, et al: Prevention and management of intrathecal drug delivery and spinal cord stimulation system infections. *Anesthesiology* 100:1582-1594, 2004.
29. Boviatsis EJ, Kouyialis AT, Boutsikakis I, et al: Infected CNS infusion pumps. Is there a chance for treatment without removal? *Acta Neurochir* 146:463-467, 2004.
30. Vender JR, Hester S, Waller JL, et al: Identification and management of intrathecal baclofen pump complications: a comparison of pediatric and adult patients. *J Neurosurg* 104:9-15, 2006.
31. Coffey JR, Burchiel K: Inflammatory mass lesions associated with intrathecal drug infusion catheters: report and observations on 41 patients. *Neurosurgery* 50:78-87, 2002.
32. Miele JV, Price OK, Bloomfield S, et al: A review of intrathecal morphine therapy related granulomas. *Eur J Pain* 10:251-261, 2006.
33. Shields CD, Palma C, Khoo TL, et al: Extramedullary intrathecal catheter granuloma adherent to the conus medullaris presenting as cauda equina syndrome. *Anesthesiology* 102:1059-1061, 2005.

Index

A

Abdominal pocket fluid collection, occurrence, 193
Abdominal pocket site, intrathecal pump tunneling, 82f
AccuRx Constant Flow Pump, 85
Acetylcholine esterase (Ach-E), 4f, 5-6
Activated partial thromboplastin time (aPTT)
  heparin monitoring, 141
  prolongation, avoidance, 115
Active drug abuse, IDDS contraindication, 50
Acute-stress response, 53
Addiction
  history, 40
    IDDS therapy, usage, 118-119
  IDDS contraindication, 50
  treatment, absence, 51-52
Admixtures, usage (guidelines), 28
Adrenergic agonists, IT therapy, 188
Adverse drug reactions, 23
Adverse event management, 164
Agents, preparation, 19-20
Algoline (polyurethane catheter), 148
Allergic reactions, 23
Alpha$_2$-adrenergic agonists
  mediation, 27
  usage, 25
Alpha$_2$-adrenergic receptors, 5
Alpha-amino-3-hydroxy-5-methylisoxazole-4-propionic acid (AMPA), 4f
  receptors, 5
Alteplase, 141
Alzheimer disease, 50-51
Ambulatory Payment Classifications (APCs)
  CPT code basis, 58-59
  ICD-9-CM diagnosis code usage, 59
Ambulatory surgical centers (ASCs), CPT code usage, 58-59
American College of Chest Physicians (ACCP), antithrombotic therapy management (establishment), 140
American Medical Association (AMA), Relative Value Updating Committee (RUC) CPT code valuation determination, 58
American Recovery and Reinvestment Act, 122
American Society of Health-System Pharmacists (ASHP) compounding standards, 22
American Society of Regional Anesthesia (ASRA), Third Edition Guidelines, 140
American Society of Regional Anesthesia and Pain Medicine, neuraxial analgesia anticoagulant guidelines, 102
Amitriptyline, 28
Analgesia
  assessment, patient ability, 39-40
  sudden loss, 106-107

Analgesia, mechanisms, 25
Analgesic perception, interference, 39b
Analgesics
  additive/synergistic effects, 25-26
  chronic intrathecal infusion, usage, 15
Anatomy, 70-71
Anesthesia, type, 79
ANS AccuRx constant flow pump, 86f
Anticoagulant medications, usage, 114-116
Anticoagulant therapy guidelines, 143-144
  hematologic factors, 143-144
Anticoagulation medications, usage, 115t
Antiepileptic medications, 28
Antihemostatic drugs, properties, 142t
Antiplatelet medications, usage, 114-116
Antithrombotic therapy, management (ACCP establishment), 140
Anxiety, 40
  disorders, 53
  levels, variation, 53
Arachnoid layer, 70-71
Arrow 3000 (Codman), 148
  catheter design, 148
Aseptic meningitis, diagnosis, 151-152
Ashworth rating scale, 163
Aspirin, usage, 115
Astramorph (AstraZeneca), 97
Atheroma formation, 114

B

B$_2$-selective antagonist, intrathecal administration, 7
Baclofen (GABA-A agonist), 18
  effectiveness, loss (causes), 169-171
  IT therapy, 189
  single-bolus IT trials, performing, 76
  trial, performing (objective measures), 72
  trialing, 76
  withdrawal, 34
Bactroban (topical mupirocin), preoperative use, 103
B-cell lineage, immunodeficiencies, 116
Behavioral observation, 39-40
Benzodiazepine receptor binding site, 3-4
Benzyl alcohol, preservative, 22
Billing compliance, 59-62
Bleeding, 102
  complications, 140
  tendency, increase (conditions), 143t
  time, predictor, 141
Blending (cocktailing), practice, 19
Blood-brain barrier permeable glial activation inhibitor, 9
Body mass index (BMI), 117
Bolus administration trial, 72-73
Bolus injection trials, 180
Bolus trials
  double-blind placebo-controlled trial, 182-183
  open-label study, 183
  retrospective chart review, 183
  single-center study, 183

Bone metastasis, 132-133
Bradykinin
  inflammatory mediator, 7
  receptors, 7
Brain, cannabis (impact), 6
Brain-derived neurotrophic factor (BDNF), 4f
  receptors (trkB), 7
Brain receptors, systemic delivery, 3
Breakthrough pain, 154
Breakthrough spasms, 160
Brief Pain Inventory, 52-53
Broad-spectrum antibiotics, usage, 103
Bupivacaine, 17
  addition, impact, 26-27
  clinician preference, 189
  elimination, 17
  morphine, intrathecal infusions (combination), 38
  toxicity, animal studies, 17
  usage, 33, 108

C

Cachexia, 150f
Calcitonin gene-related peptide (CCGRP)
  receptors, 7
  release, 7
Calcitonin gene-related peptide (CGRP), release, 17
Calcium channel, alpha$_2$delta subunit ($\alpha2\delta$ subunit), 8
Calcium channel blockers, usage, 25
Cancer, 119
  chronic disease, long-term pain sequelae, 147
  life expectancy, 132
  patients, depression, 52-53
  treatment, IDDS (usage), 38
Cancer pain
  association, 52
  consideration, 114
  IDDS, usefulness, 119
  psychological screening, 40
  syndrome, 119
  three-step analgesic ladder, evolution, 130
  treatment, 132
Cancer-related pain
  opioid medications, supplementation, 28
  opioid monotherapy, delivery, 26
  patient evaluation, 52-53
  psychological evaluation, role, 53
  treatment
    barriers, 53
    options/decisions, 52
Cannabinoid CB1 receptors, 6
Cannabinoid CB2 receptors, 6
Cannabinoid receptors, 6
Carbon dioxide retention, 117
Cardiovascular collapse, 107
Caregiver-related barriers, 53
Catastrophization, 40
Categorical Pain Relief Scale (CPRS), 180
Catheter-related complications, 105-107

Page numbers followed by *f*, *t*, and *b* indicate figures, tables, and boxes, respectively.

Catheter-related problems, 177
Catheter-tip granuloma, 105-106
  clinical presentation/management,
      106-107
  complication, 193
  prevention/risk assessment/surveillance,
      107
Catheter-tip mass, development, 107
Catheter-tip visualization, maintenance, 150
CD4+ lymphocytes, destruction, 116
Celecoxib (Celebrex), antiinflammatory agent,
      141
Centers for Medicare and Medicaid Services
      (CMS)
  intermediary, WPS Medicare guidelines, 58
  Medicare administration, 57
Central nervous system (CNS)
  GABA, impact, 3
  infections, 119
Central neuraxis, trespass, 117-118
Cerebrospinal fluid (CSF)
  aspiration, 82f
  bulk flow, 71
  continuous aspiration, intrathecal needle
      advancement, 80f
  flow, 131
    dynamics, 176-177
  hygroma, 104f
  leaks, 103-104
    incidence (decrease), tobacco sac suture
      (usage), 103-104
  space, 70-71
    distribution, 16
  visualization, 82f
  withdrawal, 34
Cervical spinal catheter, CPT codes, 61
Cervical-thoracic junction, 167
Chapter 797
  pharmacy compounding risk-level
      assessment, 21t
  standards/guidance/examples, 21
  training/certification requirements, 21-22
Chemoreceptor trigger zone (CTZ) (area
      postrema), 107
Chemotherapy regimens, 147
Children, IT baclofen (trialing), 76
Chloride concentration gradients, second-
      order neurons, 9
Cholecystokinin (CCK), 7
  receptor subtypes, 7
Cholinergic receptors, 5-6
Chronic Illness Problem Inventory, 50
Chronic infusions, intrathecal morphine
      (clinical efficacy), 16
Chronic intractable pain (treatment), opioid
      drugs (usage), 57-58
Chronic intrathecal morphine infusion, safety,
      23
Chronic low back pain, 119
Chronic malignant pain, 22-23
Chronic nonmalignant pain, treatment
      (IDDS usage), 38
Chronic pain
  characteristic, impact, 88
  elimination, 51
  management, IT therapy, 162
  spinal cord stimulation (SCS) therapy, 48
  subjective increase, 45
  treatment, 131
Chronic Pain Acceptance Questionnaire,
      50, 53
Chronic pain treatment, IDDS (reservation),
      38

Cleanrooms
  air, entry, 21
  controlled environment, 20-21
  standardization, international organization,
      21t
Clinical Global Impression (CGI) scale, 180
Clonidine, 27
  action, mechanism, 27
  alpha2-agonists, 17
    usage, 33
  analgesia, 5
  intrathecal infusion, 5
  usage, 108
Clopidogrel (Plavix)
  antiplatelet effect, 141-142
  platelet-fibrinogen binding interference,
      141-142
  usage, 115
Cocktailing (blending), practice, 19
Coding, 58-59
  trialing, 61-62
Codman 3000 implantable drug pump, 85f
Codman Archimedes constant flow pump, 86f
Cognitive dysfunction, presence, 50-51
Combination antiretroviral therapy (CART),
      116
Combination therapy, 19
Common intrathecal drug infusions, targeted
      receptors, 19t
Co-morbidities, 119
  evolution, consequences, 114
Comparative-Effectiveness Research, 122
Complex continuous mode (intrathecal
      pump), 87
Complex regional pain syndrome (CRPS),
      49, 96-97
  development, 147
  manifestation, 51
  spinal drug delivery, 152
  treatment, 133
Compounded drugs, compliance issue, 64
Compounded medications, FDA concern, 22
Compounded sterile preparation (CSP)
  definition, 19-20
  high risk-level requirements, 20-21
Compounding
  agents, usage, 22
  ASHP standards, 22
  labs, responsibility, 21-22
  occurrence, ISO Class 5 environment, 20
  risk-level appropriate compounding,
      requirements, 20t
  risk-level assessment, 21t
Compounding drugs, intrathecal use, 19
Compression fractures, 96-97
Concentration-dependent neurotoxicity,
      dependence, 23
Constant-flow pumps, 148
Constant-flow systems, 148-149
Constipation, 108
  opioid side effect, 38
Continuous catheters, usage, 167
Continuous infusion, 180
  trials, 180-181
Continuous medication, administration
      (IT trial), 72
Conus magnus snail, venom, 18
Conus medullaris, position (variation), 71
Conventional pain therapies (CPT) cumulative
      costs, IDDS cumulative costs
      (comparison), 125f
Coping Strategies Questionnaire, 50, 53
Cor pulmonale, 117

Cost-benefit analysis, complication rates
      (impact), 123
Current Procedural Terminology (CPT)
  codes, 57
  consultation codes, acceptance (Medicare
      stoppage), 60
  CPT Assistant publication, 59
  electronic analysis code, 58
  HIPAA mandate, 58
  procedure codes, 57
Cut-off score, derivation, 49
Cyanoacrylate adhesive (DermaBond), usage,
      103
Cyclic guanosine monophosphate (cGMP), 9
Cyclooxygenase (COX), NSAID inhibition,
      141
Cyclooxygenase-1 (COX-1), inhibition, 115
Cyclooxygenase-2 (COX-2), inhibition, 115,
      141
Cyclooxygenase enzymes, 6

D

Deep venous thrombosis (DVT), 114
Delta-opioid receptors (δ-opioid receptors), 6
Dementia, 40
Depressed moods, reaction, 52
Depression
  cancer patients, 52-53
  levels, variation, 53
DermaBond (cyanoacrylate adhesive), usage,
      103
Descending noradrenergic fibers, 5
Desmoids carcinoma, 150f
Device-related complications, 105
Device-related perioperative morbidity/
      mechanical failure, minimization, 97
Dexmedetomidine, 5
Diabetes, surgical site infection risk factor, 117
Diabetes mellitus (DM), 117
Diabetics, IDDS placement, 117
Diagnosis
  elements, 60b
  establishment, 70, 179-180
Diethylenetriamine pentaacetic acid (DTPA),
      injection, 170
Diffuse cancer pain, 152
Direct physician supervision, 63-64
Direct supervision, meaning, 64
Distress, high level, 40
Dorsal horn
  GABA-A receptor activation, 7
Dorsal horn interneurons, NPY location, 7
Dorsal root ganglion, presynaptic calcium
      channel production, 8
Dose-dependent allodynia, presentation, 23
Dose-dependent analgesic response, 38
Dose-dependent opioid side effect profiles,
      history (usefulness), 43
Dose-sparing effect, 188
Double-catheter technique, 73
Double-guarded array, cathodes (usage),
      133-134
Droperidol, impact, 107
Drug overdose, risks, 166
Drug-taking behavior, assessment, 51
Drug withdrawal, 34, 166
Duloxetine (SSNRI), 28
DuPen (polyurethane catheter), 148
DuPen Silicone Rubber Epidural Catheter,
      191
Dura, percutaneous approach, 80

Dural leak, persistence (risk), 80
Dural punctures, 167
Dura mater, 70-71

E

Early-line therapy, 130
Early respiratory depression, intrathecal
    morphine (impact), 16
ECRI Institute analysis, 122, 126-127
Edema, 108
End-of-life conditions, 130
End-of-life issues, 53
Endothelial Protein C Receptor (ePCR)
    database, 97
Enzyme systems, 9
Epidural blood patches, success rate, 103-104
Epidural catheter
    placement
        fluoroscopic guidance, usage, 71
        Tuohy needle, usage, 75f
    tunneling, 75f
Epidural catheterization, 140
Epidural infusion trial, 182
Epidural Port-a-Cath, usage, 148
Epidural space, intrathecal infusion catheter
    (usage), 39
Epidural trialing, opioids (usage), 45
EP subtype selective antagonists, 6
Escherichia coli, IDDS infection, 103
Ethibond suture, usage, 80
Ethylenediamine-tetraacetic acid (EDTA),
    preservative, 22
Evaluation & management (E&M)
    codes, 61-62
    levels, examination, 61
    services
        billing, separation, 62
        identification, 59
External IDDS, implantation cost, 146
External intrathecal systems, implantation,
    149-151
Externalized catheter port-a-cath systems,
    150
Externalized catheter systems, 150
Externalized systems, 147-148
    complications, 147b
External programmer, handheld device, 86
External pumps, usage, 180-181

F

Factors, half-lives, 140t
Factors II (thrombin), synthesis, 115
Failed back surgery syndrome (FBSS), 96-97,
    119, 179
    IDDS, impact, 119
    nonmalignant causes, 131
    success rates, 134-135
    treatment, 133
False-positive outcomes, prevention, 51
Fentanyl, 17
    derivatives, 17
    implantable infusions, VAS pain scores
        (reduction), 17
Fibrinolytic therapy, 140-141
Filtration, 21
    bacteria-retentive applications, 21
First Cost Study, 123
5-HT receptors (serotonin receptors), 6
5-HT reuptake inhibitors, 9

Fixed-rate intrathecal pumps, 87-88
    advantages/disadvantages, 88-89
    programmable system, 88
Fixed-rate pumps, 87-88
    advantages, 88
    batteries, absence, 88
    disadvantages, 88-89
    equipment, 88
    overview, 87-88
    pain level, change, 89
    programmable pumps, contrast, 85t
Fondaparinux, patient receipt, 142-143
Fractalkine, release, 9
Functional pain level (FPL), usefulness, 50

G

Gabapentin, IT therapy, 189
Gabapentoid receptor, 8
Galanin receptors, 7
Gamma-aminobutyric acid A (GABA-A)
    addition, 134
Gamma-aminobutyric acid A (GABA-A)
    agonist
        Baclofen, 18
        Midazolam, 17-18
Gamma-aminobutyric acid A (GABA-A)
    antagonist, sensitivity, 4
Gamma-aminobutyric acid A (GABA-A)
    receptors, 3-4
    activation, 7
    chlorine ionophore, 17-18
Gamma-aminobutyric acid B (GABA-B)
    agonists, hyperpolarization, 17-18
Gamma-aminobutyric acid B (GABA-B)
    binding, 71
Gamma-aminobutyric acid B (GABA-B)
    receptors, 4
Gamma-aminobutyric acid (GABA) receptors,
    3-4
Gastrojejunal tubes, usage, 151f
Gate control theory, 133
Generalized anxiety disorder, 53
Glia, 9
Glial cells, pain/spasticity involvement, 4f
Glutamate receptors, 5
Glycine receptors, 4
G-protein coupled CGRP1 receptors, impact, 7
G-protein coupled (metabotropic) glutamate
    receptors, 5
G-protein coupled prostaglandin receptors,
    binding, 6
G-protein-regulated inwardly rectifying K+
    (GIRK) channels, 16
Granuloma formation, 23
    analgesic effect, reduction, 176-177
    predictability, reduction, 99
Granulomas (inflammatory masses), 99
    development, 99
    guides/recommendations, 189-190
    motor/sensory dysfunction, 99
    treatment, 99

H

Headaches, opioid side effect, 38
Healthcare Common Procedure Coding
    System (HCPCS)
    HCPCS II codes, 57
        assignation, 63
    J3490 usage, 58

Health Insurance Portability and
    Accountability Act (HIPAA),
    CPT mandate, 58
Hematoma
    formation, risk (increase), 115
    minimization, 103
Heparin
    anticoagulation, advantages, 141
    monitoring, aPTT (usage), 141
Hepatic dysfunction, 143
Herbal agents, usage, 116
High-dose IT ziconotide bolus trialing,
    predictive value, 183
High-efficiency particulate air (HEPA), 21
High-performance liquid chromatography
    (HPLC)
    measurement, 18-19
    usage, 17
High-risk patient care activities, 33
History elements, 60b
Hormonal abnormalities, 108
Hormonal changes, 99-100
Hospital Anxiety and Depression Scales
    (HADS), 52-53
Hospital outpatient department (HOPD)
    reimbursement, prospective payment
    system, 58-59
Human immunodeficiency virus 1 (HIV-1)
    retrovirus, 116
Human immunodeficiency virus 2 (HIV-2)
    retrovirus, 116
Human immunodeficiency virus (HIV)
    infection, 116
Hydromorphone, 16-17
    alternative, 188
    concentrations, 149
    implantable infusion system, stability/
        compatibility (HPLC, usage), 17
    intrathecal infusions, 16-17
    semisynthetic hydrogenated ketone
        morphine derivative, 16-17
    single analgesic, 17
Hydroxyzine, impact, 107
Hypertonia
    assessment, 163
    clinical evaluation, 163
    rapid reduction, 168
Hypertonicity, reduction, 166
Hypotonia, excess, 166
Hypoxemia, 117

I

Ibudilast (blood-brain barrier permeable glial
    activation inhibitor), 9
Imaging, 71
Immunocompromised patients
    IDDS, usage, 116-117
    infection risk, 116-117
Implantable infusion pumps, coverage
    (NCD statement), 60
Implantable pain therapies, patient selection
    criteria, 188b
Implantable systems, 148-149
    constant-flow systems, 148-149
    programmable systems, 148-149
Implanted catheter/pump systems,
    complications, 44t
Implanted catheters, subcutaneous injection
    site, 191
Implanted Drug Delivery Systems (IDDS),
    costs/savings, 126t

Implanted equipment, infection, 39
Implanted infusion pump, usage, 191
Implanted intrathecally delivered medications, risk considerations, 20
Incision pain, 193
Indium I-111 DTPA (diethylenetriamine pentaacetic acid), injection, 170
Inducible nitric oxide synthase (iNOS), 9
Infection, 103, 151
    incidence rate, variation, 103
    prevention, 103
    relationship, 151
    risk, 116
Inflammatory masses (granulomas), 99
    development, 152
    neurological deficits, 99
Infumorph (Baxter), 97
Infusaid Model #400 pump, approval, 85
Infusion pumps, infusion modes, 87
In-hospitality mortality, 117
Initial evaluation, 60-61
    billing compliance, 61
    coding, 60
    documentation, 60
    medical necessity, 60
Insulin secretion, 117
    impairment, 117
Insurance companies, policies, 49
Intelligence testing, 39-40
Internal intrathecal systems, implantation, 149-151
Internal pumps, anterior placement, 150
International Classification of Diseases (ICD-9-CM)
    coding, HIPAA mandate, 59
    diagnosis codes, 57
        ASC usage, 59
        submission, 58
        usage, 63
    ICD-9-CM Official Guidelines for Coding and Reporting, 59, 62
International Consensus Conference, 132
International normalized ratio (INR)
    calculation, 140
    level, 115
Interventional pain clinics, medical efficacy, 56
Interventional pain management, 140-142
Intractable abdominal pain, 152
Intractable cancer pain (treatment), IT morphine (usage), 102
Intractable pain, IT therapy, 96-97
Intraspinal catheter, CPT codes, 61
Intraspinal drug infusion, clinical guidelines (update), 190f
Intraspinal infusion analgesia, 130
Intraspinal morphine conversion ratios, 76f
Intraspinal opioids
    drug administration, preliminary trial, 57
    preliminary trial, NCD requirements, 61
Intrathecal (IT) administration, single-bolus/multiple-bolus trials, 73
Intrathecal (IT) agents
    off-label use, 22
    pka coefficients, 22t
    solubility, 22t
    stability/solubility, 22
    usage, 15t
Intrathecal (IT) analgesia
    initiation, opioids (usage), 31-32
    long-term effectiveness, 31
    ziconotide, FDA approval, 31

Intrathecal (IT) analgesics
    infusion, financial benefit, 40
    usage, 38
        increase, 25
Intrathecal (IT) analgesic therapies
    alternative, 175
    contraindications, 39b
    cost-effective analysis, 40
    patient selection, inclusion criteria, 38b
Intrathecal baclofen (ITB)
    anticipation, 168
    assessment measures, 163
    bolus, peak effect, 163
    concentrations, FDA approval, 169
    delivery, reduction/cessation, 170
    dose, increase, 168
    effectiveness, loss (causes), 169-171
    FDA approval, 160-162
    implantation, 166-167
    long-term maintenance, 168-169
    low reservoir syndrome, avoidance, 168-169
    overdose, 170-171
    pharmacological tolerance, 170
    post-implantation management, 167-168
    procedural details, 162-163
    reservoir refills, sterility, 168-169
    titration phase, 167-168
    trialing, 76
        method, 162
    trials
        method, alternative, 162-163
        screening, success, 163
    troubleshooting, 168-169
    withdrawal
        interventions, 170b
        symptoms, 168-169, 170b
Intrathecal baclofen (ITB) therapy
    advantages/disadvantages, comprehension, 162
    effectiveness, loss (causes), 169
    long-term ITB therapy, issues, 169
    patient selection, 160-162
    role, 160
    titration phase, 168
    usage, 159, 166
Intrathecal (IT) bolus, patient positioning, 73f
Intrathecal (IT) bupivacaine, addition, 17, 26-27
Intrathecal (IT) catheter placement, 80f, 166-167
    connection, 105f
    dissection, 79f
    fluoroscopic guidance, usage, 71
    suggestion, 82f
Intrathecal (IT) catheters, 148
    access port, 148
    anchoring, 80
        photograph, 81f
    complications, 149
        illustration, 149f
    connection, 105
    contrast dye, extravasation, 105f
    dislodging, drug precipitation (impact), 149f
    displacement, 149
    exit site, localized skin infection, 150
    implantation, 166-167
        CPT codes, 62
    intrathecal placement, 149
    lateral tunneling, 150
    management, 105
    midline incision, 79f
    spinal implantation, 150

Intrathecal (IT) catheters (Continued)
    tumor compression, 154f
    tunneling/passage, 81
Intrathecal (IT) catheter tip
    dorsal placement, 106
    granuloma
        clinical presentation/management, 106-107
        development, risk factors, 106
        management, algorithm, 106f
        report, 105-106
    inflammatory masses
        development, 152
        granulomas, 99
    location, 106
    mass, development, 107
    prevention/surveillance, 107
    risk
        assessment, 107
        factors, 106-107
Intrathecal (IT) clonidine, addition, 106
Intrathecal (IT) concentrations, recommendations, 190t
Intrathecal (IT) COX inhibitors, usage, 9
Intrathecal (IT) delivery
    algorithm, 28
    handheld accessory, 168
    modes, 167f
    systems, catheter disruption sites, 169f
Intrathecal (IT) dexmedetomidine, usage, 5
Intrathecal (IT) dosages, recommendation, 190t
Intrathecal (IT) drug delivery
    codes, 57b
    inexpensiveness, 125-126
    management considerations, 152-154
    pain syndromes, 70
    technology, 147-149
    trial, indications (consideration), 72
    type, 106
Intrathecal drug delivery system (IDDS), 15-16, 131-133
    analgesic perception, conditions, 39b
    benefits, 43, 50
        frequently asked questions, 43b
    billing compliance, 59-60
    bleeding, 102
    catheter-related complications, 105-107
    cerebrospinal fluid leaks, 103-104
    coding/reimbursement, 58-59
    complications, 102
        considerations, categories, 43t
        frequently asked questions, 44b
    compounding agents, usage, 22
    concerns/pitfalls, 176-177
    consideration, 70-71
    contraindications, 39, 72
        consideration, 50
    cost-minimization models, 40
    cost projection, 126f
    cumulative costs, CPT (comparison), 125f
    device-related complications, 105
    documentation, 58
    dose, selection, 31
    dose-dependent opioid side effect profiles, history (usefulness), 38
    drug therapy, 31-33
    effectiveness, 119
    equipment, 39, 72
    evaluation process, prognostic value, 50
    expectations, 50
    expert panel (anticoagulant therapy guidelines), 143-144

Intrathecal drug delivery system (IDDS)
  (Continued)
  financial considerations, 40
  frequently asked questions, 46-47
  hypersensitivity reactions, 39
  imaging, 71
  implantation, 30-31, 84
    contraindications, 39
    financial cost, 40
    indication, 38
    peripheral procedure, 117-118
  indications, 38-39, 72
  infection, 103
    impact, 103
  initial therapy, 31-32
  interest, 48
  invasiveness, 132
  long-term mortality, 114
  long-term outcome, 48-49
  management
    co-morbidities, 114-119
    financial cost, 40
  medical conditions, implications, 116t
  medication
    FDA approval, 71, 71b
    overdose, 33-34
    selection, 31
  neuraxial hemorrhage, 39
  neuroaugmentation, direct comparison, 135t
  neurological injury, 102-103
  opioids, analgesic effect, 51
  outcome predication, 49
  outcome predicators, existence, 49
  patient management/evaluation, 74-77
  percutaneous maintenance, 39
  placement, 114, 115t
    co-morbidities, impact, 114-119
  post-implant complications, frequently
      asked questions, 46
  post-implant considerations, 46
  postoperative concerns/considerations, 46
  postoperative wound infections,
      evaluation, 43t
  posttrial evaluation, 45
  potential benefits, 49
  pre-implant preparation, 45-46
    frequently asked questions, 46
  pre-implant psychological evaluation, 48-49
  procedure, performance, 115
  psychological concerns, 49
  psychological evaluation, 50
  psychological screening, 39-40
  psychopathology, 40
  pump implantation, complications,
      151-152
  pump refill process, 46
  recommendations, 40
  removal, 115t
  risks, 44-45, 114-115
  schematic, 132f
  second-line therapy, 32-33
  short-term mortality, 114
  side effects, 114
  surgical complications, 43t, 102-105
  surgical frequency, 43t
  surgical implantation, 116
  surgical technique, 136
  systems, complications, 33
  technology, 176
  theories, 129-130
  therapy
    consideration, 49
    goals, 31

Intrathecal drug delivery system (IDDS)
  (Continued)
  therapy-related adverse events, 33-34
  treatment, 32
    usage, 33
  trialing
    history, documentation, 70
    technique, 72-73
  troubleshooting, 154-155
  usage, IV drug abuse (contraindication),
      39
  withdrawal syndrome, 34
  wound dehiscence, 104-105
Intrathecal drug delivery system (IDDS) trials
  catheter placement, 73
  contraindications, 72b
  guidelines, absence, 71-72
  indication, consideration, 72b
  medical complications, 77
  methods, considerations, 73f
  pharmacological complications, 77
  risk/complication avoidance, 77
  trial stage, documentation, 61
Intrathecal (IT) drugs
  concentrations/doses, polyanalgesic
      consensus panelist recommendations,
      99t
  constipation, 108
  device, cost, 123
  dose/concentration, 106
  edema, 108
  hormonal abnormalities, 108
  infusions
    flow rate, 106
    patient characteristics, 106
    targeted receptors, 19t
  mental status changes, 108
  nausea, 107
  opiates, 107-108
  pruritus, 107-108
  reservoir, implantation, 97
  respiratory depression, 108
  sedation, 108
  sexual abnormalities, 108
  side effects, 107-108
  urinary retention, 108
  usage, 106
  vomiting, 107
  weight gain, 108
Intrathecal (IT) drug therapy
  actuarial study, 125-126
  benefits, 43
  candidate acceptability, 42-43
  complications, 43-44
    operator error, 44
  drawbacks, 43
  efficacy, trialing methods, 44
  posttrial evaluation, frequently asked
      questions, 45b
  pre-implant preparation, 45-46
  pretrial consideration, 44-45
  pretrial preparation, 44-45
    frequently asked questions, 45b
Intrathecal (IT) Granuloma Diagnosis,
    Treatment and Prevention, 97
Intrathecal (IT) infusion
  catheter, usage, 39
  complications, reoperation requirement,
      123t
  computer simulation, 123-124
  cost-benefit studies, 123-127
  first cost study, 123
  medication titration, 152-153

Intrathecal (IT) infusion (Continued)
  problem, 123
  study (Canada), 124-125
  therapy, benefits, 43t
  usage, 122
  withdrawal, 39
Intrathecal (IT) medications
  concentrations/dosages, recommendation,
      32f
  PACC recommendations, 152, 153b
  trial, double-catheter technique (usage), 73
Intrathecal (IT) monotherapy guidelines, 28
Intrathecal (IT) morphine
  administration, 56
  clinical efficacy, 16
  dose escalation, 26f
  infusion, 6
  side effects, 44t
Intrathecal morphine therapy (IMT)
  cumulative expenditure, 124f
  side effects, incidence/management, 98t
Intrathecal (IT) needle
  advancement, 80f
  placement, 80f
    dissection, 79f
  purse-string suture, placement, 80f
  removal, 80
    purse-string suture knot, 81f
Intrathecal (IT) norepinephrine, effectiveness,
    9
Intrathecal (IT) opiate, cephalad migration,
    107-108
Intrathecal opioid (ITO)
  adverse effects/side effects, 26b
  cost-minimization analysis, 40
  delivery device, implantation, 25
  drug-related side effects, 16
  knowledge, 97
  medications, trial (success), 26
  overdose, risk, 62
  therapy
    initiation, 31
    risk, 97
Intrathecal (IT) pumps
  anesthesia, types, 79
  bleeding, impact, 152
  comparisons, 94t
  complex continuous mode, 87
  device malfunctions, rarity/occurrence,
      43-44
  device-related perioperative morbidity/
      mechanical failure, minimization, 97
  early complications, 151-152
  fixed-rate pumps, 87-88
  implantation, 150-151, 166
    infections, prevention, 103
    ITO therapy risk, 97
    late complications, 152
    technique, considerations, 78
  infusion modes, 87
  interrogation documentation requirements,
      63b
  late complications, 152
  malfunction, investigation techniques, 169
  malposition, occurrence, 152
  mechanical complications, 193
  mechanical pump abnormalities/
      programming, 170
  mechanics, 92f
  medication prefilling, 81
  motor, components (damage), 149f
  options, 85
  periodic bolus mode, 87

Intrathecal (IT) pumps (Continued)
  placement options, 166-167
  pocket seroma
    development, 152
    dissection/cauterization, impact, 193
  pocket site, preparation, 81f
  position, suggestion, 82f
  preparation/programming, CPT codes, 62
  pressure dehiscence, occurrence, 152
  programmable pumps, 86-87
  programming
    comparisons, 94t
    factors, 86-87
  pump-related malfunction, 169
  refills, technician errors (occurrence), 155
  reprogramming documentation
      requirements, 63b
  simple continuous mode, 87
  single-bolus mode, 87
  sizes, comparison, 91f
  skin covering, 104f
  stability, 22-23
  stopped pump mode, 87
  surgical technique, 79-83
  system components/function, 148
  therapy, screening methods, 125
  treatment groups, best-case/worst/case
      scenarios, 124-125
  trials, 191
Intrathecal (IT) space
  cerebrospinal fluid hygroma, 104f
  medication administration, 71, 84-85
Intrathecal (IT) therapy
  adrenergic agonists, 188
  advantages, 187
  algorithm, 32f
  application, 48-49
  baclofen, 189
  complications, 97
    avoidance, 193-194
  consideration, 15-16
  device, insertion, 23
  diagnosis, establishment, 188
  equipment, 191
  evolution, 187
  gabapentin, 189
  guidelines, 188-190
  indications/contraindications, 190-191
  local anesthetics, usage, 188
  mortality, association, 192-193
  NMDA agonists, 189
  opioids, usage, 188
  outcomes evidence, 192-193
  overdose, possibility, 31
  patient management/evaluation, 192
  patient positioning, 191
  polyanalgesic algorithm, 27t
  rationale, 50-51
  response, 38-39
  risks, 23, 31
    avoidance, 193-194
    minimization, 100
  side effects, management, 153-154
  technique, 191-192
  treatment effectiveness, 96-97
  trialing, 147
  trial procedure, 191-192
  ziconotide, 189
Intrathecal (IT) titration, requirement, 28
Intrathecal (IT) trial
  continuous medication, administration, 72
  outcome, success, 39
  procedure, 191-192

Intrathecal (IT) trialing
  adverse effects, 164
  opioids, usage, 45
  randomized trial, 125
Intravenous (IV) drug abuse, history
      (consideration), 39
Intravenous (IV) morphine, daily dose, 31
Ion channel modulators, 8-9
Ion channels, 4f
Ion transporters, assistance, 9
IsoMed (Medtronic), market removal, 148
IsoMed constant flow drug infusion system,
      85f
Itching, opioid side effect, 38
ITDSS, difference, 134

J

J codes, usage, 63
JWH015, impact, 6

K

Kainate receptors, 5
Kappa-opioid receptors (κ-opioid receptors),
      6
Karnofsky Index, 52-53
Keep it sweet and simple (KISS) principle,
      130, 130f
Ketamine, uncompetitive NMDA antagonist,
      5
Ketorolac, water-soluble COX-1/COX-2
      inhibitor, 6

L

Large afferents, presynaptic ending, 7
Lateral decubitus
  implantation site selection, 79
  position, 192
Leu-enkephalin (endogenous peptides),
      6
Level 3 drugs (highest risk drugs),
      compounding, 20
Lidocaine, 17
Limited-duration infusion trials, open-label
      study, 181-182
Lioresal Intrathecal, FDA approval, 169
Lipophilic opioid, usage, 71, 106
Liquid baclofen, placement, 167
L-nitro-arginine methyl ester (L-NAME),
      9
Local anesthetics, 17
  addition, patient improvement, 33
  intrathecal delivery, 26-27
  IT guidelines, 188
  usage, 25
Local Coverage Determinations (LCDs),
      development, 57
Localized skin infection, 150
Long-term anticoagulation, 140
Long-term intrathecal infusion, outcome
      (success), 39
Long-term ITB therapy, issues, 169
Long-term ITO therapy, 99
  effects, management, 97
  endocrine consequences, 99-100
Long-term IT therapy, 149
Long-term mortality, 114
Long-term pain sequelae, 147

Low-molecular-weight heparin (LMWH), 141
  recommendations, 142-143
  therapy, prolongation, 141
Low reservoir syndrome, avoidance, 168-169
Low-risk agents, examples, 20
Low-risk medication preparation, laboratory
      personnel usage, 21-22

M

Malignant pain
  externalized systems, 147-148
  IT drug delivery technology, 147-149
  medication selection, 147
  PACC guidelines, 153b
  relief, 38-39
  treatment, patient selection, 147
  trialing, 147
    methods, 147
Malignant patients, IT morphine dose
      escalation, 26f
Mechanical pump abnormalities/
      programming, 170
Medallion, implantable drug delivery
      system, 176
Medasys Technologies, pump design, 85
Medical decision-making, elements, 60b
Medical necessity, 56-57
  billing compliance, 59-60
  coding, 58-60
  concept, invention, 56-57
  documentation, 58, 60
  ensuring, 58
  initial evaluation, 60-61
  pump refilling/maintenance, 63
  reimbursement, 58-59
  trialing, 61-62
Medical necessity criteria
  Medicare usage, 58
  NCD statement, 57
  private payer development, 58
Medicare
  CMS administration, 57
  medical necessity criteria, 58
Medication
  adjustments, toleration, 51-52
  overdose, 33-34, 194
  problems, 23
  titration, 152-153
  trialing techniques, 72
Medication administration, 71
  IT trial, 72
  multiple-bolus trials, 73
  single-bolus trials, 73
Medication-related complications, 155
Medication-related side effects, 98-99
MedStream Programmable Infusion System,
      implantation, 176
*Medtronic Neuromodulation 2009 Product
      Performance Report Executive Summary*,
      43-44
Medtronic N'Vision clinical programmer, 86f
Medtronic SynchroMed EL programmable
      infusion pumps, 91
Medtronic SynchroMed II, 28
  programmable pump, 86f
Medtronic SynchroMed pump, focus, 56
Mental status changes, 108
Mercuries, preservatives, 22
Metabotropic glutamate receptors (G-protein
      coupled glutamate receptors), 5
Met-enkephalin (endogenous peptides), 6

Methicillin-resistant *Staphylococcus aureus* (MRSA), 149
Microbial contamination risk level, 20-23
Midazolam (GABA-A agonist), 17-18
   effectiveness, 19
Mini Mental Status Exam, 50
Minnesota Multiphasic Personality Inventory-2 (MMPI)
   personal profiles, problems, 50
   Symptom Checklist 90-R, 50
Modified Ashworth rating scale, 163
Monotherapy, clonidine (usage), 27
Mood disorders, 40
Morphine, 16
   bupivacaine, intrathecal infusions (combination), 38
   clinical efficacy, 16
   concentrations, 149
   gold standard, 16
   IDDS usage, FDA approval, 132
   intrathecal administration, 16
   intrathecal dosing recommendations, 38-39
   intrathecal medication, usage, 28-29
   intrathecal use, FDA approval, 16
   mean intrathecal morphine-equivalent dose, increase, 32
Morphine-3-glucuronide (M3G), importance, 16
Morphine-6-glucuronide (M6G), effects, 16
Morphine sulfate (opioid), 98
   IT administration, FDA approval, 25
Mortality
   IT therapy, association, 192-193
   reduction, 114
Multidimensional Pain Inventory, 50
Multimodal therapy, 28
Mu-opioid receptors (μ-opioid receptors), 6
Muscarinic acetylcholine (mACh), 4f
   receptors, 5-6
Muscle overactivity
   clinical manifestations, 160b
   clinical presentation, 160
   defining, 159-160

N

Naloxone, administration, 134
National Correct Coding Initiative (NCCI)
   edits, 61, 63
      impact, 64
   function, 59
National Coverage Determinations (NCDs)
   CMS development, 57
   medical necessity criteria statement, 57
   statement, 60
National Outcomes Registry for Low Back Pain data, 133
Natural killer cells, immunodeficiencies, 116
Nausea
   intrathecal drug side effects, 107
   opioid side effect, 38
Nav1.3 sodium channels, 8
Nav1.7 sodium channels, 8
Nav1.8 sodium channels, 8
Neostigmine, intrathecal injection, 5
Nerve growth factor (NGF) receptors (trkA), 7
Nerve root trauma, complication, 149
Neuraxial analgesia, anticoagulant usage (American Society of Regional Anesthesia and Pain Medicine guidelines), 102

Neuraxial anesthesia, provision, 80
Neuraxial hemorrhage, 39
Neuraxial procedures, international guidelines, 144t
Neuroaugmentation, 130
   action, mechanism, 131-132
   animal models, 134
   complications, comparison, 135-136
   discussion, 136
   efficacy, 132-135
   IDDS, direct comparison, 135t
   infection, risk, 135-136
   mechanisms, 134
   modality, advantages/disadvantages, 136t
   spinal cord stimulation, mechanism (schematic), 134f
   stimulation
      conductivity, 133
      usage, 133-135
   usage, indications, 133t
Neurokinin-1 (NK1), binding, 6-7
Neurological injury, 102-103
Neurologic depression, 23
Neurologic structure, structural damage, 166
Neuromodulation, placement, 49
Neuronal nitric oxide synthase (nNOS), 9
Neuropathic pain-relieving medication implementation, 117
Neuropeptide Y (NPY)
   location, 7
   receptors, 7
Neurostimulation
   modality, advantages/disadvantages, 136t
   success, 135
   theories, 129-130
   usage, indications, 133t
Neurotrophin receptors, 7
Nicotinic acetylcholine (nACh), 4f
   receptors, 5
Nitric oxide synthase (NOS), 9
   inhibitors, 9
N-methyl-D-aspartate (NMDA), 19
   agonists, IT therapy, 189
Nociceptive pain, opioid responsiveness, 38-39
Non-anatomic constraints, 78-79
Noncancer pain, 52
   opioids, usage, 114
   patients
      evaluation, 49-52
      pre-implantation psychological evaluations, 53
Nonionic radiocontrast dye injection, flow visualization, 105
Nonmalignant pain
   implantable pain therapies, patient selection criteria, 188b
   models, 133
   pain treatment continuum, 130
   patients, cost/savings, 126t
   relief, 38-39
Nonmalignant patients, IT morphine dose escalation, 26f
Nonpeptide receptors, 3-6
Nonsteroidal antiinflammatory drugs (NSAIDs)
   concentrations/daily dosages, recommendations, 32f
   discontinuation, half-lives/recommendations, 142t
   impact, 141
   usage, 115
Nonsteroidal antiinflammatory medications, 141-142

North America, diabetes rates, 117
N-type calcium channels, 8
Nuchal rigidity, 103

O

Obesity, 117-118
   definition, 117
   impact, 102-103
   surgical site infection risk factor, 117-118
Obsessive-compulsive disorder (OCD), 53
Obstructive sleep apnea (OSA), 117
   prevalence, 118
Octreotide, SST analog, 7
Office of the Inspector General (OIG)
   penalties imposition, 60
   review, 62
Off-label use, 22
Omega-conopeptide MVIIA (ω-conopeptide MVIIA), 18
Ondansetron, impact, 107
Opiates, 107-108
Opioids
   analgesics, intraspinal administration, 131
   concentrations, 149
   dose, titration, 32
   dose-dependent analgesic response, 38
   IDDS, 132
   immunomodulatory effects, 100
   incomplete cross-tolerance, 31
   infusion, 131
   initial dose, selection, 31
   initial medical care, 34
   IT therapy guidelines, 188
   local anesthetic, addition, 33
   medications, receptor action, 84-85
   monotherapy, delivery, 26
   overdose, 34
   pump failure, 22
   receptors, 6
   selective blocking, 18
   side effects, 38
   usage, 25
Opioid trials
   evaluation, factors, 76
   interpretation, subjectivity, 76
   patient evaluation, 76
   patient management, 76
      concern, 76
   patient response, assessment, 76
   success, expectations, 76
Oral opioids, treatment failure, 132
Osteoporosis
   compression fractures, inclusion, 96-97
   development, 23
Oswestry Disability Index, measurement, 123
Oswestry Disability Questionnaire, 50
Outcome predictors, existence, 49

P

Pain
   cancer, association, 52
   challenge, 146
   control
      loss, 154
      morphine infusion, 16
   coping strategies, division, 51
   disorder, 53
   increase, 106-107
   interventional management, 140-142

Pain (*Continued*)
  intrathecal therapy response, 38-39
  inventories, 39-40
  keep it sweet and simple (KISS) principle, 130, 130f
  level, VAS determination, 152-153
  management, intraspinal drug infusion (usage), 190f
  medications, preoperative management, 45
  multifactorial experience, 51
  neurostimulation, success, 135
  psychological distress, association, 52
  reduction
    IT morphine, impact, 188
    measurement, 122
  relief, opioid (impact), 33
  risk-to-benefit ratio, 130
  scores, average, 127f
  stepwise treatment, algorithms, 130
  syndromes, 70
  threshold, control-based methods, 51
  treatment, 132-133
    continuum, 130
Pancreatic cancer, 132-133
Pancreatitis, 96-97
Panel Consensus Recommendations for IT Granuloma Diagnosis, Treatment and Prevention (2007), 97
Patients
  drug-taking behavior, assessment, 51
  empowerment, 49
  evaluation, 52-53
  management/evaluation, 74-77
  positioning, intrathecal bolus, 73f
  psychological screening, 40
Patient Satisfaction Questionnaire (PSQ), 183
Pectoral region, pump implantation, 151f
Pediatric dosing, reduction, 72
Pelvic cancer, 132-133
Peptide receptors, 6-7
Percutaneous catheter insertion, CPT codes, 62
Periodic bolus mode (intrathecal pump), 87
Perioperative complications, incidence (reduction), 97
Perioperative morbidity, 97
  risk, minimization (guidelines), 97b
Perioperative mortality, 97
Perioperative VTE, prevention, 140
Peripheral inflammation, 4
Peripheral nerve stimulation (PNS), SCS adjunct, 114
Peripheral neuropathies, 96-97
Permanent catheter insertion, CPT codes, 62
Personality disorders
  incidence, 51
  severity, 40
Personal Therapy Manager (PTM), 154
  handheld device, usage, 176
  physician-programmed bolus delivery, 154
Perspiration, increase, 117
Phagocytic cells, immunodeficiency, 116
Phantom limb pain syndrome, 96-97
Pharmacological tolerance, 170
  management, 167-168
Phobias, 53
Physician-programmed boluses, PTM delivery, 154
Pia mater, 70-71
Pickwickian syndrome, 117
Plasma concentrations, 140
Platelet-activating factor, ginkgo (impact), 116
Platelet aggregation, garlic inhibition, 116
Platelet cyclooxygenase, NSAID inhibition, 141

Platelet-fibrinogen binding, interference, 141-142
Platelet-platelet interactions, interference, 141-142
Polyanalgesia, 25-26
  achievement, 25-26
  therapy, 28
  usage, reason, 26-27
Polyanalgesic admixtures, intrathecal infusion (recommendations), 20t
Polyanalgesic Consensus Conference (PACC), 189
  guidelines (2007), 153b
  IT medication algorithm recommendation, 152
  malignant pain guidelines, 153b
Polyanalgesic Consensus Panel, monotherapy (recommendation), 28
Polyanalgesic medications, 26-27
Polyanalgesic therapy
  admixtures, injection, 22
  IT therapy, 189-190
Polyurethane catheters, usage, 148
Port-a-Cath system, 191
Port system, usage, 148
Postdural headaches, epidural blood patches (success rate), 103-104
Postdural puncture headache (PDPH), 151
  avoidance, 73
  risk, 193
Posterior flank, midline incision, 79f
Post-implantation management, 167-168
Post-implant complications, frequently asked questions, 46
Post-implant considerations, 46
Postlaminectomy surgery syndrome, 152
Postoperative infection, suspicion, 103
Postoperative wound infections, evaluation, 43t
Postsurgical analgesia (enhancement), intrathecal neostigmine (usage), 5
Posttraumatic stress disorder (PTSD), 53
Pregabalin (antiepileptic medications), 28
Pre-implantation psychological evaluations, 53
Pre-implant preparation, 45-46
Premature death, risk, 117
Presynaptic afferents, N-type voltage-gated calcium channels (selective blocking), 18
Presynaptic calcium channels, production, 8
Presynaptic GABA-B receptors, binding, 71
Private payers, medical necessity criteria development, 58
Procedure documentation, usage, 61
Prochlorperazine, impact, 107
Programmable IDDS, components, 86
Programmable pumps, 86-87
  advantages, 88-89
  advantages/disadvantages, 88-89
  disadvantages, 88-89
  equipment, 86
  fixed-rate pumps, contrast, 85t
  overview, 86
  programmable system, 88
  programming, 86-87
Programmable systems, 148-149
Prometra drug delivery pump trial, results, 123
Prometra Programmable Pump System, implantation, 176
Prostaglandin E_2 (PGE_2)
  effects, exertion, 6
  increase, 9
  release, 4

Prostanoid receptors, 6
Proteus mirabilis, IDDS infection, 103
Prothrombin time (PT), vitamin K-dependent factor levels (correlation), 140
Pruritus, 107-108
  causes, 107-108
Psychiatric disorders, presence, 50-51
Psychological distress, pain (association), 52
Psychological evaluation, 52
  strategies/approaches, 50
Psychological screening, 40
Psychological tests/questionnaires, availability, 50
Psychological variables, consideration, 50
Psychometric testing, 39-40
Psychopathology, 40
Psychosocial evaluation strategies, 39-40
Psychosocial information, obtaining, 39-40
Psychosocial variables, 50
Psychotic conditions, IDDS contraindication, 50
Pump-associated complications, 148
Pump device complications, 64-65
  billing compliance, 64-65
  coding, 64
  documentation, 64
  medical necessity, 64
Pump failure, 22-23
  opioid concern, 22
Pump implantation
  CPT codes, 62
  site, 78-79
    selection, 78-79
Pump refill, 23
  documentation requirements, 63b
Pump refilling/maintenance, 63-64
  billing compliance, 63-64
  coding, 63
  documentation, 63
  medical necessity, 63
  relationship, 64
Pump-related complications, 105, 107
Pump-related malfunction, 169
Pump-related problems, 177
Pump replacement, 64-65
  billing compliance, 64-65
  coding, 64
  documentation, 64
  medical necessity, 64
Purse-string suture
  knot, 81f
  placement, 80f

Q

Quality of life (QoL)
  improvement, 122
  issues, 49

R

Radionuclide scintigraphy, 170
Randomized controlled trials (RCTs), scarcity, 122
Rash, opioid side effect, 38
Receptor-specific agents, transmission modulation, 15
Recovery Audit Contractors (RACs), government reviewers, 59
Recurrent stroke, risk, 163
Reflex sympathetic dystrophy, 134-135

Refractory cancer pain, morphine infusion, 16
Refractory chronic pain, treatment, 133
Reimbursement, 58-59
Relative Value Unit (RVU), 58
Relative Value Updating Committee (RUC),
    AMA CPT code valuation
    determination, 58
Renal failure, 143
Reservoir refills, sterility, 168-169
Resource Based Relative Value Scale (RBRVS),
    58
Respiratory depression, 23, 107-108
    avoidance, 76
    report, 31
Reteplase, 141
Rexed's laminae, 188
Risk-level appropriate compounding,
    requirements, 20t
Risk minimization, 100
Ropivacaine, 17

S

Safety, appropriateness, fiscal neutrality, and
    efficacy (SAFE) principles, 130-131, 131f
Schizophrenia, IDDS contraindication, 50
Screener and Opioid Assessment for Patients
    with Pain (SOAPP) scores, 118
Second-line therapy, 32-33
Second-order neurons, chloride concentration
    gradients, 9
Second-order spinal neurons, G-protein
    coupled CGRP1 receptors (impact), 7
Sedation, 108
    opioid side effect, 38
"See prior record" notations, 62
Selective serotonin-norepinephrine reuptake
    inhibitors, 28
Sentinel fatalities, examination, 97
Serosanguineous drainage, 193
Serotonin receptors, 6
Serotonin (5-HT) receptors, diversity, 6
Serotonin (5-HT) reuptake inhibitors, 9
Sexual abnormalities, 108
Short-Form Health Survey, 52-53
Short-term infusion, 180
Short-term mortality, 114
Sickness Index Profile, 50
Simple continuous mode (intrathecal pump),
    87
Single-bolus IT baclofen trials, performing, 76
Single-bolus mode (intrathecal pump), 87
Single continuous mode (intrathecal pump),
    87
Single-entity delivery systems, problems, 19
Single-entity salts, powders, 19
Single intrathecal bolus
    equipment preparation, 74f
    injection, completion, 75f
    lumbar region preparation, 74f
    patient positioning, 73f
    spinal needle
        advancement, 74f
        insertion, 74f
    syringe, attachment, 75f
    trial medication (injection), barbotage
        (usage), 75f
Skin incision
    intrathecal needle/catheter placement, 80f
    superficial infections, 103
Sleep disturbances, 51-52
Social Security Act, 57

Social withdrawal, 52-53
Sodium channel blockers, 19
Sodium-potassium-chloride cotransporter
    (NKCC1), 9
Somatic nociceptive pain, response, 133
Somatostatin (SST)
    peptide, 7
    receptors, 7
Spastic hypertonia (management), ITB
    therapy (usage), 159
Spasticity, 160
    benefits/problems, 160
    control, problems, 160
    interventions, 161t
    management
        individualistic model, 161f
        sequential model, 161f
        synergistic model, 162f
        techniques, 160
    modification, armamentarium, 160
    passive measures, improvement, 163
    presentations, diversity, 160
    rating scales, 163t
    reduction
        adjustment, 160
        excess, 163
    treatment, oral antispasmodics (usage),
        70
    velocity-dependent pathological
        phenomenon, 70
Spinal anatomy, 70
    fluoroscopic confirmation, 167
    illustration, 70f
Spinal canal, composition, 70-71
Spinal complications
    gender/age, impact, 143
    hematologic factors, 143
    hepatic dysfunction, 143
    patient-related factors, 143
    prevention, guidelines, 142-143
    renal failure, 143
    spinal deformities, 143
    vascular malformations, 143
Spinal cord
    alpha$_2$-adrenergic receptors, clonidine
        (impact), 5
    anatomy, importance, 71
    gray matter, division, 188
    interneurons, glycine release, 4
    receptors, 4f
        opposite functions, 3
Spinal cord stimulation (SCS), 130
    goal, 133-134
    implantation, 133
    neuroaugmentation, 133
    psychological concerns, 49
    schematic, 134f
    therapy, 48
    usage, 114
Spinal deformities, 143
Spinal drug delivery, 152
Spinal epidural abscess, 117
    formation, 117
Spinal hemorrhage, risk (increase), 163
Spinal incision, intrathecal pump (tunneling),
    82f
Spinal stenosis, 96-97
Spinal surgery/deformity, imaging, 71
Spine bleeding, 152
Stability, 22
    definition, 22
    issues, 22
Staphylococcus aureus, IDDS infection, 103

Staphylococcus epidermidis, pathogen (impact),
    193
State Trait Anxiety Inventory, 50
Sterile compounding, USP-National Formulary
    (USP-NF) requirements, 19-20
Sterile technique
    breakage, 151
    preparation, 19-20
Stimulation, conductivity, 133
Stopped pump mode (intrathecal pump), 87
Streptokinase, 141
Subcutaneous heparin, 115
Subcutaneous injection site, implanted
    catheter (usage), 191
Substance P, release, 17
Substantia gelatinosa, opioid medications
    (receptor action), 84-85
Sufentanil, 17
Suicidal depression, 40
    IDDS contraindication, 50
Superficial infection, 103
Suprapubic tubes, usage, 151f
Surgical implantation, 62-63
    billing compliance, 62-63
    coding, 62
    documentation, 62
    medical necessity, 62
Surgical techniques, 79-83
Sutures, usage, 80
SynchroMed 2 pump, sufficiency, 45-46
SynchroMed EL (extended-life) pump, 91-93
    comparison, 94t
    design, 91
    FDA approval, 70
    implantation, 91-92
        process, 92
    infusion flow rates, control, 91
    photograph, 91f
    programmable pump, 85f
    programming, 92-93
    pump model, storage, 92
    pump sizes, comparison, 91f
    system, titanium-based pump design, 91
    usage, appropriateness, 92
SynchroMed II 40-mL pump, usage, 45-46
SynchroMed II pump, 93-95
    alarm system, 95
    commercial availability, 148
    design, 93
    implantation, 93-94
        process, 94
    infusion flow rates, control, 93
    programmable delivery modes, 94
    programming, 94-95
SynchroMed Pump, FDA approval, 70

T

Tachykinin receptors, 6-7
Tachyphylaxis
    development, 17
    report, 33
Tardieu Scales, 163
Targeted receptors, understanding, 19
T-cells, immunodeficiencies, 116
Tearfulness, persistence, 52-53
Testosterone, suppression, 23
Tetrodotoxin (TTX), sodium channel blocker,
    8
Therapeutic drugs, FDA approval, 114
Thienopyridine derivatives, antiplatelet effect,
    141-142

Thoracic spinal catheter, CPT codes, 61
Three-step analgesic ladder, evolution (WHO), 130
Thromboembolic phenomena, risk (increase), 168
Thrombolytic therapy, 140-141
Thromboprophylaxis, patient receipt, 144t
Ticlopidine (Ticlid)
    antiplatelet effect, 141-142
    platelet-fibrinogen binding interference, 141-142
Titration phase, 167-168
Tizanidine, long-term intrathecal infusion, 5
Tobacco sac suture, impact, 103-104
Topical mupirocin (Bactroban), preoperative use, 103
Totally implanted catheter, implanted infusion pump (usage), 191
Toxicity scores, oncological reliance, 146
Transient receptor potential (TRP) channels, 8-9
Transporters, 9
Traumatic brain injury, 50-51
Trialing, 61-62
    coding, 61-62
    documentation, 61
    history, documentation, 70
    malignant pain, 147
    medical necessity, 61
    methods, advantages/disadvantages, 73t
    randomized trial, 125
Tricyclic antidepressants, 28
trkA receptor (nerve growth factor receptor), 7
trkB receptor (brain-derived neurotrophic factor receptor), 7
TRPA1 channels, 8-9
TRPV1 vanilloid type 1 channels, 8
Tumor compression, 154f
Tumor necrosis factor-alpha (TNF-α), 9
Tunneled percutaneous catheter, 191
2-0 Silk suture, usage, 80
Type 2 diabetes, insulin secretion, 117

U

Ultra low particulate air (ULPA) filters, usage, 21
Unfractionated intravenous/subcutaneous heparin (UFH), 141
    usage, 115
United Kingdom, ziconotide (usage), 127
United States Pharmacopeia (USP), chapter 797
    pharmacy compounding risk-level assessment, 21t
    standards/guidance/examples, 21
United States Pharmacopeia-National Formulary (USP-NF), sterile compounding requirements, 19-20

Upper extremity hypertonia, 167-168
Upper motor neuron injury/dysfunction, 70
Urinary retention, 108
U.S. health care payment system, 56-57

V

Vascular malformations, 143
V codes, bias, 63
Venous thromboembolism (VTE), prevention, 140
Venous thrombosis, spasticity protection, 168
Viral meningitis, diagnosis, 151-152
Visceral pain, response, 133
Visual Analog Scale (VAS), 123
    pain level determination, 152-153
    pain score, 181
    scores, level, 153
Visual Analog Scale of Pain Intensity (VASPI)
    score, 28, 180
    baseline, maximum improvement, 181-182
Vitamin K-dependent clotting factors
    levels, prothrombin time (PT), correlation, 140
    synthesis, 115
Voltage-gated calcium channels, 8
    transport, 8
Voltage-gated sodium channels, 8
Vomiting, intrathecal drug side effect, 107
von Willebrand factor (vWF)
    complications, 140
    glycoprotein (GP) Ib, interaction, 140

W

Warfarin, 140-141
    anticoagulant activity, 140
    clinical experience, 140
    long-term anticoagulation, 140
    usage, 115
Washington State Health Care Authority
    analysis commission, 122
    ECRI analysis, 126-127
Weight gain, 108
Well-being, decrease, 53
White blood cell (WBC) counts
    elevation, 103
    impact, 143-144
Wound dehiscence, 104-105
Wound seroma formation, 151
WPS Medicare, reimbursement guidelines, 58

Z

Ziconotide, 18-19, 27-28
    administration dose, 184
    approval, 31

Ziconotide (Continued)
    bolus trialing
        data summary, 182t
        value, 183
    bolus trials
        double-blind placebo-controlled trial, 182-183
        open-label study, 183
        retrospective chart review, 183
        single-center study, 183
    consideration, 33
    continuous infusion trialing, data summary, 180t
    continuous infusion trials, 180-181
    continuous therapy, 183
    direct receptor antagonism, 18
    epidural infusion trial, 182
    expert opinion, 183-184
    FDA approval, 31, 71
    high-dose IT ziconotide bolus trialing, predictive value, 183
    infusion trial, external pump (case report), 181
    instability, 22
    intrathecal administration
        dose-dependent adverse effects, 18
        pharmacokinetics, 18
    intrathecal therapy, 98-99, 189
    last-attempt agent, 18
    limited-duration infusion trialing, data summary, 181t
    limited-duration infusion trials, open-label study, 181-182
    long-term IDDS, 18-19
    mean ziconotide doses, 180-181
    neuron-specific calcium channel blocker, intrathecal usage, 18
    nonopioid adjuvant medication, 27-28
    nonopioid antiinflammatory drug, 98
    nonopioid intrathecal analgesic, 179
    open-label investigation, external pumps (usage), 180-181
    outcomes evidence, 180
    overdose, 34
        life threat, unlikeliness, 34
    patient management/evaluation, 180
    randomized clinical trials, 184
    selective blocking, 18
    structure, 18-19
        implications, 18
    therapy
        diagnoses, 179
        guidelines/timing, 179
    treatment, 183
    trialing
        methods, 76-77
        upward titration rate, 183-184
    usefulness, 18-19
    VASPI score, 28

Printed and bound by CPI Group (UK) Ltd, Croydon, CR0 4YY

08/05/2025

01864794-0002